MORE ALIKE THAN DIFFERENT: TREATING SEVERELY DISSOCIATIVE TRAUMA SURVIVORS

Just as the prevalence of incest and child sexual abuse was a well-kept secret until recently, the phenomenon of multiple personality – recently relabelled dissociative identity disorder (DID) – has been dismissed or downplayed. In her practice as a psychologist, Margo Rivera has found this to be no coincidence.

Confirming that the root of most severe dissociative conditions lies in trauma, most commonly child abuse, Rivera discusses the general historical and social contexts of dissociation and uses clinical theory, case vignettes, and recorded personal experience to provide practical guidance to its diagnosis and treatment. She also addresses the controversies around 'False Memory Syndrome' and ritual abuse, issues which currently divide professionals treating trauma survivors.

Rivera makes a unique contribution to the treatment of lesbian and gay survivors of abuse. She theorizes that all sexuality is a social construct, subject to change over an individual's lifetime, a reality that is nowhere more clear than in highly dissociative individuals, who may identify themselves as alternately heterosexual female, gay male, lesbian, and heterosexual male.

Insightful and provocative, this important therapeutic guide will be of interest to professionals who treat trauma survivors as well as to their clients.

MARGO RIVERA is an assistant professor of psychiatry at Queen's University, Kingston, Ontario, and co-director of the Personality Disorders Service at Kingston Psychiatric Hospital.

MARGO RIVERA

More Alike Than Different: Treating Severely Dissociative Trauma Survivors

UNIVERSITY OF TORONTO PRESS
Toronto Buffalo London

© University of Toronto Press Incorporated 1996
Toronto Buffalo London
Printed in Canada

ISBN 0-8020-0450-4 (cloth)
ISBN 0-8020-7238-0 (paper)

Printed on acid-free paper

Canadian Cataloguing in Publication Data

Rivera, Margo, 1945–
    More alike than different : treating severely
    dissociative trauma survivors

    Includes index.
    ISBN 0-8020-0450-4 (bound) ISBN 0-8020-7238-0 (pbk.)

    1. Multiple personality.   I. Title.

    RC569.5.M8R59 1996   616.85'236   C96-930991-0

University of Toronto Press acknowledges the financial assistance to its publishing program
of the Canada Council and the Ontario Arts Council.

For Raquel and Kate and Rachael
The next generations
That this world will be a better place for you

Contents

Preface

The subtitle of this book, *Treating Severely Dissociative Abuse Survivors*, could support a wide variety of perspectives. I can only offer mine.

When I was in graduate school and reading piles of theory, I often got caught up in the point of view of whatever theorist I happened to be studying. There were exceptions, of course, but usually I found a great deal to learn about in what I read. I was often bowled over by these theorists' brilliance and imagination. What I found strange and could never quite get my head around was that they did not seem to have that view of each other. Most of them seemed intent on proving that they were right. From their point of view, therefore, everyone else had to be wrong. And to me they all seemed right about so many things.

Of course, they also seemed wrong about some things. I did not lose my critical faculty just because I was awed by experiencing new ways of looking at things. Still, it never occurred to me that if my framing of experience was right, they had to be wrong. Or, because they were sometimes wrong by my way of thinking, that I should tally those wrongs rather than focus on the amazing ways in which these writers had opened my eyes.

Occasionally, this mindset was an academic liability. 'Stop incorporating. Choose a point of view, stick with it, elaborate on it and document definitively the ways it is superior to the other perspectives,' one of my professors wrote in large, exasperated letters on my paper next to a middling grade. To be honest, this put a small dent in my self-esteem. So I tried to do as he directed, but it did not make sense to me. I could not, and probably stubbornly would not, write in a way he considered appropriately academic, a way I considered exclusionary and adversarial. I ended up with a second-class standing in that class.

That is why I am warning the reader that this is my story rather than a definitive position about dissociation, treatment, or anything else for that matter. I say many things that other people have said about treating people who are suffering from severe dissociative conditions, and I say some things that are different from what other people have said, even some of the people whose work I admire most and to whom I would send a brother if he were in trouble. It is quite likely that I may disagree with some of the things that I have written here by the time the book is in print and in a reader's hands.

I look at things differently than other people do. The reader cannot help looking at things differently from the way I do. I invite you to incorporate, to digest, to mix what you read with your own experience and make it something different that is also similar. I welcome your disagreements.

When I am teaching, therapists often ask me anguished questions based on conflicts between what they read and what they experience as practical and helpful to their clients. For example, 'Do you always insist that the same personality who comes to the session leave the session?' I usually answer 'I don't think about people that way,' or 'I don't think that it is my business to control what state of consciousness a person is in when they leave a session, unless, of course, they are acutely suicidal, homicidal, totally unable to function, and so on.' The response to this is always (and this exact situation has happened at least three times) 'But Frank Putnam says in his book that whoever comes into session leaves the session, and you said his book is the classic text.'

Now, I have read that book more than once, and I have leafed through it since that question was raised, and I can't find where it says whoever comes to the session leaves the session. But there must be something that resembles that dictum closely enough that several people have made that interpretation and tried to act on it, even when it did not work for them. I do not think Frank Putnam is a fundamentalist, and I can imagine his chagrin on his work being read like the Bible.

To avoid this situation, I want to introduce myself to the reader so that you know whose thoughts you are reading. The experience of reading this book will, I hope, be more like a conversation. I say something, you reply, I elaborate, you interrupt, write comments in the margin, try something out, and so on.

I am the oldest child of a white, middle-class Irish-Catholic family. I was born in New York City ten months after my sister had died at birth so I was intensely wanted by my parents. I also had five unmarried great-aunts who lived with my widowed maternal grandmother in New York City in the winter and on the south Atlantic shore in New Jersey during the summer. They were all thrilled to have a little girl to fuss over. I spent a great deal of time with them, winter and summer, from infancy on. My paternal grandmother was both a single mother and a single grandmother. She raised her granddaughters, two girls about my age, and they alternated living on the Jersey shore and in the Adirondack mountains. I soon had three brothers whom I cared for and fussed over, and we all spent a great deal of time with our extended family, in the city, on the shore, and in the mountains.

I went to a Roman Catholic grade school, high school, and even university. I loved the nuns and the sanctuary lamp in the church, the mystery and the rituals. I payed less attention to the restrictions and the rigidities than most people I know who grew up Catholic, although I do remember being sure, after an act of petty thievery, that it was my destiny to grow up to be a robber. The love I had for some of the nuns, practically my only teachers until I graduated from high school, was one of the reasons for my relative imperviousness to the oppression that is, unfortunately, so central to a beautiful religious faith as it is practised in a patriarchal culture. There were one or two nuns who were cruel, and most were extraordinarily narrow-minded socially and politically. Nonetheless I grew to love some of my teachers both as a young child and as a teenager, and I think I heard and translated the rigid teachings through that love.

My life, like that of many children, revolved with the seasons. Summers were divided between the shore and the mountains, depending on where my paternal grandmother was living at the time. Lala, my maternal grandmother, and my great-aunts (Rene, Lorette, Kitsy, Helen, and Jule) always lived in the village of Sea Girt on the south Jersey shore from June through September. My brothers and I always spent at least a month with them, swimming in the high Atlantic waves from early in the morning until we had to go home for supper. Lunch was a hot dog from the beach pavilion, followed by a mandatory one-hour moratorium on swimming, during which we usually played stickball on the sand or imaginary games on the dunes.

Summer also meant camp for me once I was ten years old. For eight years I went to Blue Bay Girl Scout Camp in East Hampton on the end of Long Island, first as a camper and then as a counsellor. Camp came to have a special place in my life. I loved the outdoors and rituals like flag-raising ceremonies, where favourite pieces of poetry and other inspirational writings were recited each morning. Campfires burned well into the night as we sat around singing camp songs, love songs, spirituals, and folk songs. The woods where we slept in tents and the cliff-sheltered ocean bay in which we swam twice a day and often canoed were the body of the experience. The friendships I developed with some of the girls and young women who returned to camp year after year were its heart.

I developed an intense awareness during adolescence that most people did not live the privileged life that I did. I spent many hours on the school-season weekends at the Catholic Worker, a Catholic communist group that published a radical newspaper and operated a soup kitchen and clothing depot for the street people who were the principal residents of the neighbourhood (the Bowery area of New York City). In the free time I did not spend at the Catholic Worker, I fed and rocked babies at a temporary shelter uptown in Spanish Harlem. I would go home to a comfortable house and a comfortable life that felt, cognitively, increasingly uncomfortable.

As president of the student organization in my parochial high school, I organized all-school educational forums on racism, class oppression, and the ways in which we ignored these issues at our doorstep by concentrating on buying salvation for 'pagan babies' and sending missionaries to preach to people who were perfectly satisfied with their own belief systems. I was not very popular with some of the more conservative faculty, and eventually I was allowed to organize only half the monthly assemblies. The teacher who took over on alternate months organized presentations on suitably religious topics, including a particularly memorable one entitled 'Shrines of Mary Throughout the World.' Only now can I see the feminist potential in such a topic. At the time, I was overwhelmed with boredom.

My early awareness of social injustice related to the inequalities of race and class. Issues of gender and sexuality would not surface until much later. I conformed superficially – and certainly without giving it much thought – to the prevailing social norms, and went through the motions of the adolescent heterosexuality rituals as little as possible. Attendance at the occasional school dance was really all that seemed to be required. I was intensely involved with my friends, all of whom were girls. I went to an all-female high school and even college for the first two years of my post-secondary education. Although I had many experiences that, in retrospect, might have suggested that heterosexuality was not the path I would be destined to follow, I had never heard of gay or lesbian sexuality, and in some ways I was a late-maturing child.

My parents were anti-racist liberals without a great deal of money who brought us up in an affluent, conservative, racist social milieu. Consequently my brothers and I faced contradictions between the way things were presented at home and the way we were socialized in school, church, and the neighbourhood. I remember being told by the nun who taught civics class that I should go to Cuba with the rest of the Communists, because I expressed disagreement with the way the Cuban bishops were instructing Cuban Catholics to vote for particular political candidates, under threat of excommunication. A headline in a Toronto newspaper in the spring of 1994, twenty years later, 'Catholics told to pressure their Members of Provincial Parliament to vote against same-sex legislation,' startled me with its sense of *déjà vu*.

I was enthusiastic and rebellious, always pointing out unfairness to school authorities who were not always appreciative of my point of view but indulgent enough – because I got good marks, worked hard on the school paper, played sports with a modicum of skill and a lot of energy, and was basically a cheerful soul – not to insist that I shut up altogether. In university I developed more of an edge, and I was torn when I was asked to leave the Gothic, all-women college I loved for its intellectual rigour and the wonderful sounds of Gregorian chant pouring out of the chapel windows, and the parades of Ursuline nuns with black veils swinging behind them.

The school sent my parents a letter suggesting that my political activities (I was working in the civil rights movement at the time) indicated I would undoubtedly be happier elsewhere. I found out from friends who had received similar letters, as well as the few who hadn't and had remained until graduation, that the university had tried to clear out all their rebels that year (1964), and had in fact successfully evaded the campus unrest that swept North America in the next few years. One of my warmest memories of my mother is her description of her meeting with the college authorities in which she told them that they should cherish students who thought for themselves rather than demanding conformity from them.

Though my mother succeeded in persuading the college that I would be an asset, I had already decided to finish university in Canada. I came to Toronto from New York in 1964, at the age of nineteen. At that time I had only been in two cities, New York and Boston. I remember walking down Bloor Street near Yonge, looking around in amazement at the two-storey shops, thinking, 'Where is the city?' I had no idea that cities could have grass and trees that were not in parks, or neighbourhoods of family homes.

I stayed in Canada, got married, and raised a daughter and a foster son in a cult-like, psychoanalytically oriented therapeutic commune. That experience did me and people I love a great deal of harm, but it also taught me much about how to be (and how not to be) a therapist. My own psychotherapy/training analysis took place in that context, and much of what I have learned about the complexities of power and powerlessness, both personal and social, within the therapy process, I learned that context.

It was not until I extricated myself from this group, which challenged many social conventions yet held traditional gender roles and compulsory heterosexuality sacred, that I developed an overtly feminist perspective and explored the complexity and depth of my own sexuality. Eventually, I left my twenty-four year marriage and fell in love with a woman, another psychotherapist.

I began to work with people suffering from extreme dissociative conditions when I was a therapist in a sexual abuse treatment program with the Children's Aid Society in 1982. I work very differently now than I did then in some ways. Every year I seem to learn something that profoundly affects the way I do my work. Yet, looking back, although the way I now work is very different, my basic stance is much the same.

I was talking to someone recently who was asking me about my first experience of meeting the many facets of a classically dissociative client. He asked how I had felt. I told him that I remembered being really concerned about the client's little girl. This wasn't what he wanted to know. He wanted to know what the experience had been like when the different personalities had come out – the strangeness of it all.

We were not on the same wavelength. I knew what he was after, but I do not remember ever being fascinated by the phenomenology of the dissociative multiplicity, even with my first client, who was as flamboyantly differentiated as they come. The therapy process was more challenging and complex than any I had previously undertaken. I became countertransferentially entangled with my first severely dissociative client in a way that was new to my experience, but even from the first I never saw individuals with multiple personalities as very different from anyone else.

Above all, that is what I want this book to say – that treating people who dissociate to such a degree that they genuinely experience themselves as different people is much like treating anyone else – and that treating such people can teach us much about treating everyone else.

This is not a 'how-to' book. And though it is about psychotherapy, it addresses many issues that are not dos and don'ts of treatment. The more experienced I become in the practice of psychotherapy, the more I become convinced that it is the person of the therapist – her struggles, her politics (in the broadest sense of the word), her life experience and the way she wears it – that is at the heart of the therapy process.

It is not that interventions do not matter, but that interventions are chosen and made at particular times because of the values of the therapist and the influence she wishes to exert over her client. What kind of people we are determines what we value in other people, and what we value in other people is what we attempt to promote in our psychotherapy clients – sometimes consciously, often not. This is not a bad thing. It is the way it is. Pretending that we do not exert such influence simply allows us to avoid responsibility for our actions and our intentions, and that, I am convinced, is a bad thing.

I remember reading Bruno Bettleheim's *Dialogues with Mothers* (1962) many years ago, as part of my first foray into childrearing. It was written, as I remember, in question and answer format, like a manual: 'Should I physically discipline my child?' 'At what age should I begin toilet training?' And over and over again, Bettleheim would reply, 'It depends on what sort of child you want,' before elaborating on the effects of certain practices.

How we engage in our relationships, including our relationships with our psychotherapy clients, is profoundly affected by how we think, what we value, what we allow ourselves to be aware of, and what we need to block out of our awareness. Therefore, though some of the issues discussed in this book may appear to roam a fair distance from what we normally consider clinical, those are not boundaries that make sense to me. It is impossible to engage in this work and make easy distinctions between the clinical, the philosophical, the historical, the political, the poetic, and the ethical dimensions of oppression and of resistance, of horror and of healing.

Acknowledgments

There are a few people who are very much a part of this book:

Marie-Louise Bechthold, my partner and friend. It has been a joy parenting with you the little one who came into our lives the very day I began work on this book.

My mother, Dorothy Tuckey, who taught me to write my essays in grade school by beginning each one with a quotation, and who always quoted to me from the New Testament, 'To whom much is given, much will be expected.'

My father, Tommy Tuckey, who was so good at listening despite his deafness that I am sure he is listening still, even though he died a couple of years ago.

My grandmothers – Lala and Millie Burke – and my great-aunts – Rene, Lorette, Kitsy, Jule, and Helen – who all showed me women living and working together to care for each other and for three generations of children.

My brothers – John, Tom, and Steven Tuckey – all writers and/or actors and on whom, the Goddess help them, I vented my caretaking energies, from the bassinet onwards.

Marjory Old, whose no-nonsense humour and unsentimental compassion for suffering people bolstered me throughout the journey of learning to do this work. She kept me organized – despite my natural bent toward chaos – for twelve years, and, as we both foretold, I am falling apart without her.

Rafael Barreto-Rivera, poet and father of the child we have both always been crazy about.

Jean-Marc, whose growing-up years taught me more than all my textbooks combined.

Lou's brood – Mouse, Shayne, Alison, Nicole, Cory, Kyle.

Janice Ristock, comrade through the adventures and nonsense of graduate school, and the gradual and playful process of my coming out.

And all the adults and all the children who have allowed me to participate in a variety of ways in their healing journeys – for years and years or, sometimes, for an hour or two.

I thank you all for the gifts that have made their way into my spirit and therefore into this book.

MORE ALIKE THAN DIFFERENT:
TREATING SEVERELY DISSOCIATIVE
TRAUMA SURVIVORS

1

Introduction: Multiple Personality in Context

It is enough to formulate the question in simplistic terms – why have the Jews been killed? – for the question to reveal right away its obscenity. There is absolute obscenity in the very project of understanding ... Blindness has to be ... the only way not to turn away from a reality that is literally blinding ... 'Hier ist kein Warum' ... 'Here there is no why.'

Claude Lanzmann (1990)

The issue of multiple personality is embedded in the issue of child abuse, particularly the sexual abuse of young girls. A number of independent studies drawing their cohorts from individuals in treatment with a wide variety of mental health practitioners found that nine out of ten people with multiple personalities seen in clinical settings are women (Putnam et al., 1986; Ross, Norton & Wozney, 1987; Rivera, 1991).

There is some speculation that the high ratio of women to men with multiple personalities could be a sampling bias and that male multiples are more likely to be extremely violent and found in jails rather than therapists' offices, where most of the research has been done (Putnam, Loewenstein, & Silberman, 1984, Bliss, 1986). Indeed, the nine to one association is quite likely high. There are probably many undetected male multiples in jail for violent crimes, in substance abuse groups, or in the boardrooms of the *Fortune* 500 companies. However, I think, the type of violence and sexual abuse perpetrated on children who develop multiple personality is only an extreme point on the continuum of personal acts of violence towards women that our society institutionalizes, including rape and battering. Therefore, it also makes sense that this kind of abuse would occur more frequently towards girls in their preparation for womanhood.

Because as far as we know there are many more women than men with multiple personalities, I shall use the female generic (she/her) in this book when referring to persons with multiple personalities. This does not mean that what I say is not relevant to men with multiple personality, nor is it intended as a slight to the significance of their experience. Since I do not have a perfect solution to the problem of pronoun exclusivity, I shall use the female generic when I am referring to abuse survivors, unless I am specifically referring to males, and I shall also use, for the same reasons, the male generic when referring to offenders, 90 per cent of whom are male (Russell, 1986, Badgley, 1984). This is a linguistic and political strategy. It is not perfect, but it is my solution.

Multiple personality is not even officially called that anymore. In fact, it never was; it was called 'multiple personality disorder' (MPD). It is now called 'dissociative identity disorder' (DID), probably a more sensible clinical term. However, except for purposes of official diagnosis, I am not inclined to use the scientifically sanctioned diagnostic nomenclature. 'Disorder' is insulting to the people who have been all too insulted as it is. One of the most convincing protests against the use of the term disorders as applied to posttraumatic dissociation in action was a comment I received as part of a needs assessment I conducted regarding access to treatment services in Ontario:

Words are powerful symbols. I cringe each time I hear the term 'disorder'. I struggle to accept the means I used to survive absolutely horrendous sexual, physical and emotional abuse by my father and other family members. I struggle to celebrate the fact that I found a way to deal with the chaos without going crazy. Our language does not enlighten my struggle; it increases it. I am fully aware that what was once adaptive is now rather messy, to put it mildly. But I am not crazy. I am not ill. I am not a disorder. I am a human face who had to survive in a home that was totally crazy, very sick and constantly disordered. Please do not define me in terms of their behaviour.

Again and again, as I have spoken to people suffering from severe posttraumatic dissociation, I have heard the same plea – that I not collude in the ongoing process of my clients' objectification by using a word like 'disorder', which so obviously frames their way of being in the world as deviant, and implicitly justifies practices of exclusion that have been so central to the most oppressive of their experience.

For the purposes of this book, when I am referring to severe posttraumatic dissociative conditions, I will use either multiple personality, severe dissociation, severe posttraumatic dissociation, or some variant thereof, It is not very exact, but in my opinion it is more proper. Precise diagnostic nomenclature tends to reify what is actually a large and fluid category. I think it is, paradoxically, more scientific to be a bit more casual or even eclectic with our use of language in this instance than to pretend to a precision that creates the impression (backed with the legitimating power of 'science') that multiple personality or severe posttraumatic dissociation or dissociative identity disorder is more of a discrete phenomenon than it is.

Multiple personality is a way of ordering subjectivity, a way of thinking and expressing, as well as a way of not thinking and keeping silent when necessary. I will talk more about this in the next chapter. I'm mentioning it here because it relates to why I may appear to be all over the place with terminology. I recognize that all the categories I employ (or try not to employ) have consequences that exceed my intentions, and the best strategy I can think of at this point is to undermine their authority by countering each with the others.

In touching on the issue of language vis-à-vis my de-centred use of terminology, I am hinting at the basic philosophical premise of this text – that forms of subjectivity, including extremely dissociative subjectivity, do not have objective status that can be addressed in a transcendent and ahistorical fashion. Rather, they are a discursive effect. They exist always and only in relation to the discourses of social relations and power that produce them. They cannot be understood with the tools of a 'value-free' science, the concept of which is in itself an effect of a set of discourses (including medicine, psychiatry, and psychology) comprising complex networks of power/knowledge that legislate forms of subjectivity and generate normative practices based on such laws.

In this first chapter I shall address some issues that I think are crucial to placing multiple personality in context – a historical context and a social context. The first is widespread use of the physical, emotional, and particularly sexual abuse of children and adolescents in our society to disempower them and to consolidate power for those who abuse them.

Most individuals with multiple personalities report a history of child abuse, usually severe and prolonged, and, in the vast majority of cases, including childhood sexual abuse (Putnam et al., 1986; Ross et al., 1987; Rivera, 1991). Most of the data about adults with multiple personality are retrospective, but it is often possible to find independent corroboration for reported experiences of childhood abuse (Herman & Schatzow, 1987).

It is becoming common knowledge that a great many children in our society are sexually abused. In fact, the most recent prevalence studies indicate that some experience of sexual abuse is part of the childhood or adolescence of well over a third of female children and a fifth of male children (Russell, 1986; Finkelhor, 1986, 1990; Briere & Conte, 1991). With incidence this high, it becomes absurd to continue to frame the problem as one of deviancy – a few sick men going after some vulnerable, neglected children.

One of the strongest tenets of our society's liberal ideology is that we value our children, and we do everything we can to keep them from harm. The power of ideological concepts sometimes lies in their banality. Their simplicity allows them to slip by without challenge or resistance, and they become integrated into our common-sense view of reality. We speak individually and collectively about our abhorrence of the sexual abuse of children. As a society, our actions do not reflect our words.

Diana Russell's (1986) general population survey uncovered experience of sexual abuse before the age of eighteen in 38 per cent of the women, using a conservative definition of abuse that included only situations of physical contact. When she used a wider definition that included situations that most people would consider abusive – such as repeated sexual propositions by relatives the child was living with or acts of exhibitionism, such as being forced to watch an adult masturbate – 54 per cent of the women remembered at least one such incident in their childhoods. Sixteen per cent of the women interviewed were sexually abused by members of their own families, and the incest often went on for years.

Russell collected the data for this study in 1978, when the topic of incest and child sexual abuse was still largely shrouded in silence. Later research indicates that the figures – rather than being inflated, as critics uncomfortable with the implications of the results contend – are probably low. Large, community-based retrospective studies of child sexual abuse may misclassify as non-abused a significant number of individuals abused in childhood. A more recent study (Williams et al., 1993) found that abuse of very young children, for example, and abuse perpetrated by individuals with a close relationship to the victim were more likely to go undetected in retrospective studies.

Though the sexual use of children has been part of social custom throughout recorded history, a great deal of effort has been made to deny that the problem exists. Women have made some significant efforts to resist this silencing and to address the issue of the sexual abuse of children. Sheila Jeffreys, in *The Spinster and Her Enemies* (1985), unearths and examines the multifaceted campaigns of women in feminist and suffrage organizations and journals between 1880 and 1930 to protect children from sexual abuse by men. All the laws in England establishing incest as an offence and setting the current age of consent guidelines were passed through Parliament at this time.

Because of the efforts of many women, by 1930 the sexual abuse of children by men had become a legitimate issue of acknowledged social importance. It was then appropriated by the medical establishment, who appointed themselves the experts on this behaviour which they labelled 'deviant.' The extent of the problem was veiled, and the few offenders who were apprehended were treated as sick exceptions who had little relevance to men and social structures in general.

During this same time period, with the rise of the political ideology of liberal individualism, a system of psychology began to develop that, rather than viewing mental illness simply as a disease with a physiological basis, encouraged individuals to explore the emotional conflicts in their personal lives. As with many of the outgrowths of liberalism, such as so-called universal suffrage (women did not miss the irony that the term 'universal' did not apply to them and a century of protest ensued), this new dynamic psychiatry inadvertently opened up issues about the lives of women that had been previously closed to question. Women were most frequently the focus of this early psychiatric intervention, just as women are now the majority of patients in mental health clinics. One of the first issues that emerged when these women began to have an opportunity to talk about what was significant to them was their common experience of sexual abuse in childhood.

Sigmund Freud was one of the first practitioners of this new psychology. He listened to his women patients' free associations and encouraged them to communicate their memories to him, many of which, he discovered, involved incidents of childhood sexual assault. Both the detail and the behaviour and affect with which they recounted the experiences convinced Freud that they were talking about real events.

The story of Freud and his sexually abused patients has been told and retold from many points of view. In 1896, Freud presented a paper before his colleagues in Vienna, entitled 'The Aetiology of Hysteria.' In this paper, he proposed that the origin of neurosis lay in the early sexual experiences of children within their own families. In presenting what he excitedly considered to be a breakthrough in science, he was not prepared for the professional disavowal and isolation he would experience as a result of suggesting that sexual exploitation of girls by their relatives and other caretakers in apparently respectable family settings was not uncommon.

Freud ultimately retracted his 'seduction theory' and replaced it with the famous 'Oedipus complex' theory. From this point on, generations of mental health practitioners have used one version or other of this theory to reframe reports of childhood sexual assault as cases of wishful thinking of young children who are so sophisticated about the mechanics of adult sexuality and so keen to be sexually involved with the parent of the opposite sex that they are still indulging this delicious fantasy in great detail thirty or forty years later.

Freudian theory has been extremely influential in shaping the culture and the values of the twentieth century. Though some of the dogma that has evolved out of the complex, diverse, and often contradictory work of Freud has been widely challenged in the past fifteen years, it is possible, as Florence Rush (1980) says, that we have closed the barn door too late. As a society, we have taken the patriarchal practice of psychology and psychiatry and the many patriarchal judgments in Freud's own work to transform his description of the 'world historical defeat' of women and the tyranny of consciousness by the unconscious into an ideological justification for the oppression of women and children (Mitchell, 1974).

We have become imbued with the popularized notion of a personal unconscious, which relegates social problems, such as the widespread sexual abuse of children, to the realm of individual maladjustment, particularly the maladjustment of the victim. Most of the research that has been undertaken in this area has been a documentation of the shortcomings and vulnerabilities of victims and their families, particularly their mothers, that allowed the abuse to happen to them, or it has been a documentation of their manifestations of abnormality after the abuse had taken place. Little notice has been taken in the psychological literature of the wider social context in which the sexualization and the sexual abuse of children is at least ignored, and often encouraged and sanctioned. A small number of researchers attempt to incorporate a social analysis into their studies about the sexual abuse of children (Finkelhor, 1986; Russell, 1986; Briere, 1992).

Women have been trying to speak to psychiatrists about the sexual assaults they endured as children since the time of Freud, but an attitude of incredulity about disclosures of child sexual abuse continued to be the norm among professionals during most of the twentieth century. Even when it had been thoroughly documented that parents and parent-substitutes beat, scalded, choked, tied up, and physically tortured their children (Kempe et al., 1962), the notion that many men, and particularly fathers and father-substitutes, used children sexually was met with general disbelief. The 1975 edition of the *Comprehensive Textbook of Psychiatry* estimated incest to occur in one case per million in the population (Freedman, Kaplan, & Saddock, 1975).

It was not the mental health profession that brought the issue of the widespread sexual abuse of children out into the open again in the last quarter of the twentieth century. The women's liberation movement of the late 1960s and 1970s lifted the curtain on the powerful weapons that many men and our patriarchal culture were using to keep women in a subordinate position in society. One of the most vicious and effective of these has been the sexual abuse of children.

Violence against women by men was one of the salient and pressing issues that emerged from the consciousness-raising efforts of the women's movement. Rape received the first focused attention and became the paradigm for understanding other forms of violence against women. The enormous industry of pornography was cited as an expression of misogynist values that are the underpinnings of oppressive social structures. The axiom 'Pornography is the theory; rape is the practice' (Morgan, 1977, p. 92) represented the view that violence against women was not an occasional explosion by a sick individual but an inevitable consequence of what Susan Brownmiller called the patriarchal philosophy of sexual private property. And, if women are men's corporal property, then children are a wholly owned subsidiary (Brownmiller, 1975).

Social action programs responding to the needs of rape victims uncovered childhood histories of sexual abuse in many of the victims. The silence began to lift, and some of the myths that surrounded the issue – that incest is rare and that children commonly lie about being sexually abused by adults – began to be challenged. Workers in rape crisis centres and battered women's shelters listened to the women who told them about their childhood assaults. They believed these women, rather than reframing their reports as fantasy as so many mental health professionals had been doing.

By the early 1980s, an awareness of the reality of the widespread incidence of child sexual abuse in our society had begun to grow beyond the feminist community. Mental health and child welfare organizations were faced with the reality that there was a large area of child maltreatment and exploitation that they had rarely noticed and had certainly not dealt with effectively up to this point. Training sessions on recognizing and treating incest and child sexual abuse became popular and sought after for front-line child welfare workers and clinicians in mainstream social service and mental health agencies.

With growing awareness of the scope of the problem, official reports of child sexual abuse started to surface at a much greater rate than reports of other types of child abuse (Finkelhor, 1984). This awareness spread through the media to the general public. Within the past decade, the public has become aware that the sexual abuse of children is not a rare and exceptional tragedy but a part of the childhood of many children in our society.

Child abuse was not officially discovered by the social work or mental health professions until the 1950s, when Kempe and Steele made it a public policy with research about what they described as 'the battered child syndrome' (Kempe et al., 1962). Child sexual abuse took much longer to be acknowledged and was treated with the most scepticism (Goodwin, 1985). An attitude of incredulity toward victim complaints of child sexual abuse, whether made by children or by women in therapy years after the abuse had occurred, has been the norm among professionals during most of the twentieth century. After a few years of increasing openness to the reality and pervasiveness of the sexual abuse of children in the 1980s, we are seeing many of the doors that opened a little to this issue swing shut again.

The feminist movement's placing of the issue of the widespread sexual abuse of children on the social agenda and the proliferation of research that has been the result of this public awareness have gone a long way toward dispelling the myth that child sexual abuse is uncommon. Diana Russell's incidence study was only one among many. A committee to determine the adequacy of the laws in Canada regarding child sexual abuse, appointed by the Minister of Justice and the Minister of National Health and Welfare, looking at more than 2,000 Canadians, found that 34 per cent of females and 13 per cent of males had been victims of sexual abuse before they were 16 years old (Badgley, 1984). The *Los Angeles Times* study of 248 women uncovered a history of sexual abuse in 62 per cent of the participants (Wyatt, 1985).

Among the landmark research on the issue of child sexual abuse (Armstrong, 1978, 1983; Butler, 1978; Herman, 1981; Rush, 1974, 1977, 1980; Russell, 1986) was the contribution of feminist social activists, and it had an overtly political agenda. The expanded awareness of the widespread prevalence of child sexual abuse has led to the proliferation of further research in this area. Social science researchers and mental health practitioners have been scrambling to build a body of knowledge that will lead to an understanding of this phenomenon. How large is the problem? Why are certain children abused, and why do offenders assault children? What are the effects of sexual abuse on the victims? How do we treat them? Data have been gathered on many different aspects of the problem from different perspectives. Most of the research focus has been on the individual circumstances of the victims, their families, and the perpetrators, and studies have documented the long-term negative effects of sexual victimization in childhood (DeBellis et al., 1994; Trickett et al., 1994; Kendall-Tackett et al., 1993; Dent-Brown, 1993; Finkelhor et al., 1990).

Although girls appear to be more frequently the victims of child sexual abuse, the sexual abuse of young boys is a widespread phenomenon as well. However, the effects of that abuse on the socialization process tends to be very different for girls and boys. For children who are sexually assaulted, especially when they are assaulted in their homes by those whom they love and trust, the experience is often a pivotal one in terms of engraving the rules of a patriarchal culture on their developing subjectivities. Incest is one of the most powerful and intimate lessons that can be learned about power and how it is supposed to be played out in our society. Girls most frequently learn compliance and self-hatred. Their childhood lessons in sexual submission prepare them for domination in their adult lives by men who abuse them physically, sexually, and emotionally. Boys who are sexually abused themselves, or who live in homes where their mothers and sisters are the victims of physical and sexual abuse, often incorporate the values and the tactics of the victimizers as they grow up, and they, in turn, perpetrate their abuse – or the abuse they have witnessed – on others who are less powerful than they are, especially women and children.

The research about the sexual abuse of children demonstrates that, though boys and girls may both be victims in childhood, many fewer girls than boys grow up to sexually abuse children. The vast majority (well over 90 per cent) of individuals who assault children sexually are men (Russell, 1986; Badgley, 1984). It is clear that these are highly significant data, and that they have wide implications about the socialization of boys in our society and the power structures for which they are being socialized. Finkelhor (1984) proposes a model that incorporates both the psychological and sociological dimensions of child sexual abuse in a multifactor analysis addressing the complexity of the behaviour of individuals who sexually abuse children. His 'four-factor model' elucidates both the individual psychology of the offender and the social and cultural processes that contribute to the making of a child abuser. Diana Russell's (1986) study is particularly notable for combining rigorous methodology in data collection and a complex and multi-leveled analysis of the data that takes a social and political as well as a psychological perspective.

On the whole, however, research questions are posed within an individualistic framework. Who are the targets of this socially deviant behaviour? In what ways are they, and their families, particularly their mothers, vulnerable to abuse? How can we intervene in their lives so as to make them less likely to be the next targets? The same questions are asked about offenders. Who are they? What are they like? Why would they want to engage in sex with children? What techniques and technologies have we developed to rehabilitate them so that they won't do it again?

It is understandable that most of the research on child sexual abuse, generated in response to the needs of professionals to know more about our client population, is framed as studies about the sexual, social, and/or psychological profiles of victims, families, and, occasionally, offenders. But the rootedness of the perspective of mental health professionals in the day-to-day reality of our clients, plus our own day-to-day reality of trying to help them in some practical ways, is the weakness as well as the strength of our point of view. Our focus on our individual clients often influences us to concentrate only on the personal dimensions of these problems.

Professionals working with victims or offenders bring into the design of the research their own values and ideologies. Generally, underlying sexual abuse research is the axiom that the sexual exploitation of children is deviant behaviour on the part of the individuals who engage in it. It is further taken for granted that, as a society, we find it abhorrent and, now that we know it exists, we wish to do what we can to prevent it. These assumptions frame the ways in which research questions are posed, and they influence the analysis of the data as well. They are assumptions that may well prove to be unwarranted.

There is growing evidence that the sexual abuse of children is not the problem of a few deviant men going after some vulnerable and neglected children but an inevitable and widespread outcome of the power inequities that are built into our social structures. In 1975, before almost any of the research about the sexual abuse of children was done, David Gill (1975) noted:

If one's priority is to prevent all child abuse, one must be ready to part with its many causes, even when one is attached to some of them, such as the apparent blessings, advantages and privileges of inequality.

If, on the other hand, one is reluctant to give up all aspects of the casual context of child abuse, one must be content to continue living with this social problem (355–56).

Gill went on to declare: 'In that case, one ought to stop talking about primary prevention and face the fact that all one may be ready for is some measure of amelioration' (356). I am reminded of Gill's admonition when I hear professional associations bandying about phrases like 'zero tolerance' for sexual exploitation by their members.

One of the cornerstones of a patriarchal culture is the power differential between men and women, between adults and children, and between other groups of people who hold power in our society. There has been significant research about incest and child sexual abuse supporting the viewpoint that, in this society, men are generally socialized to a predatory sexuality as part of exercising their rights to power over women and children (Butler, 1978; Rush, 1980; Herman, 1981; Finkelhor, 1984; Dominelli, 1986; Russell, 1986).

Russell's (1986) study of the incidence and effects of child sexual abuse on a large random sample of women in the general population collected data about victims, families, and perpetrators; it also traces the history of the issue of incest and child sexual abuse and how it has been dealt with in our society. Her conclusions, based on her findings of widespread sexual abuse of young girls in families of all races and classes, are that the two major – and most neglected – causal factors in the occurrence of child sexual abuse are the ways in which males are socialized to behave sexually and the power structures in which they act out this sexuality. We need child sexual abuse theory and research that continues to assert the overarching truth that must be faced: '... that this culture's notion of masculinity – particularly as it is applied to male sexuality – predisposes men to violence, to rape, to sexually harass, and to sexually abuse children.' (Russell, 1984, p. 290).

My concern about much of the research into child sexual abuse and the theory that evolves from it is that it does not acknowledge this larger social reality often enough. In looking for the etiology of sexual abuse within the individual victims, families, and offenders, we are participating in a cover-up.

The sexual abuse education programs that are sweeping North America as a measure of prevention, while necessary and useful on one level, almost always obscure the basic structural problem of the unequal power between men and women and children: 'Silence is the essence of the abuser's power. Take away the silence and you make him powerless' (Institute for Family Research and Education, 1982).

This truism is a basic principle of many sexual abuse education programs to this day. However, anyone who has been involved in cases where sexual abuse has been disclosed by a child knows that the power of an adult over a child – especially when that child is dependent on the adult in some way – does not collapse as soon as she opens her mouth to protest her oppression. The economic, social, and judicial systems, in which his rights are much more firmly entrenched than hers, continue to operate, and she will be very fortunate if she emerges from the social and judicial processes that follow her disclosure less wounded than she was before she broke the silence. In fact, research findings so far indicate that there is no difference in the negative effects of sexual abuse of children whether they tell anyone about it or whether they keep silent about the experience (Finkelhor, 1986). Most clinicians and social workers, who have supported abuse victims after disclosure, have heard more than one child cry, 'I wish I had never told.'

I am not suggesting that we have any choice but to work away at changing our social structures one piece at a time, or that keeping quiet is better than speaking out, or that ignorance is safer than education. I am proposing, however, that most of our theory and research about child sexual abuse is too narrowly focused, and consequently presents a simplistic and overly optimistic perspective on the value of educational programs directed at children and their families, or on the value of knowing just which particular children in which particular types of families are most likely to be abused tomorrow. The prevalence studies are notable for demonstrating, not who is at risk, but how large and widely distributed the risk appears to be.

We live in a society that has a powerful vested interest in protecting privilege, especially male privilege, and, therefore, no child in any family is safe from sexual predation. An extremely small percentage of men who sexually assault children are ever reported to the authorities, much less charged and convicted for their crimes. If an adult wishes to sexually abuse a child, he can do so with relative impunity, sexual abuse education and street-proofing nonwithstanding. Research and theory that obscures this state of affairs, while it might be comforting and easier to digest than the truth about the situation, does not serve the cause of the protection of children.

Rich Snowdon, who ran one of the earliest counselling groups for incest offenders, portrayed them as 'ordinary guys' who used nothing more than the power any ordinary father has. The men in his group were rarely individuals with an obviously pathological profile. He quotes one of the group members saying openly what many men believe: 'She's my girl, so that gives me the right to do anything with her I want to. So stick your nose out of it; my family is my business' (Snowdon, 1982).

This is a central value in a patriarchal society. A man's home is his castle. Children who are sexually abused in these homes, or by relatives or friends of the family – and the large majority of sexually abused children know their victimizers well – are subjected to the extreme of patriarchal socialization. They are taught in an intimate and concrete way that their abuser – usually an adult male, sometimes an adult woman, teenager, or even another child who has power over their day-to-day life – is in charge of their body and their responses. They are taught that survival demands compliance.

The sexual exploitation of children does not begin when the first hand is placed abusively on the child's body. The ground has been prepared, sometimes directly by the offender who undercuts the child's sense of her own self-worth and her connections with other important and potentially protective people in her life. But it is not only the individual adult who abuses a child who is responsible for creating a climate in which children are readily exploited sexually. Many of the traditions that spring from the values that support our social and economic structures offer the same kind of messages that a sex offender gives his victims as he is preparing them to accept the assault and to accept it silently and uncomplainingly.

Picture, for example, long lines of children with their parents in shopping malls before Christmas, dressed in uncomfortable clothes and waiting for hours, so that they can sit on a strange man's lap and ask him for presents that will magically appear on Christmas morning. The same parents who proudly display the photographs of their children sitting on Santa's lap will responsibly lecture these same children about not taking candy from anyone they do not know. Which message is likely to make a deeper impression on a young child?

I went to a birthday party recently for a little girl who was three years old. Her grandfather kept touching the child on the neck, trying to get her undivided attention. The little girl shrugged him off time and time again, moving away from him to play with her friends. After this had happened at least a half a dozen times, I overheard the grandfather say petulantly to his daughter, the child's mother, '"Janie" won't pay any attention to me.' The mother shrugged and replied wryly, 'She's been street-proofed.'

She had been watching the interplay, and she was clearly feeling uncomfortable about the intrusion on her daughter's person. But she didn't think she had the right to challenge her father's territorial prerogative to touch her daughter whether she wanted to be touched or not. She could only refer to her discomfort in this oblique fashion.

This woman is not a neglectful mother. This is a caring family, doing everything they can think of within their frame of reference to protect their children. The children are at risk, not because of their personal inadequacies or some inadequacy of the family. This tiny child was already quite a register, and her mother did not insist that the little girl attend to her grandfather, as many parents would feel obliged to do in these circumstances. This child – and all our children – are at risk because we are raising them in a society that institutionalizes the excesses of patriarchal authority (Herman, 1981, 1993).

This man was old and rather frail; he wasn't doing anything overtly sexual to the little girl. It would have seemed cruel and inappropriate to most people in our society to give him a clear message, such as, 'Keep your hands off my child,' or even, 'Please leave Janie alone. She wants to play with her friends.' But, as this little girl grows older and has to put up with hundreds of such intrusions in the first few years of her childhood without any adult interference or explanation, how long will she remain sensitive to her own feelings of violation? How long can we expect her to continue to resist, even if we put a few sexual abuse prevention programs into her school curriculum?

The individual child and the individual family do not exist as separate entities outside a rigidly demarcated public space, though we all cherish that illusion to some extent. The family is established only in strict concomitance with the public sphere and is influenced in myriad ways by the material state practices that socialize its individual members and their relations and legitimize their oppression (Poulantzas, 1980). The family – and certainly not just the so-called dysfunctional family – is a central vehicle for the replication and perpetuation of the dominant norms of sexism, racism, heterosexism, and so on – patriarchal oppression in all its manifestations. Parents who have tried to bring up children with values and practices that are radically different from those of their peers and the rest of society can testify that it is a complex and difficult process, and despite heroic efforts, it rarely plays itself out exactly in the ways that are planned and hoped for.

I worked with a self-help group for non-offending family members of sexually abused children in Toronto called AFTERMATH. The members of this group were a cross-section of the population, facing the anger, grief, and helplessness that comes with discovering that a child whom they have loved, nurtured, and protected to the best of their ability has been the victim of child sexual abuse, sometimes in their own homes by people whom they trusted. They have to battle all the stereotypes they carry themselves and that are often expressed or implied by other people they come into contact with regarding the abuse, such as police, social workers, relatives, and friends.

These stereotypes declare that only disturbed and neglectful families have sexually abused children and, essentially, the abuse was their fault – or their child's fault. These parents found that one of the most powerful ways of reaching beyond these responses and of healing the wounds that were created by the abuse – their own as well as their child's – was the process of putting the pain and the rage to productive use in helping other parents and family members of sexually abused children survive the experience and deal with it creatively. They worked together with adult survivors of child sexual abuse on projects to promote social change in this area, so that other children and families might be spared the anguish they were experiencing, and society might begin to be aware that this is a large social issue rather than simply the personal problem of the victims.

The sexual abuse of children is an integral part of social structures and practices supporting the oppression of those who have less power by those who have more power, whether that power arises from age, class, race, or gender, or almost always, from some combination of these and other important differences in which power plays itself out in people's lives. One of the strengths of these social structures in a democracy is the ability to hide oppressive power relations under the rubric of ideological catch-phrases, such as 'free enterprise' and 'family values.' Those who clearly emerge as victims within these institutions, such as sexually abused children and their mothers, are seen as individual problems in a basically sound system. They are then offered treatment for their inadequacies, or are blamed for them, or both.

We need to create theory and research that does not focus only on the damage that is inflicted on individuals who are abused, but rather considers their strengths and their resistance. Though undoubtedly studies that document the long-term negative effects of child abuse and the cost to society of dealing with these sequelae generate funding for much-needed programs, concentrating exclusively on the many and varied ways individual victims are troubled after they are abused can have a stigmatizing and self-fulfilling effect.

We need to create theory and research that, in addition to documenting with rigour the incidence and effects of child sexual abuse, stresses a social analysis that recognizes that the widespread sexual abuse of children is an inevitable outcome of a patriarchal culture – as well as the intimate and painful experience of a particular child and family and the responsibility of the particular offender. Unless we are successful in building alliances that can effectively fight the sexual oppression of children on all fronts, despite our best intentions as individuals, we are in serious danger of becoming part of the problem rather than part of the solution.

Feminists who were sensitive to the needs of individual women suffering from the aftermath of rape and battering lifted the veil on the issue of child sexual abuse and identified it as a pillar of the patriarchal social structure. As well as offering compassionate help to the individual, they offered a social analysis of childhood sexual abuse, naming it – not just as a terrible problem for the children who are assaulted – but as a vicious and effective means of keeping more than half the population in a state of compliance and often even cooperation with their own oppression. This combination of understanding and intervention on the personal level and a critical social analysis that spoke out against the structural causes of the sexual abuse of women and children was crucial in building a movement that could have a significant impact in fighting the oppression of women and children, particularly as that oppression is carried out through their sexuality.

In the past few years, there has been a significant shift away from incorporating a critical social analysis into the research and practice in this area as it has moved from the margin to the centre of social awareness. Nowhere is this shift more evident than in the area of the mental health perspective on one of the most serious consequences of a history of child sexual abuse, the field of dissociation.

As women pushed the psychiatric establishment to face the reality that the early sexual traumas they were hearing about were real, terrifying experiences that had lifelong effects on the children who were forced to endure them, women who had suffered this sort of abuse began to be less afraid to speak up, and some members of the helping professions began to listen. Most of the women who had experienced child sexual abuse had developed dissociative defences to protect them from the onslaught of feeling – rage, fear, grief – that built up within them in response to the abuse, and some of them used their dissociative capacities to create full-blown separate ego-states within them to hide from and adapt to their stressful experiences.

Just as the reality of the wide prevalence of incest and child sexual abuse in our society was a well-kept secret until about ten years ago, radical dissociation has also been a reality that has been minimized. Prior to 1980, only about two hundred cases had been reported in the scientific literature (Greaves, 1980). When multiple personality has been portrayed in the popular media, it has often been sensationalized – another form of silencing. Only in the past few years, with the emergence of the issue of child sexual abuse, have people who have suffered the extreme forms of this abuse been free to speak out in large numbers, and there have been many people with multiple personalities among them.

In order to learn how to help these people who were so disturbed and distressed and who often showed such eagerness for effective treatment, therapists began to investigate the phenomenon they were observing, attempting to place it into a framework that would enable them to deal with it. In the late 1970s and early 1980s, a number of clinicians from different parts of North America independently began to study the phenomenon of multiple personality. The First International Conference on Multiple Personality/Dissociative States, held in Chicago in September 1984 in conjunction with the initial meeting of the International Society for the Study of Multiple Personality, was the first occasion in which therapists who were struggling with attempting to help these suffering individuals had the opportunity to share their experiences, their successes, their failures, and their research in a large forum organized for that purpose. This gathering was one of the formal markers of the reopening of the area of dissociation and multiple personality as a focus of legitimate and urgent scientific concern; another was the inclusion of a separate category of Dissociative Disorders in the third edition of the Diagnostic and Statistical Manual (DSM-III) (1980) and particularly the inclusion, for the first time, of Multiple Personality Disorder as a valid diagnosis.

Since that time, we have been able to help many individuals who were never before able to access appropriate treatment for their suffering. But we have largely ignored the social and political dimensions of our work, preferring to remain ensconced in a mental health frame of reference. It is my view that we retain this myopic focus at our peril.

Incest and child sexual abuse were brought into public consciousness by the women's movement as social and political issues that are manifestations of widespread violence against women and children; then they were taken up by mental health professionals. Severe dissociation, on the other hand, has always been framed in our culture as a mental health problem, and its investigation remains largely a concern of psychiatry and psychology. However, as well as being an important clinical issue, severe posttraumatic dissociation is a social and political issue as well – a feminist issue. It is about rape, battering, sexual abuse, and domination of women and children within a patriarchal society. It is also about creative and courageous resistance, the refusal by women and children to be destroyed. It is important that this reality be in the forefront of our awareness as we explore the clinical complexities of the psychotherapeutic treatment of individuals suffering from severe posttraumatic dissociation.

In summary, there are many ways in which to place severe posttraumatic dissociation in context, but the most basic way is to look hard at the historical, political, economic, social, and cultural contexts in which the inequities of capitalist patriarchy are constructed and secured. We live in a society structured so that everyone has at least one – and usually more than one – individual to blame for the abuses of power that are so keenly felt and seldom clearly seen within a system developed to benefit the privileged few. The phenomenon of widespread physical, emotional, and sexual abuse of children is institutionalized patriarchy laid bare. It is one of the most potent tools that we have as a society for creating and maintaining basic power differentials and then masking them so that they seem like an individual's personal problem, sad but certainly unintentional.

However, child abuse is not the only way that individuals are made to suffer and are diminished as a result of that suffering so that they are less likely to present an effective challenge to the status quo. Institutionalized homophobia, racism, anti-Semitism, sexism, class oppression, discrimination based on ability, size, or age – all are used to keep power in the hands of the few and deny it to everyone else.

A myth that has emerged in the past few years is the notion that abuse, and particularly sexual abuse, is the one serious problem in the world with the attendant belief that, if that is an experience a person has had, it is the cause of all emotional problems – past, present, and future. This is a point of view that decontextualizes experiences, including abuse experiences, pretending that because we are abuse survivors, or multiples, or ritual abuse survivors, that says everything there is to say about how we were hurt.

In fact, there are many ways to get hurt in this racist, sexist, classist, child-hating, gay-baiting world we live in, and some of the most painful stories I have heard – from survivors of even the most brutal and unremitting sexual abuse in childhood, as well as people who have had the good luck not to have been subjected to this kind of horror as children – had to do with other ways in which they were not heard, seen, respected, or loved. Because they didn't have white skin, or white enough skin, or they were poor, Jewish, gay, lesbian, bisexual, or transgendered. Because they were children who wore braces on their legs or a hearing aid. Because their parents drank too much and didn't act like other parents or came from another country and spoke another language and had different customs. Or because they were simply – no, never simply – children who lived in a home that looked OK with parents who seemed OK and had a life that appeared fine and even privileged, but who never felt special, never felt cherished, never in their whole lives ran in the door knowing someone was waiting there who thought they were the most wonderful, precious children in the world.

These times are some of the most exciting and most terrible to be living in. We have seen many changes in the last quarter of a century since an African-American woman, Rosa Parks, was just too tired after a long day of work in a southern U.S. city to stand at the back of the bus according to the law of that city. Since a group of drag queens in New York City had had enough of being harassed and arrested by the police and then beaten and sexually assaulted in custody, and rioted in the Stonewall bar and then out into the streets of Greenwich Village. Since the most recent incarnation of the movement for the liberation of women began to uncover, in rape crisis centres and battered women's shelters and small consciousness-raising groups throughout the world, the way in which social control is enforced on women, both through violence – especially sexual violence – and by stereotypical sex-role socialization.

Survivors of child abuse have also found their voices during this time and as part of this historical impetus. Their words have taught us a great deal since 1975 when the *Comprehensive Textbook of Psychiatry* (Freedman et al., 1975) declared incest to occur in one case in one million in the general population. Now we know that at least one in three girls and one in five boys are sexually abused before they become adults, and that many other children are subjected to all kinds of abuse, neglect, and terrorization. We are all part of a society in which the crimes of racism, sexism, homophobia, anti-Semitism, and child abuse are still rampant, but in which the victims of these crimes are now speaking up with many voices, talking back and shouting loudly 'It's not right. This country promises us better, and we won't take it anymore. It has got to change, for ourselves and for our children.

Of course there is backlash. These liberation movements have cost a lot of people a lot of power, and oppressors do not like to be told to stop. For me it helps to know that all I am required to do is the best that I can possibly do and that is what many other people are doing as well. The struggle for the rights of children and women and oppressed people of all sorts did not begin in our age or even in our millennium, but we are part of a powerful momentum just now. We may not agree with each other about everything, but we are walking on a path together, following those courageous people who broke the path before us and creating a road for younger ones to follow and to challenge and to change. Each of us, in all our splendid diversity – with our different strengths and different oppressions and sometimes very different points of view – is a vital part of that struggle.

2

Multiplicity Is the Solution, Not the Problem

One studies stories not because they are true or even because they are false, but ... in order to learn about the terms in which other people make sense of their lives; what they take into account and what they do not; what they are and are not willing to raise as problematic and unresolved in life.

Linda Brodkey (1987)

The telling of a story is shaped by the conventions available. I don't believe there is such a thing as multiple personality. But then again, I do not believe there is such a thing as medical psychiatry, or academic psychology, or white male doctors either. These are all constructs, ways of framing consciousness, experience, and practice. They do not exist in some kind of reality outside of the terms that we have created to consider them. They are all categories that are unstable and suspect.

They are not, however categories of equal power. Biological psychiatry is one of the most influential of these categories. Ross and Pam's *Pseudoscience and Biological Psychiatry: Blaming the Body* (1995) challenges the much-touted research basis of biological psychiatry as a public relations job with little firm scientific foundation – to a large extent, pseudoscience driven by ideology and self-interest. The authors claim that psychiatry suffers from an identity disorder that its practitioners are trying to cure (or more likely, in my opinion, hide) by forcing the adoption of a bioreductionist paradigm.

For me the ultimate test of the utility of a particular category is not its power but its capacity for transformation towards the realization of justice. To the degree that biological psychiatry reaches out to an underclass of citizens who are marginalized and offers them tools to live their lives more fully with less acute suffering (and there are some and maybe even many cases in which this happens), it is a useful category that I honour. When it reduces complex human beings to bags of chemicals in a way that further demeans already suffering people, it becomes a category I despise and work against.

If we are to be intellectually honest, the category that is the focus of this book – dissociative identity disorder – must be subjected to the same scrutiny as all others. Ten years ago the category MPD was a much more revolutionary notion than it is today. The very idea that it was a worthwhile endeavour to listen to people respectfully when they said they had other people living inside them who came out and took control of their bodies provided a forum for people to speak who had never been given that opportunity before. And as they spoke, many of these people found power for themselves, individually and as a group, that has allowed them to take a more just place in a society that had hitherto excluded them, or included them only when they pretended to be what they were not.

In many ways, the category of multiple personality continues to offer, ten years later, a place from which to speak the unspeakable. Some historical realities have changed, however, transforming the meaning and the value of the category MPD (or, more recently DID).

It is an interesting historical reality that the DSM-III term 'multiple personality disorder' has been changed for the DSM-IV to 'dissociative identity disorder.' There were few scientific data to motivate this change. In fact, there was little agreement among the members of the committee revising the category of dissociative disorders for the upcoming DSM-IV that such a name-change – or any name-change at all – was appropriate. On this battleground, what counts as knowledge depends on its utility for particular ends.

I happen to favour changing the diagnostic label. I think it serves a political goal that is vital at this point in history – acknowledging that dissociation in response to exogenous trauma is widespread and common, and that posttraumatic emotional symptoms are problems like any other problem. Dissociative identity disorder sounds less like science fiction, less 'other,' and more like a fuller, more elaborate form of other types of dissociation, which are not only frequent posttrauma sequelae but are part of the symptom picture of almost every emotional disturbance.

I myself am no more inclined to adopt that particular diagnostic terminology any more than I used MPD to represent all of the ways of thinking and being in the world that I refer to when I say multiple personality or dissociative condition or severe posttraumatic dissociation. Ideology functions for the individual by constituting her subjectivity for her in language, and the diagnostic nomenclature of institutional psychiatry carries a lot of baggage, much of it powerfully oppressive to the objects of its scrutiny. I still find the only way I can talk this kind of talk with any degree of comfort is to both use and undermine each label in a process of unending deferral. It does not work perfectly by any means – it does not create the miracle of situating oneself outside and above the system that one critiques – but it's better than anything else I can think of.

Generally the clinical/scientific literature about dissociation assumes the validity of the categories it then goes on to explore. It explores such questions as differences among personality states, integration of personality states, numbers and types of personality states, cognitive distortions of people who have these multiple personality states, treatment techniques or strategies for resolving some of the barriers between personality states, and so on – all without seriously considering the basic issues about the self being uncovered or constructed in this therapeutic scrutiny. Because I found that unsatisfactory, I searched for a way of addressing these issues that seemed helpful for a full critical understanding of the phenomenon of multiple personality.

And I discovered the vast, complex, difficult, and often perverse literature called postmodernism. Postmodern literature arises out of many disciplines, including literary theory, physics, and political science. I am going to refer largely to aspects of the postmodern conversation that relate directly to the area of psychology, psychiatry, and particularly to the issue of the construction of consciousness.

Postmodernism is a reaction to the ideology that has dominated the scholarship of 'modern' Western culture since the eighteenth century, when reason – and its handmaiden, science – replaced religion as the framework for delineating society's basic values. A modernist belief system holds that it is both desirable and possible – and, indeed, the highest goal of science, philosophy, and other fields of inquiry – to reveal all-encompassing principles that lay bare the basic features of natural and social reality. Such scientific knowledge – assumed to be objective and free from the prejudices and values of those who are instrumental in uncovering these truths – is seen to represent a reality that transcends the perspective of any one human being, group of people, or historical age (Nicholson, 1990).

Postmodernism offers a rich theoretical framework for feminist theorists, many of whom have launched a criticism of the norm of objectivity against the attacks of academics who used this ideal to denounce the legitimacy of an entity such as feminist scholarship, with its implication of a political agenda in the supposedly value-free sanctum of the academy. Indeed, the basic tenet of a postmodern stance – a critique of the notion of universal, transcendent, ahistorical principles – is also basic to feminist theory, as late twentieth century feminism struggles to include the many and diverse voices of marginalized people in the articulation of the values that should govern revolutionary social change. I certainly find it useful in attempting to elaborate an understanding of 'dissociative identity disorder' – what it is and how to treat it – that liberates us from some of the oppressive baggage of the discourse of psychiatry from whence its name derives.

It is interesting to me that, while every third light novel I pick up for recreational reading seems to use the multiple personality convention as a plot device, the postmodern writers with whom I am familiar, whose imaginations I would think would be fired by the lived reality of contradictory multiple consciousness, do not specifically address the issue of multiple personality at all. Despite this curious omission, their insistent questioning of the very existence of non-multiple unitary

individuality is more useful to a basic and expansive understanding of the phenomenology of multiple personality and other forms of divided consciousness than
anything in the directly and obviously relevant literature in the field of trauma and
dissociation.

The term postmodernism is applied to a range of philosophical positions, often
very different from each other. What they share is a radical critique of the humanist
notion of the coherent, essentially rational individual who is the author of her own
meanings and the agent of her own productions. They also unite in abandoning the
belief in an essential unique individual subjectivity. Postmodernism deconstructs
the object that psychology takes as pre-given: the human subject. It insists that forms
of subjectivity are produced historically in a field of power relations. The notion of
the individual has no meaning outside the socially and historically specific practices
that constitute her. This perspective has a world of potential for our understanding
of the construction of multiple personality structures and for connecting this to an
understanding of the construction of the subjectivities of everyone in this culture.

Basic to most scientific research is a modernist philosophy of science that views
the human being as the center and agent of all social production, including knowledge. This humanist perspective, our legacy from the Enlightenment, defines the
self as essentially coherent and rational. Reason itself is seen as transcendental and
universal, existing independently of the self's contingent existence. Mistakes in
socialization – conflicting and confusing stimuli – sometimes cause glitches in the
smooth and predictable running of the machinery of the person, and these need to
be set right through appropriate intervention.

This framework is applied within many diverse contexts and with widely divergent
goals. Surgeons performing lobotomies on psychiatric patients to settle them down
is one example of this philosophy in operation; feminist educators developing curriculum materials that counter the prevailing sex-role stereotypes and show little
girls in a wide variety of social and occupational contexts is another (Walkerdine,
1984). We are all imbued to a large extent with this seductive view of the world and
ourselves as orderly and knowable entities.

We also live in a time when this perspective is under attack, not only by philosophers and physicists, but by individual exposure through the popular media to a
multiplicity of experiences, values, and perspectives about human beings that are
not only fragmentary, but also competing and contradictory. That these differences
co-exist in the world is not new; that we are able – even compelled – to face them
as part of our daily lives is a consequence of evolutions in technology that we are
seeing for the first time in history.

These changes in what we allow into our field of perception have undermined –
though certainly have not destroyed – the modernist faith in a science that claims
to study objects, and claims the resulting knowledge as an object, a possession

(Gergen, 1987). A postmodern philosophy, rather than attempting to map the contours of nature and to grasp the object of study, attempts to study constructions of knowledge, using a language of verbs rather than nouns. Within the field of psychology this contemporary movement to challenge the nature of knowledge has been called the social constructionist movement (Gergen, 1985). Social constructionism views the role of psychology as one of exploring the processes by which people come to account for their lives in the world, rather than describing and explaining those people and that world.

For the modernist, for example, 'I' is the name of my identity. The postmodern assumption is that my identity is not a thing that I own but my life's project. I discover and create 'I' through practical and moral positionings and practices, and there is no 'I' to grasp and hold outside of my uttering the word.

Alice Jardine (1986) declares that the postmodern condition seems to be about not knowing, about not being sure, about having no story to tell. It also seems to be about loss: loss of identity, truth, legitimacy, knowledge, power – loss of control. Jardine notes that the responses to this loss have usually been nostalgic, cynical, or frantic. Sometimes, however, and first and most notably in France, the loss itself has been affirmed as an opportunity for exploring new conceptual tools to elaborate this strange place in which we find ourselves.

The individual/society split is part of a modernist philosophy. The notion of power as monolithic, unitary, and outside the individuals it oppresses – and the individual as the object of oppression and the agent of change – is fundamental to the humanism at the heart of modernism. The work of Michel Foucault is particularly significant in addressing this issue.

Foucault (1972, 1981, 1982) retraces the history of psychology and psychiatry within the framework of a recognition of the historicity of their development and production. In tracing the development of the social meanings of such concepts as madness and sexuality, his approach provides a starting point from which the concepts of 'individual' and 'society' are problematized, and both are seen as effects of the production that is being explored (Henriques et al., 1984).

As a postmodernist, Foucault sees language as the place where our subjectivities and our social organizations are constructed, defined, and contested. Language is a site of continual power struggles (Weedon, 1987). The notion of a 'discursive field' is part of Foucault's attempt to understand the relationship among language, social institutions, subjectivity, and power. Discourse is not simply language; it is, however, always language – language inextricably linked with social practices. Different discourses are competing ways of giving meaning to the word and of organizing social institutions and practices, offering the individual a range of modes of subjectivity. Not all discourses carry equal weight or power in a social context. Some account for and justify the status quo; others resist existing social practices.

Power operates in discourses insofar as they constitute individual subjects. For example, within the Western discourse of psychiatry, the notion of 'multiple personality disorder' refers to a mental abnormality that demands psychiatric intervention. It contains, therefore, all the conceptualizations and social practices that relate to the framing of the phenomenon in this way. Varying discourses exist around dissociative phenomena in different cultures, and the roles talented dissociators play in the maintenance of societal norms and functions within those cultures and diverse. In other cultures, and in some less mainstream religious contexts in North America, 'speaking in tongues' may be a interpreted as a sign of spiritual insight and giftedness. The individual who can take on different voices and personae at different times is considered an adept, and experiences herself and plays a particular role in society concomitant with that definition.

Discourse theory addresses, for example, women's experience by showing where it comes from and how it relates to material social practices and the power relations that structure them. It addresses issues such as desire, meaning, and the relationship of socially and historically constituted desires and meanings to the development of subjectivities and social practices. Exploring the aetiology and the social functions of the orthodoxies that feminism contests – the ways in which being a woman, as our culture defines it, seems natural – can open up our understanding of the constitution and the strategic position of a woman's place in the field of patriarchal power relations. Thus, discourse theory can be helpful in understanding and expanding the range of subject positions open to women and in understanding both the possibilities for change and resistance to change (Weedon, 1987).

The postmodern unsettling of our notions about reality and knowledge has had a profound effect on both psychology and feminist theory. While feminists all over the world were pointing to the oppression of women as a central feature of our patriarchal cultures, and North American feminists in particular were decrying Freud's theories concerning the inferiority of women, psychoanalysts in Europe, particularly in France, were reviving portions of Freud's view of psychic life and placing it within the recently developed and highly contested framework of a discipline called semiotics.

Semiotics is a metaphysics of symbols, based on the premise that reality is not knowable except through its representations in language – its signs. The structural linguistics of Ferdinand de Saussure (1974) challenged the modernist assumption that knowledge (always framed in language) reflects a reality that is outside itself – that is, that we can study and know objects. Saussurean structural linguistics asserted that there is a pre-given fixed structuring of language, prior to its actualization in speech or writing. Language, for de Saussure, was a chain of signs, an abstract system. Far from reflecting some sort of natural world outside its domain, this structure constitutes in and of itself social reality for human beings.

This notion of universal structures that construct our social reality was taken up in a number of disciplines. The anthropologist Levi-Strauss (1963) developed a structuralist theory of human society in which the incest taboo and the exchange of women by men are the universal principles that underlie the functioning of all societies. The psychoanalyst Lacan (1975) applied the principles of structuralist semiotics to the work of Freud, positing universal social structures that guarantee psycho-sexual development along certain lines. These notions of fixed and universal meanings were central to the structuralism that postmodernism grew out of, rebelled against, and transformed. Postmodernism is sometimes referred to as 'poststructuralism,' especially when noting its evolution from the philosophy of structuralism, although the two terms are only approximately equivalent.

This postmodern perspective caught the imaginations of many European feminists, who were dissatisfied with the empiricism of most of North American feminist theory, which was based on a modernist view of reality. Juliet Mitchell (1974), a British feminist, was one of the first English-speaking women to import the French interest in Freud in an effort to combat what she saw as the North American misunderstanding of psychoanalysis. Mitchell's criticism of the feminist opposition to Freud repeatedly underlines one point. She argues that feminists have misread Freud's description of the reproduction of patriarchal culture as a prescription of that culture and women's place in it.

Mitchell asserts that the wholesale disregard of American feminism for Freud's analysis is not based simply on his patriarchal framework, his personal prejudice, or the terrible misuse of parts of his work by psychiatry to further oppress women, all of which she acknowledges and laments. Rather, the distortions that are sometimes inflicted on Freud's work through a partial reading of the text are based on a distaste for the situation he describes and a valorization of some kind of empirical reality that is distinct and separate from the psychic dimension of human life. For Mitchell, this is a denial of the complexity of the reconstruction of our culture in the life history of every new member of the human race – patriarchy in the blood and bones and desires of each of us. A feminist analysis that ignores the unconscious and the importance of socially constructed sexuality, and concentrates only on external factors of oppression, is not so much anti-Freudian as pre-Freudian. Such simplification is likely to render feminism ineffective. Mitchell declares that the message of her book, *Psychoanalysis and Feminism*, is:

know the devil you have got ... We have a culture in which, with infinite complexity, the self is created divisively, the sexes are divided divisively; a patriarchal culture in which the phallus is valorized and women oppressed ... That Freud did not more emphatically denounce what he analysed is a pity (but) ... that Freud's account of women comes out pessimistic is not so much an index of his reactionary spirit as of the condition of women ... oppression has not been trivial or historically transitory – to maintain itself so effectively it coursed through the mental and emotional bloodstream. To think that it should not be so does not necessitate pretending that it is not so. (1974, pp. 361–2)

Although Mitchell's relation to the French psychoanalyst Jacques Lacan is never made explicit, much of her project follows Lacan's emphasis on the originality and totality of Freud's text and the denial of Freud's biologism. Lacan used semiotics to place Freud's work within a cohesive framework capable of addressing the construction of human subjectivity. The human animal is born into the symbolic framework of language, and it is through language that the human subject is constructed from the small human animal. For Lacan, it is the task of psychoanalysis to analyze how this construction takes place and how small human animals come to live as culturally determined, sexually differentiated human beings (Lacan, 1975).

Lacan placed himself and psychoanalysis in opposition to humanism, no less prevalent in Freud's day than it is now. Humanism – a child of the modernist faith in order and progress – espouses the belief that human beings are, or should be, more or less in control of their own actions and choices. Humanist therapeutic practise sees the client as having lost control over her true self. Lacan's human subject is the obverse of the humanist's – a being who is not the source of her own productions and who can only conceptualize herself through the symbolic order, through language. For Lacan, this necessary and universal division of the human animal within the symbolic order situates human beings in a position of constantly unfulfilled and unfulfillable desire. We desire a simplicity and a wholeness that is not within our grasp as creatures constantly being created anew in a complex symbolic order.

Ideology consists of the production of meanings in the interests of certain groups. It is done in such a way that individuals assume they create the structures within which they are constituted. They believe that they are the authors of the ideologies that are actually constructing them. Ideology conceals this uncomfortable state of affairs within an ideal of pseudo-harmony that covers the complexity of the human being's insertion into culture. Lacan includes under this rubric such elaborations of Freudian psychoanalysis as ego and object relations psychology. It is the role of Lacanian psychoanalysis to deconstruct this ideological comforter and to reveal the human being in all its divisions and uncertainties.

A group of French women, calling themselves 'psychoanalyse et politique,' have been influenced by Lacan's structuralist interpretation of Freud, but they have attempted to challenge the limitations of Lacan's closed symbolic order and to turn psychoanalytic theory into a tool in the service of liberation politics. They reject the idealist tendencies in North American feminism that separate material reality and psychic life, and they use a psychoanalytic (Lacanian) analysis of the unconscious in combination with Marxist dialectical materialism to try to understand the complex structures of women's oppression.

These women are almost all psychoanalysts; they are passionately interested in exploring the details of how women have become trapped in desires that deny them, throughout history and in their individual lives. But they are also political creatures who not only desire to understand history and culture, but also want to change it. They are not satisfied with a theory that leaves them trapped in a state of fundamental dividedness. They issue a challenge to that symbolic order in which the phallus is privileged and woman, by the nature of language, is defined as exception, *pas-tout*, the Other, and thus does not exist. 'There is no woman but excluded ... by the nature of words' (Lacan, 1975, p. 68).

In order to do this, they have built on previous critiques of structuralism, such as those of Foucault and Jacques Derrida. For Derrida (1976), there are no fixed concepts in language. He replaces de Saussure's chain of signs with the notion of *différence*, in which sounds and written images have meaning only in their relationship with each other in an endless process of deferral. Consequently, meaning is always open to constant redefinition.

Foucault's work on discourse was also influential in building a challenge to the notion of the closed symbolic order of structuralism. The meanings that are created within a discursive field in which power relations structure the subjectivities of individuals are constantly shifting and changing. This reality opens the way for refusal of and resistance to various discursive positions, including modes of femininity and masculinity.

Luce Irigaray, Hélène Cixous, and Catherine Clément are three French women whose works I will refer to in this context – although there are certainly many other women who have also made important contributions. These women are attempting to create a new writing that undermines masculine vocabularies and definitions of knowing. In these efforts to point to fissures in this symbolic order, through which transformations can erupt, they flirt with a philosophy of essences that links women with the unconscious and posits a primordial state of unity and fusion with the mother, which these feminists, in their efforts to create a new writing (*écriture féminin*) and a new knowing, are attempting to recreate (Irigaray, 1985a; Cixous, 1986).

Their works express a desire for an archaic past which pre-dates the symbolic order. The symbols of the breast and the maternal voice are privileged over the phallus. Clément (1986), in 'The Guilty One,' refers to the tradition of witches, sorceresses, and hysterics in a way that is evocative for anyone who has experienced the life of a woman with multiple personalities. The witch – and later the hysteric – embody an anti-rationalist feminine tradition that threatens the roots of the symbolic structure. Such figures 'untie familiar bonds, introduce disorder into the well-regulated unfolding of every day life, give rise to magic in ostensible reason' (p. 5).

Although their works are very different and the fierce disagreements among them are well-known, these three women all frequently reproduce the traditional dichotomy between male rationality and female corporeality, but privilege the latter instead.

"She will spring from that within – the within where once she drowsily crouched" (Cixous, 1986, p. 887).

Many particular passages in their writings can be interpreted as essentialist. However, I don't believe these women are espousing an essential femininity that exempts women from the complexities of their insertion into the discontinuities of psychic life and material reality within our culture, as some of their critics (Rose, 1983; Weedon, 1987) contend. The exaltation of woman as virgin mother (the obverse side of her degradation as whore) has been used throughout history to keep women outside the public sphere. As Clément (1986) points out, the tradition of the rebellious women she cites is anti-establishment, yet also conservative. It is anti-establishment because it revolts; it declares that some people do not fit into the symbolic system. It is conservative because these women end up being destroyed. Although they display the cracks in the closed system before they are burned or condemned to a hospital or prison, the system almost always closes in on them, and its laws are reinforced by the destruction of these wayward ones.

Clément does not, therefore, advocate an unequivocal return to an irrational or pre-rational state as possible or desirable. But she does argue that it is an important countervailing discourse to the dominant masculinist rationalist discourses, and needs to be considered when creating new subject positions capable of including an awareness of both and transcending both.

These French feminists, with their goal of not only elaborating the traps for women in a symbolic and material order created by men for men, but also challenging that order on behalf of women without simply demanding to be admitted to the order on its own terms, must play with the contradictory positionings of women. Throughout history, women have been defined as Other, surviving within a system that by patriarchal definition denies us recognition. We have accomplished this by understanding and submitting to the rules encoded in the system, while at the same time living rich and often resistance-filled lives at the edge of that culture. Much of the time, the only public expression of the hidden angers and desires of our lives has been identified in the form of symptoms and pathology. Clément speaks of the hysteric as: 'The one who roused Freud's passion through the spectacle of femininity in crisis, and the one, the only one, who knew how to escape him' (1986, p. 9).

This contradictory positioning both inside and outside the dominant culture puts women in a unique position to redefine a place in that culture for a new way of knowing, a new discourse. 'If we continue to speak the same language together, we're going to reproduce the same history' (Irigaray, 1985, p. 205). Irigaray argues that there is no simple way to 'leap to the outside of phallocentrism, nor any possible way to situate oneself there from the simple fact of being a woman' (p. 162). A simple reversal of the masculine, a 'studied gynecentrism' (ibid.) that monopolizes the symbolic order in order to benefit women – or some women – she considers an escape from the necessity of questioning the symbolic itself. This is not a denial of the symbolic order. The solidity and the continuity of social structures that have oppressed women throughout history and across cultures testify to their power and resilience despite pockets of women's resistance in every age.

These women are not discounting the complexities and contradictions that women face when pushing at the boundaries of patriarchal culture and its discourses. But they are declaring, in the face of those contradictions, that, although 'woman' does not exist, women do continue to exist, and women must continue to open cracks in the foundations of our civilization in order to create places where we can speak. The notion of *écriture féminin* is a political strategy rather than a philosophy of sexual essences (Gilbert, 1986). The overturning of culture by extoling nature is an enabling mythology, an initial countervalorization of the maternal/feminine designed to challenge centuries of patriarchal imagery that valorizes the mind, and the masculine.

The French women struggling to connect psychoanalysis and politics are offering their own challenges to the psychoanalytic paradigm, already stretched by Lacan and others since the time of Freud. They recognized that they are not starting afresh, that their discourse is, by historical necessity, connected to those which they critique, which in many ways entrap them. The struggle is, in recognizing this, to continue to push beyond their limits. Cixous comments:

For me, ideology is a vast membrane enveloping everything. We have to know that this skin exists even if it encloses us like a net or like closed eyelids. We have to know that, to change the world, we must constantly try to scratch and tear it.

We can never rip the whole thing off, but we must never let it stick or stop being suspicious of it. It grows back and you start again (1986, p. 145)

A group of British psychologists also attempted to open up the closed symbolic order. In a book entitled *Changing the Subject*, the five authors Henriques, et al., 1984) accept the Lacanian view of the human being as a socially constructed subject, caught in a web of contradictory and conflictual desires. They stress, however, the primacy of the process of the fabrication and positioning of subjects in social relations – relations of power and desire that are ever-changing – rather than within a static symbolic order. Desire and power are produced in relation to social practices. They are less inclined to speak about 'the position of woman,' as if there could be one social experience of being a woman outside the exigencies of social practices related to the individual's race, class, and sexuality, and they see all these social positionings and practices as produced rather than static.

This position opens up the social order to change, for what can be produced can not only be deconstructed and understood, but also transformed. They do not deny the complexity of the often unconscious forces that contribute to the construction of the individual subject in a range of social positionings and practices. Indeed, their individual essays on racism, for example, and on the social construction of gender, emphasize these entanglements. But they do not see the situation as hopeless. They offer a way out through individual/collective social change.

There are many powerful and telling insights on the topic of the deconstruction of subjectivity that I have found useful for understanding the phenomenon of multiple personality. It opens up the complex relations of power and domination that structure our world as a place to look for the causes of multiple personality, rather than simply focusing on the immediate causal factors of child abuse, as consequences of individual or family pathology.

It emphasizes the reality that individuals construct their subjectivities in relation to their social positionings rather than responding to oppression by constructing symptoms that can be seen and addressed in an ahistorical and universal way. These social positionings are intimately related to the specifics of their racial heritage, their class background, and the ethnic and religious cultures in which they have been situated. All of these personal and cultural realities are the crucibles within which an individual's experience is created, and who she is cannot be understood without seriously considering them.

Postmodern thinking challenges the notion of a stable coherent identity, whether that identity be 'multiple,' 'working class woman,' 'lesbian,' or 'abuse survivor,' acknowledging that all of the identities that constitute an individual in her complex, multiple, and ever-evolving identity are imbricated in one another and are vehicles for one another's construction. In this way, it points to the important similarities between the contradictory personalities and positionings within the individual who uses her dissociative capacities to create an array of clearly distinguishable personalities, and the rest of us, who are capable of pretending to a unified, non-contradictory identity and of denying our complex locations amid different discourses of power and desire. Poststructuralism challenges simple notions of 'fusion' and 'integration' as a togetherness that dissolves all contradictions, and calls into question our cultural construction of categories such as gender, sexual identity, and sexual orientation.

The history of many individuals suffering from severe dissociative conditions clearly illuminates the process involved in the construction of all human beings, not as 'unitary points of origin, but as contradictory, irrational as well as rational, capable of assertion yet constantly in the play of relations of power' (Henriques et al., 1984, p. 265).

Following the postmodern emphasis on the production of subject forms through social constructs, we can look at the ongoing creation of multiple self-states within an individual as an example of the continual production and reproduction of specific social positionings and practices. In examining the details of the construction of these subjectivities that are so clear in the manifestation of their multiplicity, we can learn more about the construction of the subjectivities of everyone in a patriarchal culture.

The notion of the unity of the self as illusion has had many proponents in philosophical and psychological thought before this latest postmodern challenge. Matthew Erdyli (1994), a memory researcher, suggests that dissociation is a ubiquitous, essential, and entirely normal mental structure, and that most of the important figures in the history of dynamic psychology (including Janet, Binet, Freud, and Jung) have essentially embraced a polypsychic view of the self. In this they have anticipated contemporary neuroscience, in which consciousness is also understood as modularistic. 'This notion of linear unified conscious experience is dead wrong ... the human brain has a modular-type organization ... the brain is organized into relatively independent functioning units' (Gazzaniga, 1985, p. 4).

Laurence Kirmayer, a specialist in cross-cultural psychiatry, describes our minds as 'shifty and full of holes' (1994, p. 103) and notes that, in a culture with little tolerance for gaps in linear narrative (such as post-industrialist Western society) we are always working hard to mend the ruptures in our experience. We shift attention when we catch ourselves daydreaming. We rationalize our behaviours and decide we know the source of our actions. We need to have conscious control over our thoughts, feelings, and behaviour, and when we do not – and most of the time we do not – we create stories about ourselves that tell us that we do.

This is one reason severe posttraumatic dissociation is so often mocked and denied in scientific circles and sensationalized in popular culture. As a society we are not comfortable with just how near to each other talented and less-talented dissociators are on the self-awareness continuum.

A commitment to the notion of contradictory, partial, and strategic identity locations both reflects and has influenced my way of understanding the self and therefore my clinical practice. I think of problematic dissociation as a disruption of the harmonious functioning of the multiplicity that makes up human consciousness. I am inclined to privilege irony as a clinical tool and to be interested in aiding people to craft some form of poetic/political unity that empowers them to live their lives vigorously and responsibly, rather than a deliberate psychological fusion of part-selves that tend to transform themselves, in any case, without any direct interference from me. I do not encourage people to pretend they are more unified than any of us can ever be, and I listen with interest and often awe to the stories my clients weave as they create with increasing confidence an evolving sense of who they are.

One of the most common questions I am asked when I speak about the issue of multiple personality treatment is what I think about integration. The questions are usually framed as if there are two possibilities – to integrate or not to integrate – or two views – I believe in integration or I do not believe in integration, with the consequence that I advance the therapy process towards integration or I do not.

I do not think about people like that. I appreciate that people with extreme dissociative defences perceive themselves to be several or many people, and, in their therapy sessions, I use that language to some degree. I also challenge it, cautiously, carefully, in order to remain in empathic connection with them while I encourage them to stretch, grow, and change.

I also recognize that most people who do not experience these kind of dissociative barriers to their thoughts, feelings, impulses, and actions think of themselves as one person in some sort of unproblematic way. I also espouse that language to some degree, in therapy sessions with clients and in all the other contexts in which I and my defensively associated friends and colleagues interact. As well as indulging a high level of defensive distortion, in myself and others, that endorses and, indeed, assumes a unitary self, in order to oil the wheels of communication, I also challenge it whenever the context allows.

In my own day-to-day life, I do not generally imagine myself to be terribly unified, and I am usually comfortable with that. Only when I cannot manage to do something I want to do in the time frame I set for myself, because of all the other things I want to do – or, usually, more viscerally, all of the other ways I want to be – do I sometimes get frustrated. Then I grumble things like, 'I wish I were a workaholic, so I could just write this book and get it finished instead of becoming so distracted by taking care of babies, falling in love, putting together albums of photographs, travelling all around, reading mystery stories and lesbian novels, and ...'

All in all, however, I figure that is how life is, and I do not think integration is the answer. I have parts of me – strong, central parts – that long to remain in one peaceful bucolic location, bake bread, tend the garden, and feed and rock the baby on a schedule as regular as the moon's. And I have other parts that climb the walls even considering such a lifestyle. Words like 'balance,' 'integration,' and 'unity' do not describe what my life is like or what I need. The reality is that my life is about coping with this multiplicity, and celebrating it, and my life is not so different from the lives of many other people I know.

I have long maintained that I do not think replacing the clearly objectionable term 'multiple personality disorder' with 'multiplicity' is a solution. When using these terms we are usually talking, if not about pathology, then certainly about adaptations that, although they were once helpful to the traumatized child, have now become problematic for her as an adult who needs more continuity of consciousness. This is why, with all of the terms that I do use to reference the notion of posttraumatic dissociative symptomatology, I do not use the word 'multiplicity.' To my mind, multiplicity is not about dissociation; it is not essentially about problems of any sort.

Dissociation is a survival strategy, useful under many circumstances. A severe, encrustated type of dissociation, like the rigidly demarcated states of consciousness that people with multiple personalities develop in response to early and ongoing childhood trauma, is a survival strategy with a lot of baggage, much of it cumbersome and even disabling. The multiplicity in multiple personality is its strength, its core of health. The repetitive and outworn dissociative defenses are the albatross that makes it difficult to manage the multiplicity with the flexibility and resilience that modern life demands.

I do not find the dissociation continuum (see Figure 1), which starts with a unified self capable of using dissociative strategies for special purposes and passes through various levels of pathological dissociation to complex, multifragmented MPD, an accurate reflection of the range of human responses to multiplicity or to association and dissociation.

A more useful illustration would start with the notion of the fragile self that denies its multiplicity in one of two ways: defensive association and defensive dissociation. Defensive association pretends to simple unity to hide fragmentation, suppression, and complex humanity in all its contradictory manifestations. Defensive dissociation acknowledges the depth and complexity of the human condition through the inter-play of a multitude of self-states, but denies it utterly at the same time through radical disconnection. The continuum moves from the fragile self to the mature, robust self, which can acknowledge its many forms and locations, where the individual struggles for consciousness about herself as she changes with each new day and each new experience (Figure 2).

This model privileges the multiplicity of human consciousness, while acknowledging the diverse ways in which it is feared, suppressed, and manipulated in the service of survival. This seems to me to be more reflective of the reality we experience in our severely dissociative clients than one that conflates multiplicity with defensive dissociation and multiple-state structures with dysfunction. The creativity and drive for health and healing so obvious even in some of the most disturbed individuals suffering from dissociative conditions adhere to the multiple part of the equation. The 'personality disorder' aspect of the condition rests in the need to defend the traumatized child and the adult she becomes against this very multiplicity with radical dissociation and many other psychological symptoms.

Laurence Kirmayer (1992) elaborates another such model of consciousness (Figure 3). This model views four broad states of mind (self-consciousness, consciousness of the external world, reverie, and automatic behaviour) as parallel modes of infor-mation processing, any one of which (or any combination of which) can be dominant at a given time. As a result of experience or temperament, individuals differ in the tendency to utilize each mode or in the style in which they shift from one mode to another. The model as Kirmayer presents it is not hierarchal. Self-consciousness is not the master mode of cognitive organization, and changes in state are seen, not as

Figure 1. Continuum of dissociation.

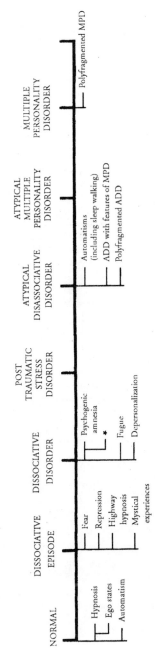

Source: 'The Bask (Behavior, Affect, Sensation, Knowledge) Model of Dissociation,' by Bennett G. Brown, 1988, *Dissociation, 1 (1)*, 4.

Figure 2. Multiplicity is the solution, not the problem.

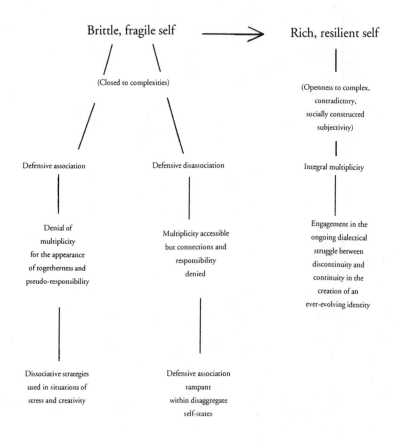

Multiplicity is the solution,

not the problem.

Brittle, fragile self ⟶ Rich, resilient self

(Closed to complexities)

(Openness to complex,
contradictory,
socially constructed
subjectivity)

Defensive association   Defensive disassociation   Integral multiplicity

Denial of
multiplicity
for the appearance
of togetherness and
pseudo-responsibility

Multiplicity accessible
but connections and
responsibility
denied

Engagement in the
ongoing dialectical
struggle between
discontinuity and
continuity in the
creation of an
ever-evolving identity

Dissociative strategies
used in situations of
stress and creativity

Defensive association
rampant
within disaggregate
self-states

Figure 3. States of mind relative to dissociative experience

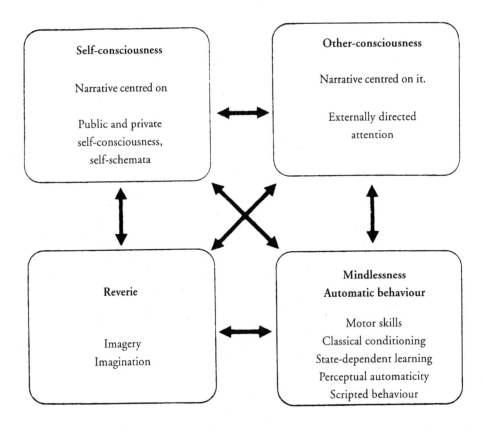

Source: 'Social Constructions of Hypnosis' by L.J. Kirmayer, 1992, *International Journal of Clinical and Experimental Hypnosis, 40 (4)*, 276–300.

the choice of some executive cognitive agent, but as the cooperative effect of parallel modes.

Consciousness is a complex affair, and even the most elaborate and complicated model does not begin to capture it. The strength of the latter two models (Figures 2 and 3) is that they are heterarchal rather than hierarchal. They priviledge the incorporation of the widest possible modes of consciousness and the most flexible use of combinations of association and dissociation (or self-consciousness and reverie, for example) rather than framing dissociation or multiple-mindedness as a problem to be wiped out by therapeutic intervention.

The notion of the multiple self evolving throughout an individual's life history – my life's project, rather than something I am or I discover or I own – is a challenge to most conceptualizations of the self, which are based on spatial metaphors: the core self; the superego, the ego, and the id; the true self buried under layers of protective socialization. Stephen Mitchell (1993) makes a convincing case that, in a postmodern world, it is more useful to look at the concept of the self through the lens of a temporal rather than spatial metaphor. He would replace the layered (spatial) conceptualization of the self with one that focuses on the evolution of the self through time.

In his extraordinary book *Hope and Dread in Psychoanalysis*, Mitchell frames psychoanalysis as a clinical tradition that continues to reinvent itself. Psychoanalysis has undergone a fundamental shift from Freud's focus on clarity, explanation, and insight and from the assumption that the analyst is outside the analysand's process as the repository of awareness, the knowledge of which he eventually, at the right time, imparts to his patient. The contemporary analyst is a product of postmodern skepticism concerning the belief in science and rationality as secure bridges to clear understanding and control, which were seen in the intellectual context of Freud's day as attainable goals.

Analysts of the late twentieth century are more likely to be concerned with meaning than with truth. They understand that the meaning that emerges from the therapeutic engagement is a mutually constructed phenomenon, and both participants are agents in the creative process (Mitchell, 1993; Stolorow et al., 1987).

As well as changes in the conceptualization of what happens in analytic treatment, there have also been fundamental shifts in emphasis in the way the conceptualization of the self – that most central and most elusive of notions– is understood. The basic questions of how people organize themselves are always explored with every new attempt to create new psychological theories and new methods of treatment. So, for example, an issue such as aggression is formulated and reformulated. Is aggression a primary biological drive, or is it a secondary reaction to perceived threat, bolstering an essentially non-aggressive self? Is aggression toward others a secondary elaboration of a primary death instinct, or is it a survival strategy of a self that perceives itself in danger of death?

Mitchell points out that, despite the enormous differences in the questions various psychoanalytic thinkers propose and the range of answers they come up with, the notion of a core self, a self that exists prior to and outside of relational contexts, is central to all of them. We are constantly struggling to find, uncover, discover, unearth, and activate this real self. We talk about being able 'to be myself with her,' and about a particular job or relationship or social situation 'allowing me to be the real me.' The notion of an authenticity buried beneath layers of socialization, framed in a spatial metaphor, is pervasive and assumed.

The ways in which highly dissociative people structure their consciousness offer a challenge to this archaeological image of the self, but generally clinicians avoid the challenge by interpreting the multiple-state structure simply as pathological. Glass (1993) carries this to an extreme to make his quite valid point that the romanticization of fragmentation ('libidinal freefall') of some postmodernist thinkers (Deleuze & Guattari, 1977; Baudrillard, 1988) discounts the palpable and intense suffering of real people suffering from conditions of ego fragmentation such as schizophrenia and multiple personality. Though his outrage at the victimization of hospitalized women suffering from severe dissociation whom he has interviewed is palpable, and his compassion for their torment is understandable, he seems to end up interpreting their divided selves as pure pathology (though, he understands, adaptive and imposed pathology). He frames their experience as radically different from other women's and declares that clinical understandings that may be relevant for women with relatively 'normal' psychological and sexual development mean nothing to the severely abused girl:

The abused daughter possesses no psychological avenues enabling her to create a seductive fantasy about the relationship; she has no internal space from which to construct out of the father's presence a fantasized object of love and affection. He lives in her mind as a stark reality ... There is no attraction, no life instinct, just fear of pain. (p. 69)

Nothing of the French feminist's celebration of the feminine exists in the multiple personality (p. 54). [W]hatever is multiple in the self's 'being' as identity is symptomatic – not a sign of possibility in the feminine or the maternal relation, but a sign of the domination of the father, his force and will. (p. 72)

In my experience, women who manifest their multiplicity in severely dissociated states have found ways of celebrating their womanhood, of preserving the life instinct and of protecting possibilities of all sorts, despite the 'domination of the father' in all his guises. It is true that they suffer and that they are degraded, and that they sometimes degrade themselves. It is also true that the fragmentation that revictimizes also protects, and that it is not necessary to deny the multiplicity to heal the fragmentation.

For Glass, the choices seem to be between some unproblematic (and undefined) type of solid self or a self in a state of fragmentation and unmitigated terror, between a fixed identity or a multiplicity rooted in brutality and terror. The notion of dialectical development in which contradictions are held, challenged, resolved, and then held again on a different level in the creation of an ever-evolving self is not even considered.

This is not uncommon in psychological theory. Finding the core of the person – with the implication that we shall find the true and real self therein, and can then begin gradually to rope all of the extraneous part-selves into its embrace – is often either explicit or implicit in the theoretical formulations upon which clinical interventions are based. I think it is a misguided effort on the part of those of us who strive for a high degree of self-consciousness, and who tend to the defensively unified portion of the association/dissociation continuum, to tame the shifting nature of the self and render experience – our clients' and our own – more manageable.

The idea that the self moves in time rather than being constructed in space is congruent with a postmodern science and sensibility that understands that we can never stand entirely outside the field we wish to observe and disconnect ourselves from our knowing. The awareness that all knowledge is perspectival, constructed, and rooted in its social and historical context has arisen within the disciplines of physics, neurophysiology, psychology and philosophy in an interactive fashion. Accepting the notion of a self constantly shifting over time – organized, disorganized, and reorganized as it moves within its constantly changing relational context – makes much more sense in today's world than the wrestling to ground of a final and true version of the self that is then named 'me,' and considered real and authentic.

This way of thinking about the self has obvious implications for the way a therapist approaches the treatment of someone suffering from severe dissociation. It influences how we think about personality states, for example – what they are and are not.

They are not a slice of past selves; the three-year-old alter personality is not an isomorphic re-enactment of the client at the age of three, who had to hide beneath the more recently developed older selves. Without really fully conceptualizing it, therapists often assume that their clients' minds are like something out of *The Lord of the Rings* or *Watership Down*, a hobbits' village or underground rabbit warren in which a plethora of little people, teenagers, adults, demons, or animal creatures are waiting for the psychologically appropriate time to emerge and take their place in the ongoing life of the client.

Self-states or personalities are ways of being in the present; they are not frozen aspects of the past. This does not mean they are not related to the past in any way. They are aspects of the individual – including cognitions, feelings, ways of behaving, or even physiological characteristics – that evolve from psychological structures that were organized in the past and are still functionally effective in an ongoing way in the individual's life, or remain available to be mobilized under special circumstances. This way of thinking about a two-year-old alter personality who tries to throw the paint around the art therapy room makes a considerable difference to a therapist's approach to such a situation.

If I believe I am dealing with a two year-old – even a cryptogenically reborn two-year-old – I am going to be much more likely to encourage tantrums that are developmentally appropriate for a two year-old, if not actual paint-throwing. If, on the other hand, I think that throwing tantrums continues to be useful for my adult client, either regularly or occasionally, I am going to help her understand the ways in which she thinks this is the only way she can survive or communicate or get her needs met, with the immediate goal of helping her find other, more sophisticated and functional ways of accomplishing these goals.

This is no way means that I lecture my client, while she is in her toddler frame of mind, about not being a brat. I am more likely to be warm and patient or at least firm and even-tempered (depending on the behaviour that is involved) until she is able to muster a state of mind in which she can engage in useful dialogue. But I do not think that bringing up clients through all their developmental stages in a literal-minded way through age-appropriate interactions with child personalities is neces-sary for an effective therapy process.

Sometimes this happens (fingerpainting with a three-year-old alter, reading a story with a message to a six-year-old alter, sitting quietly and saying soothing things while a preverbal baby personality sobs in grief), and it can be helpful. This is not because these are babies or children from the past, however. Rather, this is the only way, at this point in time, that this adult knows how to express herself creatively, to receive constructive input, or to allow her grief to surface. If I do not understand that these alters are a way of denying as well as expressing present-day emotions – if I collude with my client in seeing them as literally separate entities – I am engaging in a kind of re-parenting that is much more likely to encourage disempowering regression rather than growth and independence.

Multiplicity is not a problem; it is a wonderful thing, individually, socially, and culturally. That an individual can be alternately loving, aggressive, playful, sensual, stubborn, relaxed, creative, and methodical testifies to the depth and breadth of humanity's emotional reach. The problems from which multiples suffer do not derive from the existence of their personality states, their many ways of being in the world. That is their strength. The difficulties arise from the way in which the defensive dissociative barriers between these states are rigid; management of the self, in all of its diversity, consequently becomes a terrible burden, and for many an impossible one.

Some who experience themselves as many, therefore, have a powerful and des-perate drive to rid themselves of their multiplicity – in effect, to become just part of who they are. People in the early stages of therapy often state as their goal 'to get rid of the voices,' or 'to make the others go away.' A beleaguered sailor in the middle of the ocean, in a boat carrying a rich cargo and with a large hole in its side, may well start frantically pitching the cargo over the gunwhales, thinking to lighten the load and thus slow the process of sinking. However, unless she finds some effective way of mending the hole, cargo or not, eventually she will go down.

The focus of treatment for those with multiple disaggregate self-states should not be whittling themselves down to size so that they become more like people who suppress their multiplicity for the sake of control. The therapy process should facilitate the exploration and nurturing of all aspects of themselves, with the purpose of making it possible for all of who they are to participate actively in the creation and maintenance of a productive and fulfilling life.

The adoption of this approach – which not only appreciates the adaptive function of radical dissociation in the face of trauma, but also privileges a high degree of multiplicity in the organization of the self as a rich resource – has significant implications for the type of intervention a therapist would utilize with clients experiencing disabling dissociation.

For example, one of my clients, who holds a responsible position in the field of medicine, has created a state of consciousness called 'the woman in the lab coat.' In this state, the individual is completely focused on work-related matters, is warm and empathic with patients, exact about procedures, and can work long hours without loss of productivity or concentration even when generally tired and/or disturbed. For achieving the goal of maintenance of stability and efficiency at work, this self-state organization is perfect. Not only would I not attempt to interfere with its relatively autonomous functioning, I think I can learn something from this person's capacity to create a barrier against stimuli that would ordinarily interfere with the ability to concentrate on complex and important tasks.

As this individual's therapy process moved into the resolution stage, 'the woman in the lab coat' developed an awareness of the more personal aspects of the individual's life. The ability to step back from a situation and examine it objectively expanded from strictly work-related matters to all aspects of life, and became less personified and situational. This was a gradual process; no hypnotically-facilitated fusion ceremony dissolved the distinctions between 'the woman in the lab coat' and all of the other parts of this individual. Neither the client nor I even noticed the progression, only the result. In calling to change a session time, I realized, one day, that I was talking to my client at work in a natural, casual way, and I wondered when the change had taken place. 'The woman in the lab coat' had always spoken to me previously when I had called my client's workplace; the communication had always been stilted and abnormally functional – like talking to a computer.

The images that individuals healing from dissociative conditions use to designate particular aspects of themselves and various strategies for functioning may remain the same after resolution of the dysfunctional aspects of dissociation without any implication of dysfunction:

I got off the telephone from this argument that made me very upset, and I had to call on the woman in the lab coat to see the next patient. In fact, I didn't think about the argument again until I left the hospital that evening.

They may also change.

I was so upset when I got off the phone that I knew I had to do something if I was going to be able to give my next patient the care she deserved. So I closed my eyes, took a deep breath and took all those feelings and put them away. I got a picture of my patient and of me talking to her. Then I could go out and see her. I didn't think about the argument again until I was driving home from work.

Although the first formulation is a more concrete way of thinking about experience, both are equally healthy and effective. In fact, many – perhaps most – individuals who resolve the problems that fueled their radical dissociative symptoms stop thinking of themselves as many people, even metaphorically. What was a necessary survival strategy – the complex and cumbersome system of self-states – gradually dissolves when it is no longer needed. Generally, this occurs with no instruction, suggestion, or assistance from the therapist. Therapeutic tools or relaxation images that evoke a sense of internal separateness may well be inappropriate for the recovering multiple. The image of the inner child can resonate differently, and not particularly helpfully, within the imagination of someone who has once thought – quite literally – that she was inhabited by many children. This does not mean, however, that the there is anything more psychologically evolved about more abstract conceptualizations about the self, or that some people who once used radical dissociative strategies for organizing consciousness defensively will not find that such images work for them, even when they understand them differently.

People with multiple personality should not be taught in therapy that, because they had previously used dissociation in a way that caused enormous problems for themselves and others, it was the multiplicity or even the dissociation that was the problem. Multiplicity is a rich resource; dissociation is a strategy that everyone struggling to cope with a complex and stressful environment must utilize effectively to some degree a great deal of the time.

Therapy is not, therefore, the process of helping a dissociative individual to become non-dissociative, or a multiple to become one person. It is a process of helping a person with a disorganized, rigid, chaotic, unhappy life use both her multiplicity and her dissociation skills (in conjunction with all her other resources) in an increasingly constructive fashion in the service of a productive, fulfilling life. How that finally plays itself out – what kind of images people use to think about themselves, the style in which they talk to themselves, or the techniques they use to modulate their feelings and their behaviour – will be as varied as the people themselves.

I talk – to some degree – to many severely dissociative individuals in the early stages of their therapy (and this can mean for three years), as if they are different people. I try to stop using this type of metaphorical language as soon as it is possible to maintain a meaningful and healing conversation without doing so. And even in the early stages of therapy, much of my language assumes more unity than I assert. I attempt to facilitate as much control over the behaviour of the whole person without insisting on a unity of the self.

It is crucial that the client who experiences herself as different people feels heard. It is also crucial that the client and the therapist do not create a precious and encapsulated communication – like twins in a playpen creating a language that separates them from the world beyond the nursery. This comfortable and comforting *folie aux deux* can enable the client and the therapist to collude in the avoidance of the most difficult and essential task of psychotherapy: dealing with the mundane problems of building a constructive life and cultivating, as Freud named the signs of maturity, the ability to love, the ability to work, and the ability to bear frustration.

I have spoken to trauma survivors with extensive therapy histories who claim integration and talk glowingly about abreactions and fusion rituals and other specialized therapeutic experiences. Some of them appear to be having great difficulty maintaining the most fundamental stability; others carry a distorted and inflated sense of themselves that is making it hard for them to develop relationships with anyone except other individuals with similar self-perceptions. Therapy for these people, as they describe it, has been an unending reliving of horrors from the past in combination with the cultivation of an engorged sense of entitlement that increasingly diminishes their motivation and their ability to struggle with making a constructive contribution as a responsible adult. This re-enforcing of the cult of the victimized – whether in therapy or in other social situations – is a form of disempowerment and revictimization, however well-meant.

Richard Kluft, a pioneer in the field of dissociation, used to joke that when you complete the multiple personality part of the treatment and the person has achieved integration, you are then dealing with a person with single personality disorder. My clinical experience has shown me that many of those 'single personality disorder' issues can be amenable to intervention in the early and middle stages of therapy. If the major focus of the treatment, rather than trauma and dissociative phenomena, is issues like attachment, responsibility in relationships, modulation of affect – the same kind of issues that anyone wrestles with in therapy – the radical dissociative structures evolve gradually into something less cumbersome and more effective in terms of day-to-day functioning.

In order to accomplish this, I use whichever language my client can communicate within. For someone with classical dissociative identity disorder, that language may need to be imagistic and concrete. One of my clients, for example, was increasingly reawakening many feelings that had been blocked off since her abuse as a child. Until, as part of her therapy process, she had started to become connected with the intensity of her feelings, she had been an A student. Her sense of self-esteem was bound up in success in school. Her success as a student, however, was predicated upon her ability to dissociate most of the time from any and all of her feelings, past and present. Consequently, her opening up to a wider range of affect was creating problems in her functioning at university.

One solution to this type of problem would be to encourage the client to take some time off in order to ensure that she can do the work she needs to do in therapy without creating more life problems for herself. For some people in some situations, that is necessary and appropriate. If their work situations are dangerous to them, or their difficulties are endangering others, or if the degree of disorganization is great and cannot be contained by the therapy, it may be necessary for individuals to take some time off school, work, full-time care of children, or other responsibilities. On the whole, however, I do not think this is the best solution, and, with the help of the therapist, individuals suffering from severe dissociative conditions often have the resources within them to create other alternatives.

In the case of the student who was in danger of failing because having feelings was so new and so destabilizing that it was interfering with her ability to concentrate on her studies, neither she nor I ever considered her taking time off from school as a viable solution to the problem. Instead, we worked together to restructure her dissociative strategies to address the current problem. I do not start playing around with tricky dissociative strategies until I have tried to solve problems in more mundane ways. In this case, we had worked together on the issue of coping with school for a number of months, and this individual had done all of the obvious things to give her the support she needed to get through the school year. She had developed a group of helpful friends who studied together and played together. She structured her time and prepared at home for all classes, labs, and tests. She worked as hard as she had ever worked in her life. Still, she would get flooded with feelings and forget everything she knew.

Towards the end of the school year, when she was beginning to wonder, for the first time in her school experience, if she had the capacity to pass her final exams, we focused on her self-system, and she created a different dissociative strategy that enabled her to both feel her feelings and concentrate on her studies. A part of her that was previously only a guard – its function being to observe everything that went on in her life for the sake of self-protection – was enlisted to do the academic tasks at any time when the part of her that usually fulfilled this responsibility became flooded with feeling. In this part of herself she had all the information needed already from its function as a guardian/watcher, and it was simply a matter of widening its function. This part then began to serve in a way that was similar to 'the woman in the lab coat' of the other client.

Both of the student and the medical person developed dissociative strategies that enabled them to maintain a high level of vocational functioning while engaging in a gruelling and sometimes rather destabilizing therapy process. These techniques are not magic – though they sometimes seem so in the way they enable an individual to do something on Tuesday she felt completely unable to accomplish on Monday. They do not take the place of hard work, understanding the dynamics of stressful situations, challenging cognitive distortions, building affect tolerance, or learning affect modulation – all the things anyone must do to grow and change. But the enhanced capacity to dissociate and thus to compartmentalize feelings from function can be used as a coping strategy in the present as it was in the past, but with more conscious control and without the global, undifferentiated zoning out that makes defensive dissociation in response to trauma almost as much of a problem as it is a solution, even in the short run.

Learning the language of multiple personality and gaining clinical experience in working effectively with individuals suffering from severe dissociative conditions not only enables a therapist to treat abuse survivors who have built up these types of defenses with the skill this treatment demands, it also opens up avenues for more effective and imaginative treatment for everyone else the therapist sees.

Sheldon Kopp (1972) defines the role of the therapist as 'being where they ain't.' People who live within the reality of multiple severely dissociated self-states need help in making connections between states, owning all of what they think, feel, and express as theirs. People who do not have multiple personality often deny altogether those thoughts, feelings, and impulses that severely dissociative people may acknowledge, but designate as 'not me.' Most people cannot bear the cognitive dissonance that comes from expressing what they cannot understand, integrate, or take responsibility for. The distancing techniques that highly dissociative trauma survivors learned at an early age can be useful to many people attempting to come to terms with ego-dystonic material in a therapy process. The ability to look at one's self from the outside can make it possible to face what previously had to be denied: 'I was shocked when I heard "the bitch" talking to my five year-old. No wonder the poor child is so scared half the time. "The bitch" has one nasty mouth on her.'

This type of compartmentalization – in its extreme form so pervasive in the thinking of highly dissociative individuals – can facilitate the exploration of shameful or ego-dystonic material. An individual can acknowledge the content of the material without becoming immediately overwhelmed by taking full emotional responsibility for it. This is an unfamiliar luxury for most not-so-dissociative people, and it can make the difference between a failed or a successful treatment.

This does not mean teaching non-multiples to become multiple, nor encouraging the avoidance of personal responsibility. It does mean helping clients who are blocked in accepting aspects of themselves to find concrete ways of distancing themselves enough from their thoughts, feelings, and behaviour so that they can develop the strength to look at issues that they had previously had to avoid. A basic goal for everyone in therapy is to make the changes that are necessary and desired at a pace that is possible. These kind of dissociative techniques – which put some distance between individuals and their most feared thoughts and feelings – can, with certain caveats, be taught with good results to people who are not severely dissociative.

Just as a therapist encourages someone with multiple personality gradually to take more responsibility for the thoughts, feelings, and behaviour that they have encapsulated in their disaggregate self-states or alter personalities, it is important that not-so-dissociative clients who learn to imagine part-selves do so gradually and in a way that enables them to integrate the material into their sense of themselves, so that they are able to take full responsibility for it. Whether or not individuals continue to use the language of the separate self as a useful shorthand is not the point; what is important is that the therapy helps people accomplish what was previously out of their reach.

The metaphor of the inner child is used this way in many forms of counselling, particularly in the field of addictions treatment, to enable people to acknowledge and tend to the more vulnerable aspects of themselves. It is generally easier for people who do not see themselves positively, except in their most adult high-functioning states, to learn to treat themselves with warmth and tenderness – or at least tolerance – when they visualize themselves as a child.

Severely dissociative individuals create inner child images as part of their defensive disavowal of traumatic experiences ('It happened to that other little girl, not me'), and eventually they elaborate this process as a way of managing all kinds of experiences ('She picks up men and has sex with them; I would never do that because I think sex is disgusting'). In therapeutic work with individuals who use dissociation extensively in a way that creates serious problems for themselves, the therapist works within the framework of the client's inner imagery to help her talk about issues that are difficult and conflictual for her. The imaginative way someone with multiple personality can both work with painful material and also back off from it when necessary to maintain some degree of stabilization can teach a therapist a great deal about how to help clients who are very closed, both cognitively and affectively, to acknowledging frightening, ego-dystonic material. Simple inner child work can be expanded to deal with many other issues that some people find intolerable to process in much depth, such as anger and sexuality.

This is certainly not a new idea in the field of psychotherapy. Psychosynthesis and gestalt are two types of therapy that make use of learned dissociation as a central part of their practice. Hypnotherapy, in the context of intensive psychoanalysis or for pain control or surgical analgesia, is carried out by teaching the patient how to dissociate. Dissociation – whether consciously learned or happened upon as a less deliberate psychophysiological response to extreme stress – serves the same basic functions, among which are an escape from the constraints of an intolerable reality and the isolation of unmanageable experiences or feelings. The dissociative process enables an individual to accomplish tasks with more efficiency and economy of effort than would be possible if the individual were not in a state of focused attention. Individuals are also able, on some level and for some time, to resolve irreconcilable conflicts when in a hypnotic or dissociative or focused state.

Self-hypnosis or dissociation can be a valuable tool if it remains largely under the control of the person who is using it. For young children who dissociate crudely and globally in response to terrorization, dissociation quickly evolves from an almost magical, life-preserving solution to a serious, often life-threatening problem. Unfortunately, information that is necessary for understanding and defending oneself against future assaults – as well as just figuring out what is going on in a multitude of more mundane ways – can be lost in the process of mentally hiding from the experience that originally could not be understood and survived. It is important that therapists working with highly dissociative clients and teaching dissociative strategies to others understand thoroughly both sides of the wonderful/terrible phenomenon of dissociation. Like the splitting of the atom, it has fearsome potentialities if not properly harnessed.

The basic tenet of the model of multiplicity that I am proposing is that each facet of the crystalline structure of the consciousness of a person is precious. When the basic and abiding value of all parts of a person is finally appreciated, the damaging psychological effects of a painful life history have been wrestled with successfully in psychotherapy, and significant psychosocial changes have been made and consolidated, the multiplicity can exist in a different form from the rigid and disjointed system that evolved, in part, to defend against knowing itself. The different voices with different perspectives no longer have to be silenced or devalued. The individual, who is now in a position to bear an awareness of the depth, breadth, complexity, and contradictory nature of her life experience, can now call all of those voices 'I,' accepting none as the whole story, but embracing them all.

This is the multiplicity at the heart of all of us. It transcends categories such as 'sexual abuse survivor,' 'ritual abuse survivor,' 'multiple,' and all of the other ways in which individuals have come to identify themselves by reference to a particular aspect of their experience. The evolution of the identity of 'survivor' (meaning one who has managed to survive particularly brutal circumstances, such as 'Holocaust survivor,' 'psychiatric survivor,' or 'abuse survivor') has been part of the opening up of the issue of the widespread violence against women and children in our society. Creating an identity category that allows an important aspect of an individual's experience, hitherto unspeakable, to be named and proclaimed has been a liberating strategy for a great many individuals. It has carved out a discursive space for people who had previously assumed that they were outside the boundaries of socially-sanctioned, generally acknowledged reality, a space in which they can declare, 'This is an experience that constituted me. It is an experience that has been important, even central, to making me who I am, and I refuse to be forced into silence about it (and therefore about myself) any longer.'

However, a strategy that can be legitimating and liberating can also be limiting. To say, 'I am a multiple,' tends to reify the category of dissociative identity disorder. Multiple personality is not a thing. The experience of understanding oneself as a variety of different people – with all its physiological, psychological, and sociological correlates – always and only exists within the ongoing construction of an individual's personal consciousness. It varies significantly from one person to another, and at different times in the life cycle of one person.

In the context of the prevalent polemic of the poststructuralist essentialist/constructivist debate, identity politics (and I include the identities of 'survivor' and 'multiple' as two of the identities that have a political meaning and purpose) are often framed as a reinforcer of a liberal humanist idealism that limits the subject to a fixed definition, a thing that, by definition, is different from other things in a way that is referenced by the identity label. The creation and dissemination of a category such as 'survivor,' can be part of constructing a discourse that allows the unspeakable to be spoken for the first time. The security of operating from within a discursive structure that is meaningful to more than one person can empower people whose experience has been marginalized by offering them a language that is resistive and challenging to the status quo which, up to this point, has outlawed their freedom of expression.

However, as well as providing a vehicle for liberation, the creation of a discourse of identity can have reactionary effects. The discourse that has created terms such as 'survivor,' 'multiple,' and 'ritual abuse survivor' is an example of a language that can be radically empowering to a group of people who have had little power and also and at the same time limiting to those very people.

'Multiple' and 'survivor' are not stable and universal categories, and they are invested with very different meanings in different contexts. Even within one context at one time, many meanings may adhere to a single term. The pathologizing that is endemic to the medical model of treatment has become attached to the notion of dissociative identity disorder, very obviously, but it also echoes through the use of words that were created in opposition to the constrictions of mainstream mental health ideology, like 'survivor.' Lists of survivor issues, safe houses for survivors, survivor groups, self-help books for survivors, all potentially practical tools, also contribute to the increasingly common assumption that survivors are a category of people who are essentially different from non-survivors and like one another – as multiples are very different from non-multiples and like one another, and people who report childhood histories of ritual abuse are qualitatively different from those who don't and are like one another. These can be comforting notions; they can even be true in some ways. They are also not true, and in many significant ways profoundly unhelpful.

They are not true insofar as they ignore the ways in which an individual's subjectivity is continually constructed along many dimensions. Experiences of race, class location, ethnicity, religion, and the many other influences on the developing individual are likely to be as powerful in the evolution of who she comes to be in the world – her values, her perceptions, the way in which she creates relationships, even her physiology – as her experiences of traumatic incidents of abuse. All of these factors mediate her response to such trauma and therefore its effects on her development.

Anyone living in our society is significantly influenced by the structures of capitalism and patriarchy and, to varying degrees, by the sexist, racist, classist, homophobic oppression that is central to its evolution and maintenance. This is in no way to deny the depth of the painful, frightening, and dehumanizing experience that childhood sexual abuse represents. It is to say that such abuse is not an "it", not a thing. As they are lived out, experiences of abuse are embedded in many other experiences that are, in turn, embedded within a particular personal, social, and historical context that renders them meaningful in a different way for each person who carries their legacy.

Identity categories like 'survivor' can also contribute to an individual's continuing oppression when they endorse a currency of victimization that is constraining to an individual's growth. Many of the people I know who have engaged in and completed a healing process in which they emancipated themselves from their most significant emotional shackles eventually felt constricted by identity categories that were initially liberating. This does not mean that they deny their history of childhood abuse, but that those oppressive experiences are no longer as central to their conceptualization of themselves once they had resolved most of the ways in which their abuse experiences still held them captive.

Support groups, formal or informal, can be invaluable at times. However, when individuals create their entire life around issues and people whose main focus is a particular victimization, there is a danger that they will be forced at some point to choose between their friends and support networks and their own need to grow into a person who no longer feels comfortable being named in her deepest and most authentic identity as 'abuse survivor.'

A model that espouses multiplicity as the solution rather than the problem and conceptualizes a variety of limited and limiting ways of associating and dissociating as problematic to a wide range of individuals – and probably to some degree to all individuals socialized in a culture such as ours – acknowledges the specificity of the difficulties of individuals suffering from severe posttraumatic dissociation, but does not claim – explicitly or implicity – that these problems are the only ways in which a person can construct her consciousness in order to defend against full knowledge, full feeling, and full responsibility. Individuals who experience themselves as radically divided selves are in some ways in a much better position to unmask the fiction of unproblematically unitary identity than are most of the rest of us who need our comforting fictions in our own journeys as survivors of one sort or another.

The interplay of the different personality states is the quintessential postmodernist drama. Each state has its point of view, which competes with the perspectives and the demands of the others. However, the individual suffering from the ongoing constrictions and torments of a life attacked and diminished at an early stage in its development does not wish to be a play. She usually wants a life – and a peaceful, productive life at that. All too often she is persuaded that her only choices are either a disorganized, fragmented identity that is multiple in character, or an identity of simple unity.

It is my message – to her and to all of the rest of us, including myself – that this is not a choice any of us have to make. We all have the choice to wrestle and to play with an identity constructed in heterogeneous and heteronomous sites, to be creatures who live in the always-changing spaces between the binary – the 'I' and the 'not-I,' the together and the fragmented, the old and the new subject positions, the constructed and the constructing. We have the choice to celebrate, if sometimes uneasily, our multiplicity.

3

Learning the Language of Dissociation

What constitutes the outrage of the Holocaust – the very essence of erasure and annihilation – is not so much death itself ... but the fact that death is radically indifferent ... people die as numbers. In contrast, to testify is to engage in the process of finding one's own proper name, one's signature.

Shoshana Felman (1995)

When one cannot turn to a 'you,' one cannot say 'Thou,' even to oneself.

Dori Laub (1995)

The claim of many so-called sceptics regarding the existence or the utility of the diagnosis of dissociative identity disorder – that if you ignore the symptoms, they will go away – is true in a particular way. If you are not willing to talk to someone in their own language, they will either try to talk in your language or they will go away and not talk to you at all; often they will do both. The phenomenon of hypnosis bears this out. Individuals suffering from severe dissociative conditions are highly hypnotizable and therefore, by definition, highly suggestible when in a trance state. And it does not take much to induce a trance state in an individual who is highly hypnotizable.

No formal induction is needed to encourage a highly hypnotizable individual to slip gears and go into a trance state. Diminishment of the critical faculty and compulsive compliance are central characteristics of the trance experience. Social influence phenomena, such as a doctor who has clear opinions on the subject of multiple personality, are enough to influence an individual to intensify her concentration and modify her peripheral awareness such that she is in a trance state without any conscious awareness of this fact on her part or on the part of the doctor. She could then be inducted to admit to any number of things, including that she is fabricating her dissociative symptoms and her abuse history.

Obviously, this works both ways. If I have an agenda to diagnose every highly hypnotizable person I come across as suffering from a full-blown, classical dissociative identity disorder, I simply have to focus a great deal of intense attention on such people, ask them suggestive questions that point them in the direction I want them to go, and it is very likely that I could induce a trance in many of them and get them to comply with my demands to produce certain types of responses. This does not mean I have created multiple personality any more than suggesting to a person with DID that she does not have this condition in such a manner that she agrees cures her of the problem. People suffering from severe dissociative conditions can be highly suggestible. There is no doubt that if a therapist wants clients to stop express-ing their radically dissociative symptomatology in obvious and concrete ways, most clients will do so, at least in the presence of said therapist. The question remains whether this is helpful to the client.

I agree in some respects with those who say multiple personality does not exist. What they often mean is that the individual claiming to have separate people living in one body is wrong – she or he is only one person like the rest of us. Basically – with some significant, but in this context perhaps not terribly relevant caveats about the degree to which any of us can claim to have a unified self – I think that is true. True, but not a communication that the individual who experiences herself as radically divided can understand and therefore benefit from.

Colin Ross noted that multiple personality is an illusion with measurable corre-lates. The personality states that experience themselves as separate people sometimes have documented differences along a number of psychological and physiological lines – different allergic responses, memory banks, pain thresholds, galvanic skin responses, EEGs, laterality, needs for prescription lenses, and so on (Putnam et al., 1982; Braun, 1983). Despite their singularities, however, these self-states, with their often obvious and pronounced differences, are all aspects of one person. To be helpful, a therapist must engage with both aspects of this paradox simultaneously.

This is not such a unique notion. The concept of stepping into a client's world so that the therapist can understand the client's frame of reference sufficiently to engage in meaningful dialogue is a basic principle of all interpersonal forms of psychotherapy. If a woman comes to see me with a black eye that she says was inflicted by her husband and then tells me she stays with him because he loves her so much, I am unlikely to be useful to her if I say, 'Loves you? Are you nuts? He is going to kill you one of these days.'

I may be absolutely right. But being right is different from being helpful. I cannot offer her the support she needs to begin to see the situation from a different point of view, and then make some changes in her life, if I am not able to let her express herself about the situation as she experiences it. I must also allow myself to understand the situation from her point of view enough that I can talk her language. That does not mean I agree with her, or that I pretend to agree with her. It means that I get inside her skin enough that I understand deeply what it is like to be her and that I reflect that back to her so that she does not feel alone with her experience, that she knows that I understand. That is the first step. Without that step, any other steps taken are unlikely to be useful.

With people who experience themselves as radically divided, part of the therapist's first step in learning to see their client's situation from their point of view is learning to speak their language. A therapist learns the language of multiple personality or of other forms of dividedness in the same way she learns anything else about her client, by listening to what her client says and then asking sensitive questions or making empathic responses that indicate that she 'gets it,' thus encouraging the client to say more and to show more. As the client says more and shows more, the therapist understands more what it is like to be that person under those particular circumstances, and the therapist can then speak to the client from within the frame of reference of that understanding.

This empathy is not the same as identification (colonizing a person's experience and claiming it for one's own), or sympathy, or a clinical understanding – as we often speak of that concept – of standing outside a phenomenon and figuring it out intellectually. Rather the therapist moves inside the experience of the client; she tries to 'walk a mile in that person's shoes.'

As well as entering into the client's experience, the therapist, in order to be helpful, must remain thoroughly grounded in her own experience, her own language. It is difficult to express notions that contain contradictions in a discourse that usually does not even attempt to wrestle with the contradictory nature of human existence, that is, the discourse of psychology and psychiatry. But psychotherapy is as much art as science, and art has no trouble acknowledging and even celebrating paradox.

Therapists often identify their client's experience as being the same as their own (or, as it is more commonly labelled, 'identify with their clients'), or may be cognitively preoccupied with fitting what the client is saying into a typology learned in graduate school or the latest conference. They may become overwhelmed with sympathy for the client. When mentally and emotionally travelling down these distracting paths, therapists are unable to engage in the stance of sustained empathy that is a prerequisite for deep therapeutic communication.

As a therapist, I should be able to be clear and separate enough from my client so that I can allow myself to merge with her experience deeply enough to enable me to truly understand it, and also be able, simultaneously, to stay thoroughly grounded in my own experience of reality. From this position I can combine my ability to experience how my client sees a situation with a talent for showing her how to glimpse the situation from a slightly yet radically different slant, for opening up a way in which she can move a little without giving up everything.

Clinicians who need people to be multiple or not to be multiple for their own reasons will not be able to place themselves within the client's experience, for the distraction of the therapist's need will create a barrier between the client and the therapist. They have their own road they need the client to walk and their own talk they need their client to talk. It does not matter so much what that walk or talk is. It is not the client's own, and therefore it cannot make out of her experience a meaning that heals.

Highly dissociative individuals are as different from one another as anyone else is different from any other person. True, it can be helpful to know that most people who suffer from severe dissociation experience states of consciousness that seem developmentally younger than their actual biological age, and it may make it clearer when a client who is known to be very explosive says, 'Anger? No, I never get angry,' that she is not lying but simply not in touch with the discrete states of consciousness that hold her anger.

It is useful to know that many hear voices in their heads and experience time loss as one state communicates with another or takes control of the awareness and behaviour of the individual. Knowing about these things is useful if it helps the therapist ask sensitive questions that enable clients to tell their stories without fear of being thought crazy, strange, or stupid. It is not helpful if the therapist reifies these categories in such a way that clients have to distort their experience so that it fits into the therapist's conceptual framework. Learning the language of dissociation is a new task with each person who speaks that language.

Another helpful aspect of thinking about the expression of the dissociative experience as a language is that it can lead us to useful conclusions regarding appropriate responses. Professionals in a variety of settings come upon individuals who experience themselves as different people in one body and are flummoxed as to how to behave with that person in a way that is compassionate, ethical, and sensible – that is, in the way they wish to behave with anyone else.

For example, a shelter worker is confused about how to respond to a situation in which a child personality emerges every evening when it is time for the woman to do her evening chore, the dinner dishes. The child cries, says she can't reach the sink and that she wants to play blocks with the worker. The staff is divided over the appropriate handling of the issue. The first night it happens the worker on duty takes the woman to her office where she plays with toys that are kept there for the children in the shelter. The second night, another worker becomes irritated, mutters something about manipulation and leaves the woman alone in the dining room while she pitches in and helps the other residents clean up the kitchen. At the staff meeting the next day, a heated argument takes place about how the situation should be handled. The discussion becomes quite personal, opinions become polarized, conflicts exacerbated, and eventually the talk wanders far afield from the original issue of what to do about the woman who turns into a child when it is time to do the dishes.

This is not a unique scenario. Individuals who express themselves in a way that is so concrete and at the same time so oblique can often be a catalyst for the expression of feelings in others that breaks through long established boundaries between individuals and in group settings. It can lead to catastrophe, destroying relationships and organizations, if the dynamics that emerge are not faced, opened up, and understood, both regarding the client and other issues that may have been suppressed but have been driven out from under cover in the course of addressing the complex and emotional issues that trauma survivors often present.

Take the dishwashing situation and the different workers' responses to it. What does it mean? Certainly it is not simply, as the woman with multiple personality experiences it, that she is no longer an adult but a three-year-old. To the degree that the first worker responds to this situation in this way, she is identifying with the resident's distortion and re-enforcing it. On the other hand, the resident is not simply pretending to be a three-year-old to get out of doing the dishes, as is implied by the second worker's attribution of manipulation as the explanation for the state switch at chore time.

The only way to get out of the impasse of placing the resident in the equally disempowering roles of helpless child/victim or malingerer is to look at the action as language and to deconstruct it by engaging in a conversation with the resident so as to understand what she is trying to say. The woman in her child state is likely to respond to clear, quiet, non-judgmental questioning as to why she came to the dining room at this particular time. If all she can say is I wanted to play blocks, it is simple enough to respond that there may be time for her to play blocks later in the evening after the dishes are done, but it is time for Sandy to come back because it is her turn to clear up the kitchen. When the switch to Sandy is facilitated, it may or may not be helpful to see if Sandy knows why she shifted into a child state at that point – or it may be enough just to say casually to a confused-looking woman something like, 'You seemed to have left us for a few minutes there just as we were about to start doing the dishes.

Depending on why the dynamic occurred, more talk may be needed in the moment to get the situation back on track. Often, in these settings, mundane household events such as chores or meals or children's bathtime, can trigger reactions to earlier experiences that were imbued with sinister meaning. In this woman's family of origin, for example, the beginning of doing the dishes may have been the signal for the mother to leave the scene, the father to take over, and the abuse to begin. Shifting into a child state and declaring that she is too small to reach the sink and therefore cannot be expected to go into the kitchen and do the dishes is indeed an attempt at manipulation – manipulation in the service of self-preservation. Only when the language is unpacked can a helpful intervention be made.

Such intervention will take into consideration both the past and present reality of the resident, helping her to bracket the past so that she can behave in a responsible adult way in the present, while at the same time acknowledging the importance of that past in shaping her feelings, impulses, and behaviour in the present. If, for example, rather than simply saying that she wants to play blocks – in response to a question as to why the child state appeared just as the dishes were about to be washed – she bursts into tears and cowers behind a chair, saying 'Don't push my head in the sink,' there is more information being provided about what the state switch meant.

This is not the time to engage in a complicated and intense abreactive session; it is time to do the dishes. However, in order to get the woman into a state of mind in which she can accomplish the task reasonably expected of her as an adult resident of the shelter, it is necessary to engage as quickly and efficiently as possible in a communication with her that allows her to calm down and to distinguish the shelter kitchen from that of her childhood home.

Talking to the individual in a way that she can comprehend when she is in a child-like state, the worker could say, 'You do not have to go into the kitchen. You can go into the safe place that you and your therapist made and stay there all safe and sound until you see your therapist on Monday and then you can tell her all about this. Is that OK? OK, you are now safe and secure, and it is time for Sandy to come back.' Depending on what state Sandy is in, she can either just get down to doing the dishes or she may need to get oriented for a few moments by talking about her experience of what happened, also with the direction to talk about it more fully with her therapist on Monday.

This type of communication sounds exotic, and it sounds like it would take a long time, but neither needs to be true. Many workers say that they do not want to talk to alter personalities because it is beyond their area of competence (as a shelter worker, child protection worker, or housing social worker, for example). But all of these professionals consider it their job to communicate with the people who look to them for help in a way that will enable them to hear what they have to say. Certainly, in a shelter for abused women, if a woman panicked at the dinner table because she was suddenly flooded with recollections about the way she and her children were beaten during suppertime, it would be entirely appropriate to facilitate her talking about her reactions briefly, either at the table or privately if there were children or vulnerable adults at the table, so that she could stabilize and eat her dinner.

A child protection worker would not be likely to say to her client, 'I only want to talk to the part of you who is mature and cares responsibly for your children,' but that is essentially what she is saying when she says to a woman who experiences herself as radically divided, 'Only bring your host personality (or adult self) to meetings with me. It is not appropriate for me to speak with any other part of you.'

A Children's Aid worker does not have to do therapy with her client to take into consideration the important reality that when this woman leaves her children alone or yells at them or hits them, she is not responding from her adult, responsible state, and it is quite possible that if the worker insists on talking only a 'we're all adults here' language with her client, she will only get confabulation, which will be totally useless in helping either worker or parent understand what is going on. There are some situations in which this can be not only unhelpful but downright dangerous, and child protection situations are among the most risky.

Psychiatric hospitals, in which suicidal patients are placed for their own safety, can also be situations where it is very common for a patient to be given the message, 'Talk our language; if you regress, we will increase your medication, place you in isolation, and you will never get out of here.' The result of these instructions is that the parts of the individual who were suicidal, homicidal, or disoriented – and need to communicate the problems underlying these behaviours that landed her in the hospital and for which, presumably, she should be treated – are driven underground. Again, confusion covered over with confabulation, in which the patient attempts to figure out and provide the 'appropriate' responses, is the final product, and nothing useful gets communicated.

Some of this lack of communication is not particular to highly dissociative people. There are some, perhaps many child welfare offices, hospital settings – any context where the healing capacity of the facility is often overwhelmed by the social control aspect of its mandate – in which the message, 'Just tell me what I want to hear and it will be easier for both of us,' is the order of the day for everyone. Highly dissociative people are no more shut up or shut down than anyone else. But there are mental health and social service settings in which a person with a relatively integrated consciousness will be encouraged to express as many aspects of her thoughts and feelings as she possibly can; the notion that you would say to a client, 'When you come to my office, I expect you to be mature, calm, and well put together, and any expression of vulnerability, fear, or anger is unacceptable,' would sound ridiculous and unprofessional. Yet professionals who would never think of giving these kind of suppressive directives to most of their clients appear to be able to say righteously to someone with multiple personality, 'Just talk like an adult in my office; I'm not interested in the rest of that histrionic nonsense.'

I think the root of this problem is the professional attachment to the notion of the unified, cohesive subject – both in others and in ourselves – and a need to defend against the performance of highly dissociative people, whose self-presentation not only speaks to their own perceptual distortions but also to the reality of a de-centred self. This de-centred self is more similar to the way most of us experience the world than we are comfortable seeing. The conversation that takes place between a professional and someone who is floridly dissociating has an uncanny air. It is often a discourse that can be foreign, unfamiliar, different from the way we usually talk about things.

When I first started to work with clients suffering from multiple personality, I would sometimes look up and around in the middle of the conversation with my client, suddenly self-conscious about how odd the talk would seem if some else were listening. Most of the time it did not seem odd to me at all, but I think that is because the kind of talk I had long been most comfortable with was pretty uncanny. I went to girl scout camp for eight years, and we sang songs and recited poetry constantly. My friends and the teachers I loved in high school were writers and artists. At college a group of us regularly spoke a combination of poetry and Gregorian chant. We would sing the statement 'Iamgoingtothedininghallforlunch-doesanyonewishtojoinme?' in plainsong, and then during the long leisurely meals, our conversations would be dotted with scraps, and sometimes fairly long passages of poetry.

This was neither self-conscious nor precious. Music – particularly the church music that we heard across the small Gothic campus from the chapel for a hour five times a day and which most of us had heard throughout our entire, intensely Roman Catholic, pre–Vatican II childhoods – and poetry, others and our own, were at the very centre of our lives at that time, and we expressed ourselves through them very naturally. It was only when I arrived at the gigantic University of Toronto, and my peers stared at me strangely when I would respond to a question with a quotation, that I began to see the uncanniness of the type of communication I had previously taken for granted. In fact, one of the things that most attracted me about the man who became my husband were his identities of poet and Latino, which expressed themselves through unCanadian behaviours like walking around the university campus creating poems aloud, occasionally stopping other students, usually strangers, to ask them if they thought that a particular group of words constituted 'a good line.'

My graduate training was in psychology, but when I tried to become a registered psychologist in the province of Ontario, I discovered that having an undergraduate degree in English and philosophy was not only not considered an asset, as I had always assumed it to be, but might well stand in the way of my becoming a full-fledged member of the science club. In fact, I always knew I wanted to train for some profession like psychology, but I took my undergraduate studies in literature and philosophy because I thought I was much more likely to learn about human beings and how they communicate (which I considered and still do consider to be central to psychology) from the literature and the sacred books of the world's peoples than from basic social science textbooks.

People who talk multiple personality as a way of communicating their experience of feeling divided in this world are like poets in the middle of an accountants' convention. This is not to say that the source of their defensive dividedness is not the need to distort and the need to distance, but almost everyone divides and distances to some degree and then covers this reality with mundane talk that hides rather than reveals this state of things. Indeed, people suffering from full-blown dissociative conditions divide internally more than the average de-centred individual who has not needed to embrace the extremes of dividedness to survive, but they also – if we have the ears to listen to their language – acknowledge that state of dividedness at the same time that they deny it utterly. The language of multiple personality has a poetic quality that opens up the uncanny aspect of the paradoxes of their existence in a way that enables us to catch a glimpse of the many levels of meaning that adhere to each action, each word.

Paradox is at the heart of the multiple personality experience. This making of the multiple is through the process of the double bind, the contradiction that cannot be spoken. 'Your father loves you; your father rapes you; your father never touched you, and if you say or even think he did, he will hurt you again harder until you learn that he never hurt you.'

Learning the language of dissociation does not mean buying into all the contradictions that are central to its defensive use. The woman who turns herself into a little girl because she is afraid of doing dishes is not literally a little girl in the way she perceives herself to be. But that is not the point. If a worker tries to persuade her that she is really an adult and not a little girl – 'Look in the mirror. What do you see?' – she may get her to agree that she is not a little girl, but she will not truly comprehend that concept of responsible unity that the worker is trying to convey when she says, 'You are not really three years old. You only feel young, but you are indeed an adult.'

What is most likely to happen is that the communication between the worker and the woman will be damaged, because though the woman with multiple personality cannot tell the worker everything about her experience when she switches states, she is trying to tell her something. Insisting that she be able to understand it all and tell it all will only result in a communication impasse – she will be able to tell nothing.

This does not mean that the language of multiple personality is the language the client must speak forever. If the therapist becomes so enraptured with the evocative aspect of the multiple personality rhetoric and the way it deconstructs much of what is usually hidden in our society – the way it sometimes shatters mundane reality and supplies a surplus of meaning – she is in danger of being fascinated rather than helpful. A genuine understanding of the language of radical dissociation includes a comprehension of its limits, of the ways in which it constrains the client's understanding as well as allows her to speak the unspeakable, and traps her in contradictions as well as frees her to express the forbidden.

Learning the language of radical dissociation within a therapeutic context in such a way that the learning will be helpful to the client means understanding the discourse well enough to be able to help the person, who could only speak certain truths in the language of multiple personality, gradually – incrementally – expand her capacity to interconnect the discourse of dividedness with the discourse of unity.

This does not mean replacing the discourse of exaggerated dividedness with one of exaggerated unity, though that is the more socially sanctioned discourse. Generally, in our society, we talk the talk of unity, while simultaneously behaving in ways that contradict the content of our conversation. Simply encouraging individuals who experience the world through the lens of a kaleidoscope to pretend that reality is a fairly obvious unidimensional affair is to do them a great disservice. However, to help them construct a language for themselves that is just as rich but not as rigid, that takes into consideration the complexities and contradictions of reality, past, present, and continuing, and also enables them to incorporate themes of unity, leitmotifs that can connect one passage to another – this is truly to be helpful. It enables an individual who has had to disown significant aspects of her experience, and consequently her behaviour as well, to develop a more refined and workable sense of personal responsibility and a wider range of personal freedom to talk her own talk and know, even when it is complex, confusing, and contradictory, that it is hers.

We all live in language. It is the central and invaluable insight of postmodern thought that the person is not outside her language. She does not learn a previously wrought language. She is her language. To the degree that we deny individuals who speak the language of multiple personality the right to talk their language, to the degree that we refuse to listen to them respectfully, we are unlikely to catch a glimpse of them as they are creating themselves.

Healing is made out of changing the narrative of facts into the narrative of transformation. In engaging with the client's ongoing expression of her life as she experiences it, the healer falls under the client's spell as the client tells her story. This compelling aspect of her storytelling allows the client to create meaning out of the broken pieces of her experience, and also binds her in a spell that limits her capacity to make changes in the narrative flow. It is the client's ability to mesmerize the healer with her interpretations and her identifications that enables the healer to 'get it,' to understand to some degree, to catch a glimpse of the client as she continues in the process of creating herself with each new telling of the tale.

It is the therapist's task to allow herself both to be spellbound and to step out of the story and break the spell. This movement in and out of the story enables the therapist to create an empathic bond with the client, and thus to experience the story from the inside out. It also enables the therapist to interpret the story from another perspective, to perceive different ways of seeing the story and to communicate these to the client with the sensitivity that only one who is both entirely in the story and entirely outside of its strictures can manage. This communication – which contains both the empathy of one who knows what it feels like and the objectivity, disinterest, and clarity of one who is not spellbound – is what allows the client to challenge, a little bit at a time, the self-constituted view of reality that anchors her in a semblance of safety, the only safety she has known, and yet constrains her every day of her life.

The process of moving in and out of the narrative happens in a variety of ways, depending on the context in which the healing takes place. Themes are spoken as they relate to the mundane realities of daily life as the client lives it, and out of which she weaves her story. For example, the woman in the shelter who regresses when it is time to do her chores has created a theme of inequality, dependency, and eventually anger in the story of her relationships with other women. She says that women are caring and concerned about her when she first meets them as she comes to depend on them for help, and then they turn on her in anger and she is rejected again and again. She does not know why that is. There must be something basically and deeply wrong with her that behaves in the same ways other women do and yet always she draws anger to her.

The creativity in the work of the shelter staff is shown in the ways they manage to create space for the individual and her needs and feelings and, at the same time, for the needs of the group for stability and structure. This dialectic between the individual and the group – between freedom of expression and the need for order – is not only the result of practical necessity, but also a representation of the dialectic between the needs of the individual and the needs of others, between the rights of the individual and her responsibilities. That is a central issue in everyone's maturation process and is a particularly thorny and core issue for the survivor of severe childhood abuse.

Within this context, if the shelter workers are able to hear both the stories the woman tells – the story of the woman in a child state who is terrified of doing the dishes and the story of the woman in her adult state who wants to do her share – they can find the space between, the place in which the two stories intersect, or do not quite intersect but play off each other to create the possibilities of a new story that is not quite either and more than both. Thus the compulsive pattern of telling and retelling the same stories with slightly different facts but always the same endings of failure and betrayal can be interrupted, and room can be created for change.

Learning the language of the individual with a multiple state system should not be about collecting as much data as possible about the elaborations of each discrete state of consciousness. This map-drawing, in which the therapist tries to figure out all of the intricacies of the system, can, in fact, have the effect of reinforcing multiple-mindedness rather than moving the client in the direction of a more integrated way of being in the world.

This does not mean that the therapist should discourage the client from using whatever method works for her in attempting to gain more knowledge about her own self-system, so as to get more control over her daily life – whether this is journaling, creating maps, making lists, painting portraits of alters, or all of these and more. The therapist should attempt to keep her own focus on process rather than on content, so that she learns more and more about themes, about patterns in the way the client operates in the world, rather than collecting masses of data about alter personalities that makes the job of helping the client to create some order in her daily life increasingly overwhelming.

If the therapist, as well as the client, takes literally the client's perception that there are sixty-seven adult states of consciousness that must participate in any decision, plus one hundred and forty-two child states whose very diverse needs must be taken into consideration before any changes can be made, plus a host of demons who will destroy any accomplishment – then the therapist would be completely unreasonable and unrealistic if she did anything but throw her hands up in despair and agree with the client that the situation is, indeed, hopeless.

If the therapist, on the other hand, understands that the complexity of the system signifies the multidimensional nature of postmodern adult life, with its complex demands overridden with the fears, needs, and angers of a particularly unsatisfying childhood – a situation perhaps more difficult and complicated in degree, but not different in essence, from everyone's struggle to build a constructive adult life while dealing with the ambivalence derived from unmet childhood longings and unexpressed childhood fear and rage – then the therapist is much more likely to be able to give her client – and herself – a constructive message: the struggle is a difficult one, and there are no quick solutions, but if one step at a time is taken, she can get where she wants and needs to go. The grounded therapist can help the client understand that, in changing one word of the story, she is that much closer to the transformation she most desires.

The key to unlocking the language of radical dissociation is understanding that it is not so different from the language of any human being. The tools that the therapist brings to her work with the individual who experiences herself as utterly divided are the same tools that she uses to work creatively and effectively with other clients who are struggling with their less radical dividedness. They are the same tools, essentially, that she brings to her own struggle. The more therapists have deconstructed their own stories, the more experience they have had in wrestling with their own demons, confronting their own ambivalence, and comforting their own inner children, the father along on their own journeys of self-discovery they have travelled, the more skilful they will be in understanding the language of multiple personality or other forms of radical dividedness.

As well, the more professional experience therapists have had, the more people they have guided through an in-depth therapy process – especially if many of these people have suffered greatly in their lives – the more familiar they will be with the human themes that play throughout everyone's life song when it is sung in all its keys with fullness and some degree of freedom. They will then have the capacity to interpret the unique and concrete way individuals with multiple personality express themselves in the light of these experiences, rather than referring the expression of the multiplicity back on itself.

Therapists often ask me questions like, 'What should I do when an angry alter comes out and says he has fantasies of wrecking my office?' Most questions that begin with the phrase, 'What should I do?' are usually the wrong question. Almost always the question that needs to be asked first is, 'What is going on?' or 'What is being said?' or 'How do I understand this situation?' When those question are thoroughly explored, the answer to the question, 'What should I do?' is usually pretty obvious.

The situation of the angry alter that is threatening to trash the office, for example, needs to be assessed. Is this a threat at all, or is talking about fantasies of damage to property simply the only way this individual knows to express what is the sine qua non of an effective therapeutic alliance, the negative transference? If it is indeed a threat, is it a threat made by someone who has a history of acts of physical violence and damage to property? Is it a test to see if you are able to be clear about the parameters of acceptable behaviour? If so, then clearly stating the limits about violent behaviour is an entirely appropriate intervention and likely to result in a more secure client who knows you respect yourself and will insist on that level of respect from her.

On the other hand, it may be that talking about thoughts of breaking up the therapist's office – or the therapist, for that matter – is the first sign of the erosion of the dissociative barriers between the part-selves that are compliant and co-operative and those that are mistrustful and enraged. In that case, treating such an expression of feelings as an actual threat and talking about guidelines regarding physical violence and damage to property would be a breach of empathy that would clearly communicate, not the therapist's self-respect, but fear of the expression of anger.

Thus, the same story can have very different meanings in different contexts. By definition, individuals with highly discrete dissociative states, which they understand as separate personalities or even separate people, are individuals who express themselves in a very concrete fashion. When initially accessing and bringing into the therapy milieu a threatening emotion, such as anger, they may well revert to their most regressed level of communication and, like a young child, be able to see and speak only in terms of enactment. 'I want to break your window,' is like to mean 'I am full of explosive anger.' It may or may not mean that there is any likelihood of the words being translated into action; an accurate assessment of this likelihood is one key to an appropriate response. The same intervention that would make one person with one set of problems secure enough to take the therapy process to the next level would induce deep shame in another person and reinforce the dissociative barriers to honest communication.

Multiple personality is one of the most vivid illustrations of the postmodern notion that a signifier is only meaningful in reference to its context. The act of an angry alter exclaiming with intensity that she wants to grab the therapist's chair, break the window with it, and then hurl the chair and the therapist out the window can be deconstructed to mean any number of things. The accuracy and the relevance of this deconstruction is what opens the process up and allows the client a little bit more space to move, a little less need to deny and dissociate.

The client who knows that the therapist will not tolerate abusive behaviour has then the opportunity to look for ways of processing frustration other than physical violence, and she also knows that if her own limits are not terribly reliable, her therapist can be counted on to set clear limits within their relationship. The client who sees that her therapist can tolerate her fantasies about hurting her without necessarily taking them literally, being priggish, or retaliating with anger of her own has the opportunity to face the reality that she is not simply compliant and coop-erative, although she may be those things as well, but that she carries a great deal of anger, and there may be room for her to know about this anger without destroying everything constructive she has built for herself.

The more people I talk to who are extremely dissociative, the more I am struck by how much this consciousness-structuring that we have been calling multiple personality disorder – and are now calling, officially at least, dissociative identity disorder – is not the problem. This does not mean it is unimportant, or that we do not need to comprehend its intricacies. But we need to understand it the same way we need to learn to understand the way anyone we care about thinks and talks, what it is they mean by what they say, the way we struggle to understand art and dreams – creatively, deeply, and always partially. We need to see the structure as pointing the way to what we really must understand if we are to help.

Through her fantasy life, the growing child creates cognitive structures that explain the world to herself. Some contemporary psychoanalysts (Ulman & Brothers, 1988) believe that the core of the psychological damage of child abuse is the shattering impact of traumatic occurrences for that fantasy life. They understand symptoms to be the various ways in which the child (and later the adult) attempts to compensate – to re-build on a damaged foundation. The complex fragmentation of consciousness that we see in severely dissociative people is, for me, just that – an attempt to create meaning where meaning has been eroded or destroyed, an attempt to make order out of threatening chaos using the elements of the chaos, of meaninglessness itself. Its purpose is to create a language to speak about the unspeakable.

The dissociative symptoms have to be plumbed, not cured. The richness that they give up in the context of an empathic connection with a therapist enables the survivor and the therapist to develop a bond within which all of the significant aspects of the client's life experience – including but certainly not exclusively the most obviously traumatizing experiences – become activated, incorporated into an evocative transference relationship, and eventually transformed.

Jane's problem is not that she has a part of her called Jean who compulsively picks up abusive men and engages in sexual encounters with them. Or that she has a part of her she calls Jan who rages constantly and has been known to become assaultive when provoked. Or that she has a part of her called little Jeannie who curls up in the closet and sobs for hours on end. We do not know what Jane's deepest problems are when we know these things about her, but we will come to know, as will she, if Jane, Jean, Jan, and Jeannie all find their voices in the context of the empathic connection with the therapist.

Gradually, the client and the therapist will come to understand together what it is all her part-selves are telling us, if we both listen and encourage openness and self-revelation and also give her as much room as she needs to retreat from the telling into the fragmentation. To the degree that we give people the freedom to use those structures of revelation and of hiddenness as fully and as freely as they need to, gradually they will be able to speak in a language less divided about a struggle much more central.

At this point, what is called the problem – this multiple-mindedness – will begin to appear to be resolving itself. Separations in consciousness, in memory and in identity will become less obvious. But if we are paying close attention to the process, we will be less focused on the devolution of the structures of radical dividedness and more aware of the longings, terror, and rage of an individual who could previously escape into her fragmentation but must now face these realities whole. When these feelings resonate in the therapist as a result of her empathic connection with her client, it becomes increasingly clear how the multiple personality structuring of consciousness is not the problem. In fact, compassionate and sensible therapists often find themselves teaching an overwhelmed client how to use less radical methods of dissociation so as to avoid exposure that is too intense and a consequent rebuilding of defenses.

Multiplicity is not the struggle. Dealing with dissociation is not the core of the struggle. The struggle is trying to live a life that was truncated and damaged, trying to express what was silenced under pain of death, trying to build on the ruins a new and a just existence.

4

Assessment: A Joint Endeavour

The goal of the diagnostic process is to strategize revolutionary social change from within.

Laura Brown (1994)

In any therapy regimen, assessment is an ongoing process that begins before a therapist meets the client and continues until termination. When an assessment is requested of an individual displaying signs of a high level of dissociative behaviour, what is often sought is an opinion as to the degree of dissociation, usually asked in the form of, 'Do you think this person is suffering from multiple personality disorder (dissociative identity disorder)?'

What focus one takes in an assessment depends on the context in which the assessment is requested. I always want to know who wants the assessment and for what purpose before I agree to facilitate the assessment procedure. Sometimes people want assessments for very limited and practical reasons, such as confirming the diagnosis for hospital records or for disability insurance. Other times the assessment request is more like a request for consultation. The clinician may be pretty clear that what she or he is seeing is a dissociative condition but is unsure of how to think about it or what to do.

An assessment requested particularly to address the level of dissociative behaviour should consider the following general areas:

1. Degree of dissociation
2. Awareness and control in present-day life
3. Strengths and vulnerabilities
4. Personal and social supports

These are not separate categories that can be probed discretely. Questions about each often follow logically from the others. It is important, however, for the assessor to ensure that basic information about each of these areas is gathered by the end of the interview.

In referring clinicians are in a position to administer the Dissociative Experiences Scale (DES) and the Structured Clinical Interview for DSM-IV Dissociative Disorders (SCID-D) or the Dissociative Disorders Interview Schedule (DDIS), then I encourage them to do so before the assessment interview. I review the results before I see the client. The Dissociative Experiences Scale (Bernstein & Putnam, 1986) is a 28-item self-report measure of dissociative experiences. It takes about ten minutes to complete and is useful for screening large numbers of people to flag high levels of dissociation for further screening for a possible dissociative disorder. The SCID-D (Steinberg, 1993) is a 250-item interview that takes up to 90 minutes to administer. It rates the severity of the five dissociative disorders and shows great interrater reliability in differentiating dissociative disordered from non-dissociative disordered patients and normal control subjects. Interestingly, the Dutch translation of the SCID-D (Boon & Draijer, 1991) has yielded almost identical symptom profiles for Dutch subjects, suggesting a degree of cultural continuity in the expression of dissociative symptomatology (Krippner, 1994). The DDIS (Ross, 1989), a 131-item measure that takes approximately 45 minutes to complete, is faster and simpler than the SCID-D and it shows an interrater reliability of .68 and a low false positive diagnosis rate in clinical populations (Ross, 1991). It also yields DSM-III-R diagnoses for borderline personality disorder, somatization disorder, and depression.

The main reason I request that referring clinicians fill out the diagnostic questionnaires themselves, if possible, is a practical one – to save clients the money it would cost them to have the data collected in my office. However, I have also found it to be clinically useful at times. Many therapists have reported that, when they administered the questionnaires as per my instruction – that is, in a systematic way, without processing the replies therapeutically beyond clarifying any questions the client does not understand – they gleaned information about their clients that they had not previously revealed in the course of the therapy. Sometimes issues are raised in the structured interviews that the client was uncomfortable about bringing up spontaneously, or that neither the client nor the therapist thought to address. Opening up such issues within the context of a battery of questions that are simply supposed to be answered rather than felt or processed can sometimes break the silence around aspects of history or behaviour that the client had previously deemed taboo.

Looking through the client's completed structured interview while she is sitting with me enables me to refer matter-of-factly to issues that might be difficult to reveal for the first time to a stranger – issues related to abuse history, self-destructive behaviour, past therapy experiences, and any other aspects of the client's life history that may be immediately relevant. For example, 'I notice from the questionnaire that you and your therapist filled out that you cut yourself sometimes. Can you tell me about that? How often you do that, and what it is that makes you feel like doing it?'

After I have looked over the results of the tests, maybe asking a question or two for clarification and maybe just storing the information for use in structuring the interview, I encourage the client to talk to me about her life in the present, her level of functioning at home, with intimates and friends, at work if she is employed, and so on. I weave in questions about dissociation as they seem relevant, so as to get a feel for the way dissociative experiences affect her day-to-day life and how much awareness and control she appears to have over her behaviour.

After getting a sense about the individual's present-day functioning, I try to glean more information about the degree and kind of dissociation she is experiencing. If, for example, she has mentioned being distracted by hearing voices in her head in response to a question about how well is she able to concentrate at work, I get as much information as she can give me about the voices. Are they familiar; that is, do they sound like anyone she knows? Are they male voices or female; adult or child; angry, judgmental, or soothing; clear and distinguishable or all jumbled up? Sometimes the client can tell me very little except about her sense of being distracted and her immediate effort to put them out of her mind. More often, she has some awareness about the tone or content of what she hears and/or images connected to the auditory hallucinations.

If an individual identifies many dissociative symptoms (that is, amnesia for events most people remember, time loss in the present, auditory hallucinations, fugues, blackouts, radical changes in handwriting style, watching herself do things but experiencing no control over her actions, frequent depersonalization and/or derealization experiences), I will investigate further to see if it is possible to communicate with her in an alternate state of consciousness.

This involves encouraging the individual to relax and allow another aspect of herself to emerge and engage in conversation with me. By paying attention to the information provided about the voices the client hears or the types of behaviours she experiences as ego-dystonic or does not remember but have been reported to her by others, I can often make the request for an autohypnotic switch of consciousness in a manner most likely to ensure success. For example, 'Just relax and breathe deeply and allow any part of you who is willing to do so to speak with me,' is a general invitation that is likely to be responded to by only the client most ready and eager to reveal her dissociative process. Alternatively, 'Just relax and step back and allow the part of you that you perceive of as a teenage boy (or who sometimes tells the boss to bugger off) to come forward and talk to me.' Pause, and then shift to speaking directly to the part of the person being elicited: 'I don't want to control you but I think that, since you seem to be in charge of many of the activities that Susan is not very aware of, it would be very helpful if you would be willing to speak with me,' is likely to give the message that you are not just a nosy professional but that you have some knowledge about and respect for the particular aspect of the individual with whom you are requesting communication.

In most circumstances, it is important when requesting access to usually hidden aspects of the individual's self to take a one-down position in terms of power and control. Requests made with the assurance that you know you cannot force this communication, but you think that the input this part of the person has to offer is likely to be valuable, are less likely to be perceived as crude assaults on the defence system.

Sometimes issues related to power and control have to be dealt with on a number of levels before direct access to the dissociated self-system is provided. The presenting aspect of the self often needs to express her profound dis-ease with the letting go of control that is implied by allowing the therapist to communicate directly with other self-states or personalities. Fear that states of consciousness perceived to be more assertive or stronger will gain control and entirely take over the day-to-day functioning of the individual is common. Empty reassurances are worse than useless in responding to these fears; they must be given the serious consideration they deserve. Asking how this dyscontrol occurs day-to-day is often helpful in allowing the client to further explore the ways in which the control she perceives herself to be preserving is actually marginal. It may help her to see that giving up some of the more superficial aspects of control of her consciousness is a step toward the goal of developing more appropriate controls in her life.

The exploration of control issues will also provide crucial data about the alter personality states that will be useful to the therapist in gaining their cooperation. Which alter personality or personalities should be evoked in an assessment session is an important clinical decision. If a variety of voices are mentioned, it is usually wise to attempt to call out the aspect of the personality system that is most likely to offer some immediate additional strengths to the individual in her daily functioning as well as useful information about the whole personality system. If a roaring demon, a weeping child, and an angry young adult who thinks therapy is stupid and who 'controls them all' are mentioned by the client when she is asked to describes images associated with the voices she hears in her head, it usually makes sense to ask to speak to the latter.

Alters with the most obvious and significant survival strengths are often framed by the presenting personality as 'the angry part' or 'the bitch,' and fears are often expressed about allowing this part of the person any rein in the presence of the assessor because of the kinds of inappropriate social behaviour this personality state has been known to manifest in other situations, particularly with authority figures.

These states of consciousness tend to represent the resistance of the individual to the oppression that has been so pervasive in her life. They are the states in which the individual's suspicion is stored, and they are on the lookout for further danger and exploitation with the goal of protecting the individual from revictimization. Initiating an open communication with this part of the person allows the therapist to make it clear that the role this personality state plays – protecting the individual from further harm, including harm from the therapist – is crucial to any therapy process that will be at all useful. I emphasize the reality that I not only do not want to rob the client of the help she gets from this part of her, I know she (or he) can help in ways that I cannot.

In order to facilitate communication with this aspect of the individual, I find it helpful to enquire whether this part of the person knew that the assessment session was going to take place and if so, to ask what she or he thought about it. This often brings out into the open the anger and/or contempt in which the mental health profession in general and/or I in particular am held. These perceptions and opinions are often seen as socially unacceptable by the presenting part of the client, and one of the reasons that she is reluctant to allow access to alternate aspects of herself is her fear of saying something rude or embarrassing. Reassurance that all parts of her are free to express their opinions to me, and that I will not take them personally or hold them against her, are often accepted by the presenting personality and also resonate throughout the client's self-system. Some of the most seemingly antisocial parts of a person turn out to be eager to communicate as soon as they come to understand that the therapist will not exercise judgment and censorship over their communication.

For example, I might say 'From what you have told me, I understand that there is a part of you who doesn't think much about your efforts to get professional help for yourself and also thinks it was pretty stupid to come here today. Even though he (or she) doesn't have a very high opinion of mental health professionals, I would be very grateful if he (or she) would come to speak to me for just a few minutes. I know I don't have any control over you (shift of focus to speaking directly to the part of the person being elicited) and you certainly don't need to stay for very long, but I would find it very helpful if you would tell me your point of view on the matters we've been talking about so far (or some particular matter).'

This type of invitation both addresses, by way of hypnotic suggestion, the presenting personality's fear that another part of her will stay in control once it emerges ('you don't need to stay out for very long'), and it also gives the part of the person who is often feared and denigrated by the presenting personality (and has also had many experiences with mental health professionals who are not open to listening to any communication that is not framed deferentially) a respectful message from the assessor about the worth of its perceptions and opinions. Creating a direct and respectful working alliance with the part of the person who has a deep and abiding suspicion for the structures of systemic patriarchal oppression, including and often especially the mental health profession, offers an immediate source of strength to a process that will need all the resources that are available.

Attempting to communicate with a feisty, rebellious part of the person in an assessment session – rather than or prior to communicating with more vulnerable parts of the person – not only gives the client more immediate reinforcement of the survival attitudes and skills that these types of personalities represent, it is often easier to accomplish. An individual carrying around a lot of resentment and contempt (much of it justified) often cannot resist an invitation to express some of it to an authority figure who both represents the previously dismissive authority figures and also has shown some signs of being different, in that she has recognized these attitudes and invited their communication. An individual who has been struggling, possibly for most of her life, to hide alternate aspects of herself will naturally be quite anxious about revealing them directly for the first time, but the vulnerability of the person is much less great when revealing a more feisty, protective attitude than in opening up more vulnerable states.

When a client talks in an assessment session about 'the angry part' it is important to ensure, before requesting direct access to that part, that the personality being referred to is of the type I have been describing. While most clients, when offering such a description, exaggerate the negative power of these parts of themselves, others may be in fact pointing to a level of dissociated rage that is very different from a sarcastic protector who is angry about past mistreatment, but eager or at least cautiously willing to consider, when approached tactfully, a pro-social alliance with the therapist.

It would be foolhardy to invite out-of-control anger into an assessment session, and it is the assessor's responsibility to determine what it is a client is talking about when she says, 'I am afraid, if I stand back and let you talk to that part of me, terrible things will happen.' Most clients are afraid of any expression of feeling, and they overstate the risk of acknowledging volatile emotions, especially anger. Other individuals, however, may be trying to warn the therapist about out-of-control rage that certainly should not be toyed with for the stake of assessment – except occasionally for very particular reasons, usually related to forensics, and in a more secure setting than most therapists' offices provide. The individual's history regarding violence is a particularly significant indicator of what the person means when she says, 'Oh no, you don't want to talk to Joe. He hates therapists.'

The alternate modes of expression that personality states embody often manifest themselves in terms of polarities. For example, a presenting personality may talk something like this:

I try so hard to do everything that I am supposed to do but things just seem to get worse and worse.

My husband says I scream terrible things at him and sometimes even hit him. I would never do those things, but I can't believe he would lie about something like that.

My doctor gives me all these drugs. They don't seem to do much good, but I would take them except that I am always losing them.

I appreciate you seeing me, Doctor. I've seen eight doctors this year about my problems. It costs a lot of money and doctors don't seem to have a clue about what to do.

No, I don't drink. I sometimes find liquor bottles in the garbage and my little boy brought a bottle to Show and Tell and his teacher called me. I told her I don't know where he got it because I don't drink. My parents were both alcoholics, and I've always said that my children would not go through what I did as a kid.

I am very tired, my head hurts, and no disrespect intended, Doctor, but I am having a hard time staying awake while you are asking me all these questions.

When the teenage alter emerges, the individual may communicate in a very different style:

Not another doctor. What a joke!

Of course I drink. What red-blooded Canadian guy doesn't have a few beers when he watches the hockey game. No, I don't drink gin; that's Ginny. She puts away plenty every night so she can sleep. Pretty funny about her kid finding that gin bottle and bringing it to kindergarten, wasn't it?

It's gross, the things that guy she lives with wants to do. Just like her dad, and it scares the life out of her. Of course, I come out and tell him off, and if he doesn't listen, well I just have to hit him. She may be a wimp who can't figure out whether she's coming or going, but it's my job to protect her. She's such a basket case, anyone could take advantage of her if I didn't keep my eyes open.

Yeah, I keep an eye out for the little ones too, but Ginny is the one who takes care of them. I just make sure no one hurts them ever again.

Yeah, there are times when we all feel really down. I go around stirring up a bit of shit here and there just to snap myself out of it, but sometimes even I don't want to bother.

If at all possible, it is important to communicate directly with dissociated aspects of an individual's mind (alter personalities) before rendering a diagnostic opinion vis-à-vis degree of dissociation. States that are amorphous – more like the inner-child states that most people are able to experience – may be very useful to engage in communication in the therapy process, but they are not particularly indicative of a dissociative identity disorder. Individuals with a full-blown multiple personality condition have ego states that are more fully developed in terms of differentiated access to memory, cognition, or behaviour, and there is always a significant degree of amnesia between these states as they alternate control over the individual's functioning. Without communicating directly with the individual in an altered state of consciousness, it is difficult to determine the degree of dissociation and to comment on it responsibly.

Many therapists, in these litigious days, are discontinuing the use of anything that resembles hypnosis in the clinical setting for fear of suggestion and contamination. Unquestionably, only professionals well-trained in the use of hypnosis or other hypnotic techniques should consider using them in the assessment and/or treatment of trauma survivors, and they should use hypnosis judiciously and certainly not automatically. Individuals who are truly highly dissociative, however, move into trance states with or without guidance. To pretend that our communication with them is not a hypnotic one simply robs the therapy context of our skill in directing the process in the direction of healing rather than letting it drift.

It is not hypnosis or other types of adjunctive trance-facilitating and guiding therapeutic techniques, such as focusing or guided imagery, that cause individuals to become wedded to inaccurate versions of events. It is the demand characteristics of the interpersonal situation in which the therapeutic experience takes place that has the potential to create the powerful suggestion. If, for example, I have a stake in influencing a client to believe her troubles are a result of abuse from a particular source, I could aid her in interpreting the images that emerge in her mind under hypnosis in that direction. I could tell her that hypnosis is like a truth serum, and no one lies or is mistaken in that state, or I could neglect to correct her entirely mistaken understanding that this is the case. If I have a stake in getting her to retract allegations of abuse, I could do the same thing. A trained and ethical therapist will not use hypnosis or any other therapeutic tool in this way.

Also, hypnosis and the other trance-facilitating therapeutic techniques are not tools that should be used automatically in cases of suspected dissociative conditions. There are many assessment situations in which the type of hypnotic communication to which I have been referring is not appropriate. For example, if an individual talks about her dissociative symptoms in a way that leads me to suspect that the degree of dissociation is not particularly great, or that there are secondary gains that she is deriving from seeing herself as someone with multiple personalities, I often treat the dissociative symptoms as a system rather than facilitating a trance state, even in my usually casual style. I do not ignore the symptoms, but I do not encourage them to emerge in bits and pieces either. It behooves us as clinicians not to encourage people to own up to problems they do not have or to exaggerate those they do have. This will not help them solve their own very real problems.

It is better to be diagnostically conservative rather than promote the notion of a level of dissociation that may not be an accurate reflection of a particular client's reality. Indicating in an assessment report, 'This individual uses a high level of dissociation (or some degree of dissociation) as a coping strategy. Full blown dissociative identity disorder is not ruled out, but also was not confirmed in this assessment interview' is a more responsible way of communicating suspicions of classical multiple personality, so that the possibility will not be overlooked as the treatment process unfolds, while not confirming something without the appropriate data to back up the confirmation. It is important to note in such an assessment report that the exact degree of dissociative behaviour – whether some variant of dissociative disorder not otherwise specified (DDNOS) or clearly elaborated dissociative identity disorder (DID) – is not nearly as important a clinical issue as the ways in which dissociation is used by this individual – both constructively and in a way that undermines her functioning – in her day-to-day life.

Increasingly, I do not focus particularly on the issue of dissociation in an assessment process with a client that I am likely to be seeing in an ongoing way, either individually or in a group program. I find that the degree of dissociation becomes obvious and incorporated helpfully into the therapy process in a much more natural way if I simply converse with the person about her problems as they affect her day-to-day functioning. Severely dissociated people generally present various aspects of themselves without my poking around for them, and there is much less danger of reinforcing any factitious elements of an individual's condition that might be present when I do not place any particular emphasis on the dissociative phenomenology per se.

In fact, an assessment issue that has become increasingly important as the diagnosis of dissociative identity disorder has become less of a rarity in the past five to ten years, depending on the jurisdiction, is that of distinguishing a severe dissociative condition that began in early childhood in response to a traumatogenic environment from a factitious disorder or from a condition that is frankly iatrogenic – or some combination of these three.

A factitious disorder is one that is created by the client for reasons of secondary gain. There are a variety of factitious conditions that might present themselves as a dissociative identity disorder. For example, one of the most obvious is the deliberate imitation of severe dissociative symptoms to escape the consequences of criminal behaviour. Less conscious creation and/or exaggeration of dissociative symptoms are sometimes found in hospital settings or other residential programs, where people suffering from dissociative conditions are seen to get a degree of helpful attention that is appealing to other patients.

Most clinicians consider the possibility of malingering when facilitating forensic assessments. And some of the factitious disorders I occasionally see are just that – people taking on the trappings of severe dissociation, more or less consciously. Even when the faking is not entirely planned and willful, the use of the semblance of the condition to get something that would not be given freely (hospital stays, excesses of nurturance, the illusion of specialness, escape from adult responsibilities) – something different from arduous, challenging psychotherapy with the goal of building a responsible life – and the demanding and hostile style of communication and interaction have much of the flavour of the classical malingerer.

Some people presenting at hospitals again and again with extraordinary physical (and secretly self-induced) symptoms – or harming their children and then present-ing in medical settings asking for help for the child – may well be high dissociators, but their multiple personality presentation is often atypical and a cover (conscious or not so conscious) for the Munchausen dynamic. Focusing on the plethora of dissociative symptoms these individuals offer up to the therapist – either in the assessment or in ongoing treatment – will not be helpful. Having had the desired effect of increasing focused nurturing attention and deflecting the appropriate chal-lenge to adult responsibility, the symptoms will increase and multiply. Colin Ross (1995b) found that patients with the profile of factitious DID tended to score in the very highest ranges of the DES and the DDIS regarding dissociative symptoms, presenting a picture that looks like 'faking bad,' a term psychologists sometimes use as shorthand to describe unrealistically elevated levels of pathology reported in testing, usually considered an indication that the test-taker is either extremely his-trionic or a malingerer.

Other individuals presenting with a factitious dissociative disorder are more empty than sociopathic. Suzette Boon (1995) tells the story of a woman who begged her for a diagnosis of multiple personality disorder. 'You are my last hope. If you rule out multiple personality disorder, I am nothing.' Ross (1995b) is compiling data from a large sample of inpatients at a dissociative disorders specialty unit about different pathways to a dissociative identity disorder presentation. He has found the following four routes to an eventual diagnosis of dissociative identity disorder, with some patients developing a condition which feature an admixture of these influences: (1) childhood trauma; (2) childhood neglect; (3) factitious; and (4) iatrogenic.

The word iatrogenic derives from the Greek *iatros*, meaning physician or healer.

An iatrogenic condition is, therefore, one that is created by the therapist. Ross notes that some individuals with a history that features significantly more childhood deprival than extreme physical and sexual abuse develop a relatively simple dissociative system, and that successful treatment in these cases involves working with the system as a whole, rather than communicating with it in parts and encouraging an elaboration and exaggeration of symptoms. We need a great deal more data about both incidence and clinical outcome before we can do more than speculate in this area, but the evidence strongly suggests that we cannot ignore the reality that some people – deliberately or not – imitate the symptoms of a dissociative condition, and that others come to treatment with relatively simple conditions and elaborate them in response to the suggestion and encouragement of peers, therapists, or other cultural influences, such as books, made-for-TV movies, or talk shows – what Richard Kluft labels the 'Oprahgenic factor' (Kluft, 1995a).

We have, unfortunately, in the past fifteen years, created some significant social problems in our struggle to create appropriate services geared for people with severe abuse-related problems. We have occasionally made it seductive for some who have very little in their lives to claim this special condition – one that is interesting, attracts therapists who talk instead of medicate, gets you admitted to certain support and self-help groups as an equal, and offers a language to say how bad you feel. In fact, many severely dissociative trauma survivors are intelligent, creative, and energetic, as well as tormented and disoriented. Having been badly hurt themselves, they can be eager to extend a hand to others with similar problems. This may appear to be an attractive peer group to be a part of if you have a history of neglect, maybe abuse, certainly not love and nurturance, or if you are limited, exhausted, and depleted, and have never been able to meet conventional social expectations and find a place for yourself in this demanding world.

People in this state can be vulnerable for developing a superficial kind of dissociative structure, in response to their own needs and distorted perceptions. They would also easily fall victim to naive therapists, who are not cautious about suggestions, who make it clear that severe dissociation, ritual abuse reports, or some combination of psychological symptoms and abuse allegations are the bait to catch their interest. In such cases, the dissociative structure would be a combination of factitious and iatrogenic. Such a combination, in some cases added to a perfectly respectable and undramatic DDNOS configuration that might well be amenable to sound treatment, is a not terribly rare scenario, particularly in settings where more severely dysfunctional clients are treated.

The single published study comparing genuine and simulated multiple personality (Coons & Milstein, 1994) found many similarities between the two groups. The authors note that although some factitious or malingered cases can be quite obvious, others are extremely difficult to discern, even for the experienced clinician. Reports of childhood abuse and of the classical symptoms of dissociation, such as amnesia, auditory hallucinations, time loss, and handwriting changes, do not distinguish one group from the other. The two most significant differences were the incidence of *confirmed* reports of child abuse (genuine, n=50, 85%; simulated, n=11, 0%) and symptoms/behaviours common to factitious disorders in general, such as *pseudologia fantastica* (genuine, 8%; simulated, 100%), highly dramatic presentation (44%; 100%), inconsistent work history (24%; 73%), *la belle indifference* (34%; 73%), refusal of collateral interviews (0%; 55%), and persistent lying (10%; 55%).

Some individuals with factitious disorders presenting as severe dissociative conditions may be open to tactfully and non-judgmentally expressed recognition from their therapists that their dissociative symptoms are an overlay upon their real and very genuine problems, which need treatment, but not the same kind of treatment as severe dissociation. They may appreciate diagnostic clarity (especially when mild factitious elements were reinforced in earlier treatments, and the individual has a genuine and easily accessible desire to solve their problems), and they may remain in therapy and resolve their difficulties, thus benefiting both themselves and the health care system. Others will leave in denial and anger and re-emerge in another setting in the not-too-distant future. In any case, it is unfair not to be as rigorous with this group of people as with those suffering from posttraumatic dissociation in offering them an honest and accurate appraisal of their situation and the chance to get the help they need.

Recognizing and dealing with the complexities that have accrued from a diagnosis changing status from rate to relatively common in fifteen years does not make the dissociative disorders field anything out of the ordinary in mental health. In the hospital setting, I see cases of factitious schizophrenia – and factitius/iatrogenic schizophrenia – in individuals who are eventually accurately diagnosised as having personality disorders. The treatment of dissociation does not hold a monopoly on complexity, confusion, and mistakes that need to be set right, and individually and as a field, we are also, needless to say, not exempt from them either. There are misdiagnoses, factitious disorders, conditions that are iatrogenic, and combinations of all of the above in every mental health category, and it often takes us too long to turn around an assessment or treatment process that has gone awry. The challenge to be rigorous and subtle in our assessment of complicated and unique human beings is faced by every practitioner in the art and science of therapeutic treatment, and not one of us accomplishes it perfectly.

The purpose of a discrete and formal assessment is to provide signposts that will lead to effective treatment. The final diagnostic opinion is a result of conclusions drawn from the data gleaned from psychological testing, information provided from collateral sources such as hospital records or therapists' reports, and from the clinical assessment interview itself.

Such an assessment is not always necessary. Many clients are assessed in an ongoing fashion as part of their therapy process and this is, in many cases, not only sufficient, but also a much more organic process for addressing the issue of symptoms that need careful attention. If an individual is working successfully in a therapy process and showing significant improvement in daily functioning, there is not necessarily any reason to provide this kind of specific assessment interview. The purpose of accurate assessment is simply and only to point the way to appropriate treatment. If appropriate and effective treatment is already occurring, imposing what are essentially crude and reductionistic diagnostic categories on the individuality and the complexity of a human being's way of being in the world is completely unnecessary.

An important part of the assessment process is communicating with the client and then to the referring professional about the findings. This is usually done in a number of different languages. An explanation that is helpful to a psychiatrist will not necessarily communicate anything of value to the client. I often say something like the following to a client who is not particularly versed in psychiatric jargon:

You have a serious problem that used to be called multiple personality and is now called dissociative identity disorder. This means a number of different things.

It means you are not crazy, not psychotic, when you think you hear voices in your head.

It means you divided your mind up into separate compartments when you were a little kid. You did this for a number of reasons – to feel better, not to remember things that you didn't want to think about, basically to try to cope the best way you knew how.

There is good news and bad news about this condition. The good news is that it is treatable. Many people who have this problem get completely better. The bad news is that the treatment takes a long time and is very stressful.

You need a primary psychotherapist who has experience treating people with your problem. You also need to begin, with the help of your therapist, creating more stability in your everyday life. Treatment for this problem is often a grueling enterprise and you need as calm and structured a life as you can make for yourself and a few supportive people in your life to give yourself the greatest chance of treatment success.

I speak differently to the referring professional depending on their level of experience with dissociative conditions. For example, I might speak in the following way to a professional who has not had much experience in this area about a client with a confirmed history of abuse:

Your client has developed a dissociative defence structure to cope with traumatic experiences as a very young child. She divides her mind into compartments with fairly rigid amnestic barriers separating them. This process causes her to have only intermittent access to certain memories, feelings, and so on.

This was once a somewhat adaptive coping strategy, but it has become generalized and elaborated over time so that now she believes that there are other people living in her body and controlling her actions. She has some serious problems, such as regular episodes of amnesia, a tendency to think rigidly, a repetitive pattern of unstable explosive relationships, and ongoing self-destructive acts, such as abusing alcohol and self-mutilation.

Her severe symptoms of depression may have a significant biological component and may be responsive to medication. However, until a regimen of therapy is initiated that enables her to stabilize, it is hard to tell whether the meds she is taking are part of the solution or part of the problem. In any case, medication is always adjunctive to the core of the treatment, which is long-term intensive psychotherapy.

For a hospital chart, I might note:

The primary Axis 1 diagnosis is Dissociative Identity Disorder

with significant Axis 2 psychopathology (Borderline Personality Disorder)

Co-morbidity in the area of substance abuse disorder; rule out possible underlying major depression.

I am aware of the objectification, diminishment, and occasionally even abusiveness that adheres to much of this language; it pigeonholes rich and complicated individuals. If I do not perceive it necessary, I do not use it. I am also aware that neither my choices or my clients' choices are unlimited, and I make the decision as to what language to speak each time I do so. To my mind, ethics is a pretty contingent affair. I look at the issue of using language in the same way I make other decisions – asking myself the question, not which action is right and which is wrong, but what good is likely to come out of this action and what harm. I then weigh the two against each other. In the case of using sanctioned diagnostic terminology to categorize human beings, the advantages of providing a familiar framework to legitimize needs and access resources often seems to outweigh the damage of using such inadequate and dangerous language.

Issues related to dissociative symptoms are not the only, or even necessarily the most important, aspect of the assessment, although they are often the focus of the referral. The area of radical dissociation may be the most unfamiliar to the referring professional. It is important that the assessor integrate other issues of clinical relevance into the assessment interview and report.

Dissociation is only one of the consequences of a childhood history of severe interpersonal trauma that cause ongoing problems for people suffering from dissociative conditions. Others relate to the profound effects of having as role models individuals who are disturbed and destructive enough to cause terrible harm to small children. Individuals who report experiences of being ritually abused in cult settings talk about the way in which they were trained to believe that what society generally considers good is evil, and what is generally perceived of as evil is good.

This may be more deliberate than the training in values and human relations that many abuse survivors receive from their abusers, but it is not necessarily more effective conditioning. There is an equally insidious quality to the socialization inflicted on a child by a parent who conforms in superficial and sometimes exceptionally rigid ways to conventional social and religious dogma and demands that kind of conformity from his children, while at the same time abusing and exploiting them in ways that are explicitly forbidden by the very codes preached and enforced.

This is only one of the many ways in which children can be socialized into extreme distortions in thinking, feeling and relating to other people. Basic issues central to everyone's ongoing life struggle, such as, 'How do I balance my right to get my needs met with the rights of others?' are often seen through the filter of adult behaviour that is destructive and psychopathic. This lens is then focused on every other interaction the child has throughout her life and may influence her in obvious ways, such as a repetition of the very behaviours that were inflicted on her, or in more convoluted and self-punishing ways. In any case, the ability to take a healthy and balanced stance towards basic issues like self-respect and respect for others is usually severely damaged.

Some children are abused outside the home, or by relatives or other caretakers, and their parents have no awareness of the torment that is being inflicted on the children. Although this is an incredibly confusing situation for the young child, who assumes parental omniscience and omnipotence, this child may at least receive significant non-abusive care, nurturance, and socialization, which can go a long way to modulating the effect of the abuse on the developing value system.

. Other children appear to have had no significant contact with adults who are not either abusive or neglectful. This terrible circumstance can place these children in the position of having very few values and behaviours but the offending adults' to incorporate into their developing character structure, at least until they are exposed to extra-familial influences, such as school, neighborhood, or church, somewhat later in childhood.

Though there are many differences in the ways in which children incorporate the values of their abusers, the reality that malleable children exposed to toxic adult behaviour must make some use of those influences in developing their belief systems is one of the most far-reaching consequences of a history of child abuse, whether physical, emotional, or sexual.

There are many symptoms, such as anxiety, depression, somaticization, problems with work, with eating, with abusing substances, sexual difficulties, and problems with intimate relationships, that are often the legacy of a history of abuse in childhood. Any and all of these, in combination with high levels of dissociation and character and value distortions derived from formative contact with abusive or neglectful caretakers, can be incorporated into the behaviour of individuals suffering from severe dissociative conditions. How these difficulties play themselves out in the day-to-day life of the client are as significant indicators of the type of treatment regimen that should be initiated and the prognosis for treatment success as the degree of dissociation. In fact, they are often more significant.

Assessment is not only the responsibility and the prerogative of the professional. Although the therapist has the training and the experience that give her more responsibility for the effectiveness of the treatment, it is crucial that the client not lose control over what is an extremely important aspect of her life. Therapy is always a partnership, and unless both partners respect the roles and responsibilities of both themselves and the other, the relationship is likely to undermine the client's strengths rather than contribute to her growth.

For the client, this means a number of things on a practical level. It is ideal if the client can shop for a therapist and can interview several possible therapists until she finds one that seems not only to have the necessary qualifications and experience, but also with whom she is comfortable. What the appropriate qualifications are is an issue on which there is more than one opinion. My experience has been that there are psychotherapists with many different levels and kinds of academic and clinical training that have proven to be skilled at the complex and difficult treatment of people with dissociative conditions. Having a degree in medicine or an advanced degree in psychology is no guarantee that a clinician is competent to offer such treatment, and I also do not think that a master's degree is the minimum level of education necessary to do this kind of clinical work responsibly. I have conducted training seminars and provided case consultation to literally thousands of clinicians and, in such contexts, I have heard both success and horror stories from therapists with every level of professional accreditation and from their clients.

Though there are no foolproof guidelines for locating a therapist who will be able to offer competent assistance, a consumer approach is the most likely to result in success. Referrals or recommendations should be solicited from people whose judgment the client trusts. An initial assessment session should be set up for both the client and the therapist to determine the suitability of their working together. In my opinion, before a person is placed on a waiting list for a particular practitioner such an interview should take place to avoid the eventuality of waiting six months for treatment and then finding out that it is a bad match. The degree of freedom to choose to quit at that point is often very small and long, counterproductive entanglements can result. I also think keeping long waiting lists for people in acute and extreme distress can be unethical. The advantage of knowing that in eighteen months there may be a space in an experienced practitioner's caseload is often outweighed by the disadvantage of going without treatment for so long. Obviously, accessing effective treatment is often a difficult endeavour, and there can be many practical constraints on creating an ideal or even a reasonable process.

Prospective clients have the right to ask any questions that seem relevant to the type of service they expect or hope to receive from a therapist, such as qualifications, experience, practical matters such as fees and time available, issues that the therapist feels comfortable working with, and therapeutic attitudes and approaches. Questions of a personal nature, relating to age, marital status, sexual orientation, experience raising children, views about religion – any issue that may be important to the client in making a decision about engaging a therapist – may all be considering appropriately relevant by the client and should be asked if they are important aspects of the decision to hire one individual over another. It is also important for the client to respect the therapist's decision to answer or not to answer questions of a personal nature. Quite often, it is the general sense that the client gains from the conservation about some of these important issues that determines whether a therapist seems suitable, rather than any one factor.

Once a client has contracted with a therapist for treatment, the responsibility for ongoing assessment of the process has begun in earnest. It is very easy, when one is feeling overwhelmed – as people in the early stages of therapy often are – to give over the responsibility to assess the process to someone else, especially someone who seems willing to take it on. Maintaining an appropriately central role in the ongoing assessment of the treatment does not mean that the client does not solicit and is not respectful of her therapist's opinions. What would be the purpose of hiring an experienced professional and then disregarding her perspective? It does mean, however, that the client is also respectful of her own reflections on the effect the treatment seems to be having on her life and that she recognizes that she is the only one who lives her life day to day and that she therefore has information to which no one else – including the therapist – has access.

People with dissociative conditions often have parts of themselves who can offer a great deal of helpful input into the therapy process if they are encouraged to do so. Therapists who are both confident in their own abilities and open to the full participation of the client in the ongoing structuring of the treatment will provide a framework for the respectful incorporation of the client's perspective. Many clients and many clinicians have been socialized within a restrictive medical model that privileges the doctor's opinion and invalidates the patient's, and this conditioning must often be tackled directly from the first day of therapy.

When a client makes self-deprecating remarks like, 'Well, you must know, you are the one with the degree. What use would my untrained opinion be?' I make it clear that, although indeed there is much that I do know, and therefore I can probably be helpful about many things, there is also much about her life that I do not and cannot know, and that she must bring her expertise about her own life to the sessions or we will be playing with half a deck. Usually it does not take much time to change the attitude of 'doctor knows best,' and with it the subservient (and passive-aggressive) stance of 'fix me.'

Many clinicians and researchers have made the point that non-psychotic individuals with serious problems in interpersonal relationships – the ones who tend to get labeled borderline personality disorder in psychiatric settings – realize their worst potential in their ongoing interactions with mental health and medical professionals. Dawson and MacMillan (1993) make a good case for the proposition that in our attempts to nurture, protect, and treat these people, we often add to – and, in fact, cause – some of their most outrageous and dangerous behaviour. The social contract between doctor and patient or therapist and client, defined through tradition and various codes of legislation governing the actions of the professional, creates the parameters of the relationship, in which one party is viewed as sick and therefore exempt from normal social responsibilities (Parsons, 1951). In adopting a caring professional role, the physician or non-medical therapist (or mental health/social service worker of any kind) assumes responsibility for the individual's self-definition, well-being, and behaviour.

Even professionals who resist the mandate to name their clients' experience (feminist or humanist therapists who refuse to use official diagnostic nomenclature) find it difficult not to take on the most basic responsibilities for their clients – whether their client carves pentagrams into her flesh, rubs oven cleaner into her eyes, or decides to live or die. In fact, some of the most non-traditional professionals get particularly mired in struggles with their clients over these issues, for the very reason that they try especially hard to respect their clients' perspective and attempt to meet their needs. Unfortunately, in reaching out with caring and compassion, without having thought the issues through in such a way as to be capable of creating clear and implacable boundaries against being constantly put in a no-win caretaker's position, they create a positively charged emotional context without helping that individual develop the affect tolerance skills and self-reliance to use the situation in her interest. The result can be ever-increasing suicide threats, attempts, and near-successes, acts of increasingly dangerous self-harm, dramatically decreased competency, and increased helplessness.

If we are supposed to be helping people and this is the outcome, it is our responsibility to assess whether our help is at all helpful even if there is no other program or practitioner willing or able to take this client into treatment. Something is not necessarily better than nothing. If a person is starving and all I have to offer is poisonous to that person, I am not only not obliged to offer the poisonous substance, I am ethically obliged not to do so.

I do not consider myself responsible for anyone's decision to live or to die, even though I have some fairly well-defined legal responsibilities as a mental health professional if I am of the opinion that suicide is imminent. Most of the people I work with are at least profoundly ambivalent about living, and a great many of them struggle with pressing suicidal impulses for years. Many of them also do serious damage to their bodies by way of self-mutilation, eating disorders, drug and alcohol abuse, neglect of basic medical care, and so on. Though I recognize that I have no control over their behaviour, I do have the capacity and the responsibility to assess whether or not the treatment I am providing is helping them. If I see that symptoms such as life-threatening behaviours not only do not abate as a result of treatment, if only slowly and gradually, but rather increase in frequency and intensity, I communicate to the client that I clearly am not providing her with effective help. If she cannot change the pattern of seriously self-destructive behaviour, I will not continue as her primary therapist. Although I have no control over her behaviour, I do have control over my own, and I choose not to engage in relationships – therapeutic or otherwise – in which the currency of communication is threats and acts of self-destruction.

I have also not signed on to do psychological hospice work. If someone has decided to kill herself, I personally believe she has the right to do so. However, if she wants a therapist to accompany her as she prepares for or works herself up to suicide, she needs to engage someone else. I explained my point of view to a client regarding this issue, and she responded, 'So your support is not unconditional?' I assured her that she was absolutely right. As a human being, I wish her well in whatever (basically ethical) way she chooses to conduct her life. My support as a therapist, however, is contingent upon her struggling to engage in the therapeutic process that I offer, and that process involves choosing to live, and to live honestly and with courage, facing whatever needs to be faced rather than escaping from it by acts of serious self-destruction.

The process is not always steady and there may be acts of self-harm once a person initiates therapy. But I will not repeatedly hospitalize a person for suicide attempts or seriously damaging acts of self-harm. If an individual has such a need to externalize her conflicts that she is compelled to act them out constantly in a way that demands non-therapeutic intervention, then I assess it as unlikely that she has the discipline and ego strength to engage in the rigorous process of long-term, dynamic psychotherapy. I am, in theory, willing – maybe, sometimes, even obliged – to hospitalize without consent, once. I make it clear that I see a second time as a pattern, and I will not engage in a pattern of distorted interpersonal transactions ('Help me get in touch with my feelings. I am so overwhelmed when I feel anything that I have to kill myself') under the guise of psychotherapy.

Rich Loewenstein quotes the Kenny Rogers song, 'The Gambler' as particularly relevant to ongoing assessment issues in the treatment of individuals with dissociative conditions. The words of wisdom handed on from the older (and clearly broken-down) gambler to his younger train-riding companion are good for both the therapist and the client to keep in mind as they journey together:

If you want to play the game, boy,
You've got to play it right.
You've got to know when to hold 'em,
Know when to fold 'em,
Know when to walk away,
Know when to run ...

I have engaged in consultation sessions with therapist/client duos who should have divorced each other months or years previously. Their enmeshed and clearly counterproductive relationships may well have been salvageable, or a great deal of time and heartache might have been saved, if either had been able to pay heed to the gambler's undoubtedly hard-won advice.

In saying this, I am not encouraging facile disconnection in therapy relationships that are going through a difficult time, or implying that any time a client thinks she is not making enough progress fast enough that the answer is to change therapists. Some therapy relationships have a powerful and obvious negative transference element in them almost from the first session, and such relationships – though very difficult to endure for both client and therapist – can be as successful a treatment ground (gauged by concrete changes in the individual's functioning capacity, not by positive reports about the therapy process) as smoother relationships where the client experiences the therapist as generally nurturing and only occasionally threatening or awful.

However, if a client feels generally uneasy in the therapy relationship or process, she should address her discomfort to her therapist, difficult as that may be. The therapist should be able to encourage this expression of dis-ease and help the client feel free to explore such feelings without discounting them. If a client implies she is considering terminating treatment, the therapist should give the client lots of room to consider this as a viable option. It is only when clients feel that the therapist will not be angry, hurt, or offended by the prospect of their ending the relationship – nor assume that such thoughts or even actions discount the positive aspects of the relationship or the good that has been accomplished in that context – that many clients feel at all empowered to assess the therapy process fully from their point of view.

In a relationship with an inherent power differential, the client's power to walk away, limited as it can often be by many factors, including her own need for treatment of some kind, should be considered inviolable by the therapist, and the client should be encouraged to explore that option without being influenced by a barrage of insight from the therapist about why she might be considering such a self-destructive alternative. In general, I have found that people I consider to be doing well in therapy do not leave as a result of being given every opportunity to do so, even when they are having a difficult time seeing that the benefits of the process outweigh the difficulties. This kind of experience makes it easy for me to encourage clients to keep their options open, but even if this were not the case, even if I saw people leaving therapy whom I felt strongly could benefit from it, I still think it is an ethical imperative to leave the door open as a bottom-line power balance.

Some therapists let go too easily. They take their client's defensive fears or anger personally and literally and withdraw in response to the onslaught of feeling usually central to the healing process of anyone who has experienced a childhood history of maltreatment (and many other people as well). It is an art to convey consistently to an individual who has been rejected many times that I am committed to playing my role in her healing process for as long as it takes to accomplish the goals we have agreed upon without giving the similar but altogether different message, 'I will always be here for you no matter what.'

There are many reasons why a therapist might have to terminate therapy with a client. Some of them are personal and practical, or outside the therapist's control, such as illness and death. Others involve life decisions on the part of the therapist that are not directly related to clients but affect them profoundly nevertheless. Changes in professional circumstances, pressing mental/emotional needs of the therapist or the therapist's family for a change, or the desire for a move to another geographical location may necessitate terminating the therapy of clients, who were responding well to the treatment, and transferring them to another therapist when they would undoubtedly be better off continuing the treatment with the original clinician. Most therapists, although they would agonize a bit in these circumstances (particularly when there is no other adequate treatment available for the client) would not consider it unethical to terminate treatment. Many of the same therapists, however, find it almost impossible to terminate the therapy of a client with whom they do not appear to be working effectively. They justify continuing the treatment on ethical grounds, referring to the client's desire to remain in therapy as the basis for deciding to conduct a treatment that is ineffective at best and abusive at worse.

I always make it clear to my clients that they and I are both entirely in charge of their therapy, and, although I do not discuss this unless it is directly relevant in a particular case, this includes termination. Each of us not only has the right but the responsibility not to do anything that we think is harmful in the course of the treatment. My client can ask me to engage in practices that I consider – in her case or sometimes in any case – to be countertherapeutic. I will listen to her as she explains to me why it is she thinks she needs what she is proposing, and maybe, if I glean something from her explanation that I did not understand before, I will change my mind. But I will not do anything I think is wrong or unhelpful to her, no matter what pressure is exerted, from her or from other collateral sources. That is not only my right but my personal and professional responsibility, and I could not continue to do this work if I made compromises in this area.

This is not only my right and responsibility, but my client's as well. If we disagree about the course of treatment, I will do my best to communicate my belief that she must act responsibly on her own behalf. If she thinks that she can only get well if she has a therapist who will call her each day, provide sessions in her home when she cannot leave, allow her to self-mutilate in the office or waiting room, or promise never to admit her to the hospital or always admit her to hospital at the first sign of distress – or if influential family members or social service personnel make these demands – then it is up to my client and her support people to make a decision about the suitability of a primary therapist who will not engage in these practices. Power struggles – overt or in the guise of offering a thousand anxious explanations about why we do some things and cannot do others – are pointless and counterproductive in these situations.

The bottom line is that I only wish to work with people who can make some level of commitment to the type of treatment I have to offer. I understand and accept ambivalence as an ongoing part of a gruelling and scary enterprise. Who would not be ambivalent when faced with such a project? But ambivalence is different from making a decision not to participate in a particular type of treatment and then coming to every session in the hopes of persuading the therapist to be someone she is not or to engage in practices she thinks are wrong. In such situations, I hope to persuade the client – who truly does not want what I have to offer – to make the decision to terminate with me and to engage another therapist. If she cannot or will not do so, after a good try at initiating treatment that I feel comfortable doing, I will terminate the relationship myself.

Although I have not as yet had to walk away from a treatment process that the client wanted to continue, I do walk away from many situations before they begin. Assessment, it is important to remember, begins before the therapist meets the client personally; the first contact with the client is not usually a face-to-face meeting. Most therapists first meet their clients over the telephone, through a referral from another professional, or through exposure to the case records. For therapists to say blithely, 'I never look at the records or solicit anyone else's perspective before I see a client because I do not want to go into the first interview with a contaminated point of view,' is to deny themselves rich sources of information that can facilitate an expeditious and full assessment process.

Of course, therapists should not accept every conclusion they read or hear about an individual, and of course first impressions are only that, first impressions. But records, initial telephone conversations with prospective clients, and referral conversations can and should be mined for every ounce of wealth they can produce, both about the client and about her circumstances. Much time can be saved in disentangling countertherapeutic misalliances by paying attention early on, in and before the first interview, to clues as to what it is an individual requesting therapy wants and is able to manage.

In an inpatient unit or residential program, many of the same issues need to be considered as part of the assessment procedure, as well as some additional ones that relate to daily living as a member of the program community. The emphasis in a community treatment program, as in group outpatient therapy, should be on self-care and social interactions rather than the specifics of the dissociative symptoms or trauma history. Particularly in group settings, an excess of such an interest can create all kinds of iatrogenic problems, such as fierce competition for numbers of personalities, most intense symptoms, or the ability to recount the most horrible childhood experiences.

These are clearly not the kind of norms a program wants to set out for status among peers, one of the most reinforcing aspects of group treatment. Generally speaking, it makes sense that talking in detail about trauma experiences be reserved for private sessions with staff. Group meetings and peer interactions should be focused on the here and now. This does not mean trauma will not be mentioned, but it should not be excavated or processed in group settings except to illuminate cognitive distortions and behavioural problems that affect present-day functioning.

Inpatient programs and intensive day programs, which are always short-term compared to the duration of therapy, must place the greatest emphasis on symptom management, stabilization, and concrete changes in the patterns that make it difficult for individuals to function in their communities. A program stay that uncovers all kinds of new material and leaves the person further destabilized is a program that has failed. No matter how boring, slow, or gruelling creating changes in the direction of responsible behaviour may appear compared to the intensities of processing the past, it is the heart of the treatment. Without it, treatment will not only be ineffective, but can be extremely harmful.

The following is an assessment model for a residential or day hospital program for severely dissociative trauma survivors.

The initial assessment is carried out in four steps:

1. by the program staff before the participant arrives (speculation, through examining the intake information);
2. in an initial interview with the participant;
3. in a post-interview staff assessment meeting; and
4. at an initial group meeting with all program participants.

Each assessment meeting should address the following issues:

Degree of Dissociation

What are the most obvious behaviours that adversely affect self-care and social interactions? What seem to be the triggers for these behaviours? How much awareness and control does the individual seem to have over her states of consciousness and her behaviour?

Strengths

Every possible strength (practical – 'makes good chocolate chip cookies;' interpersonal – 'good listener;' intrapersonal – 'figures out what triggers her quickly') should be noted and emphasized. They will be needed.

Vulnerabilities

A concrete and non-judgmental list of problems that make self-care and social interaction difficult should be made. In staff meetings when the individual is not present, and especially before the staff know the participant, this list is obviously hypothetical. During assessment meetings where the participant is present, she should first name her own difficulties. Other participants and staff should work hard to frame their observations and challenges constructively, so that the participant can understand them. She can then be invited to develop goals towards making incremental and measurable change.

External Resources

Family and community supports (including treatment resources) should be assessed for both strengths and vulnerabilities. The program is an opportunity for the participant to assess these connections and learn how to utilize them effectively and appropriately, including learning about personal boundaries. All social learning in the program should be consistently connected to plans for change in ongoing relationships after graduation.

Recommendations

Clear goals (personal, social, medical, spiritual, – long-term, short-term, and immediate (with built-in monitors and consequences, when applicable) – should be set at each assessment interview, including concrete ways of implementing these goals.

Once group meetings with all program participants are initiated (step 4), the emphasis should be on problems that affect present-day functioning. The initial group meeting is the prototype for an ongoing progress assessment and an opportunity to monitor change and set new goals with the input of the other program participants and the staff. Such occasions should take place weekly – or at least biweekly – over the course of program participation.

Each meeting should be structured so that the participant clearly states her goals for the weekly or bi-weekly time period and asks for specific help in implementing them. Creative input from staff and other participants can ensure that these goals are both realistic and relevant, and are concrete enough that progress can be easily assessed. It is important that there be at least one goal that has every chance of being achieved in the course of the immediate time period, as well as one or more that are much more difficult to meet. These goals should be written down during the meeting and both the participant and her primary nurse/therapist should keep a copy for reference over the course of the week.

This strategy provides a systematic survey of each participant's improvement and the areas on which she needs to focus. It also offers compassionate, powerful and unremitting feedback in a secure context that is seen to be central to the healing process. To be effective and not unduly threatening, the structure must be carried out in a completely even-handed manner (weekly or biweekly assessment meetings and consistent accountability for everyone). This structure reinforces for both the individual and the group some basic standards for interpersonal relationships that are key to both their problems and the potential solutions to these problems.

Many inpatient and day hospital programs become so involved with a combination of crisis interventions, teaching sessions, and enrichment activities that a time-consuming structure like the one outlined above – that should only be initiated if it can be carried through with consistency – can seem unworkable. However, most explosions, either internally directed or attacks on others, are messages of desperation that the individual perceives no other way of communicating. This type of structure has the potential to reduce crisis-management interventions to a minimum, by placing the need for the development of other, less self-destructive vehicles of self-expression out in the open as goals the participant has a right and a responsibility to struggle towards with the help of the other group members, most of whom know her experience intimately.

Generally, when each individual is surrounded in this way, the ability of all members of the program community to profit from the treatment experience is exponentially increased. Therefore, I think that some such structure should precede classes and activities in terms of program planning priority. Enrichment activities can then be added to a program with a solid grounding in the individual and group commitment to each individual's healing, and the degree to which each participant can profit from these activities can be assessed. Activities like art therapy and other expressive therapies, assertiveness training, psychoeducational groups about managing symptoms, and many other creative and useful programs can then be more clearly tailored to the needs of a particular group.

This kind of structure makes it simple to be clear about limits and bottom lines, always an issue in group therapeutic programs. Essentially, the same general limit that makes sense in individual therapy applies to group treatment as well. If a person is not getting better as a result of participation in the program, then I assess it to be possible that the program is not appropriate for her. If an individual consistently fails to meet the goals she sets – and, in fact, her symptoms get more volatile and out of control as she participates in the group – then I ask her to consider the possibility that leaving the group would be a less self-destructive option than remaining and continuing to deteriorate. When faced with these alternatives, many individuals find the resources within them to contain the acting out of their symptomatic behaviour. If it is not possible for the person to make the choice of getting better, a group program will probably continue to do her more harm than good. As well, her presence will be distracting and discouraging to the other participants.

Any therapeutic group re-creates for its members the dynamics of the family of origin as well as other earlier group experiences. This is one of the ways in which the context evokes feelings that are then accessible for therapeutic attention. Individuals with a history of severe trauma almost invariably have had a great deal of experiences in groups, including but not exclusively families, that have been chaotic, rigid, and radically unresponsive to the needs of their members. Residential and day programs, which are often situated within larger structures like hospitals, suffer almost inevitably from some degree of chaos and rigidity. It seems to come with the territory. It is extremely important, therefore, that programs geared for highly dissociative individuals minimize as much as possible the ways in which the operation of the program replicates in the present the dynamics of a dysfunctional and abusive family so as to ensure that the good that is accomplished over the course of the residential treatment outweighs its retraumatizing effects. Structures such as the one suggested here can create the combination of caring focus and consistent boundaries that characterize stable, nurturing homes.

Richard Kluft (1995b) has developed what he terms the Stabilization Plus model of hospital treatment. He frames inpatient treatment as boot camp, a training ground for the long and difficult task of outpatient therapy for the severely dissociative trauma survivor. This model involves the accomplishment of the following eight tasks to enable the individual to leave the hospital with the best chance of completing her treatment in a community setting:

1. Develop a workable safety contract
2. Detoxify emergent material
3. Manage uproar and/or rejection in the individual's life
4. Enhance coping re destabilizing events that led to admission
5. Attend to co-morbidity concerns, such as substance abuse, depression, eating disorders, etc.
6. Neutralize triggers
7. Attempt to minimize damage or fallout from the admission and its precipitants
8. Ensure that outpatient therapy is established and well-grounded

The process of active assessment of these eight areas of psychosocial functioning and the initiation of effective treatment in all these domains is more effective than a quick inpatient stabilization that allows the individual to leave the hospital at high risk for readmission.

When day program treatment is available, many individuals can often get the intensity of therapy that they need without suffering from all of the disadvantages of a hospital admission in terms of the disruptions in important relationships and the regression that a total-care program often promotes. A day treatment regime can, therefore, be of considerably longer duration without creating secondary problems of institutionalization and regressive dependency. In either case – residential inpatient or day treatment – these intensive programs should be time-limited and goal-oriented, with the aim of enabling the participant to cope in a community setting with a greater degree of independence and a less protective support system.

The process of assessment – whether by therapist, client, or a program community – is an ongoing one, and it is at the heart of an effective therapeutic treatment. In my own training analysis, I was encouraged to look at my own dynamic of growth and change, and resistance to growth and change, as 'a young scientist.' This always sounded pretty unlikely and irritating to me as I wrestled fitfully with my demons. But the directive – which, in retrospect, was undoubtedly put forth with some irony – has always stuck in my head, and I try to encourage that attitude in my own clients.

Socialization to the therapy process makes all the difference to the likelihood of treatment success. Individuals who must grapple with a history of maltreatment and all of the psychological fall-out of that history will be better able to bear the process with grace if they can develop the ability, and the habit really, of moving from a place of intense and often overwhelming engagement to a vantage point from which they can look at the process with some detachment.

People who are highly dissociative have the personal skills to do this; they are using their ability to detach all the time. It is the therapist's job to help them learn how to harness these already highly developed skills in the service of a stance of active and creative assessment of their own healing process. This does not mean that they will always know exactly what is going on in their own healing process or be entirely secure that the process is on the right track. That degree of objectivity is very rare in anyone's in-depth psychotherapy. They will understand, however, that it is their right and responsibility, as well as their therapist's, to address the issue in an ongoing way.

5

Constructing the Healing Process

The test of a first-rate intelligence is the ability to hold two opposing ideas in the mind at the same time, and still retain the ability to function.

F. Scott Fitzgerald (1945)

There has been a great deal of optimism, both in clinical settings in which individuals suffering from dissociative conditions have been treated and in abuse survivor circles, about the prognosis for complete healing. The earliest outcome study (Kluft, 1988) found that more than 90 per cent of the individuals followed after a period of two years or more of stable integration did not relapse, and not only no longer suffered from multiple personality but showed substantial improvement in most areas of their functioning. Most clinicians who have treated a number of individuals suffering from severe dissociative symptoms have had the gratifying experience of watching people who had floundered through years of fruitless treatments and had endured high levels of acute difficulty that appeared impervious to therapeutic intervention, gradually become stable and productive. There is no doubt that once these individuals receive an accurate diagnosis and effective treatment, their chances of getting better increase astronomically.

However, the initial optimism that greeted the first treatment successes in this field has been tempered as a wider range of individuals have been diagnosed in a wider range of settings. As part of a demonstration project funded by Health and Welfare Canada to create and test a training model for professionals to enable them to recognize the symptoms of multiple personality and severe dissociation in their clients (Rivera, 1991b), 2,500 Ontario professionals received basic education in the assessment of severe dissociation. Many of these individuals have since facilitated the diagnosis of multiple personality disorder (DSM-IV: Dissociative Identity Disorder) or DDNOS in several clients. There are now many more individuals in Ontario who are aware that one of the sources of their difficulties is a dissociative condition.

However, although more individuals know they need treatment, there are still few mental health workers who have the skill and the experience to treat them successfully. Even those who would be capable of offering effective treatment are often precluded from doing so by the mandate of their agencies to engage in only short-term treatment. A needs assessment funded by the Ontario Ministry of Health (Rivera, 1992a) documents the lack of accessible treatment for this population in Ontario, Canada. There is no reason to believe that resources are dramatically different anywhere else.

The advantage of high levels of optimism about prognosis is that it offers hope to both survivors and their therapists that previously intractable symptoms can be understood, contained, and eventually ameliorated. The downside to this frame of reference is that myths are quickly created and proliferated that lead to disappointment, frustration, and even suicidal despair.

One of the most pervasive and most dangerous of these myths applies not only to the treatment of severe dissociation, but presents particular dangers in the therapy of highly dissociative people: 'If you uncover and deal with your childhood trauma, you will be healed.'

As with most myths, there is some truth to it. People suffering from multiple personality as an outcome of child abuse do not usually get much better without processing their trauma history therapeutically to some degree. However, the cognitive error of taking a part and misidentifying it as the whole is extremely common in the field of abuse treatment. Abuse survivors who experience intense dysphoria understandably latch on to the notion of a straight and uncomplicated solution to their difficulties. It is very common for a client to begin therapy with the goal of 'getting back my abuse memories' or 'working on my abuse issues.'

When someone asks me to see them for the purpose of helping them uncover memories, I ask her why she wants to do this. The usual reply is along the lines of, 'I think maybe my father (uncle, brother, and so on) sexually abused me but I can't remember it.' I often inquire as to why she would spend time and money trying to remember something so unpleasant. Eventually she begins to talk about the difficulties in her day-to-day life – constricted relationships, job problems, parenting difficulties, sexuality problems – all of which she thinks may be a consequence of her forgotten history of child abuse.

I am not dismissive of her conclusion. It may turn out to be true. However, neither of us knows at this point, so I try to be helpful. I tell the individual that my understanding of therapy is that it is to help people have a better life, and if abuse experiences are part of the problems that are standing in the way of her having as full, rich, and rewarding a life as she deserves, then that will undoubtedly be part of the therapy. But in the meantime, we need to start by exploring her life in the present.

If a person remembers a history of abuse, it is equally important not to collude with her notion that, if she simply focuses on her abuse, before long she will be better. Recent trauma experiences in the lives of basically emotionally stable people can often be dealt with in this direct fashion, in what is essentially a desensitization process. However, when an individual has a history of severe ongoing childhood trauma, immediately delving into the experiences with powerful therapeutic tools, such as hypnosis and guided imagery, is unlikely to be helpful and may quite possibly be destabilizing and dangerous.

In-depth exploration of the trauma may occur at some point in the therapy process. However, the building of ego strengths, the management of disruptive, symptoms, the establishment of a solid therapeutic relationship, the exploring of the most obvious ways in which formative experiences are being re-enacted hurtfully in present-day life, and the creating of personal and social supports that will be reliable when the therapy becomes increasingly volatile and painful – all these mundane interventions are the heart and soul of the therapy process.

Focusing on the trauma work as the centre of the therapy process would be similar to focusing on the heart transplant in a patient who is suffering from cardiac problems. Imagine a situation in which a patient sees a heart specialist and says, 'Doctor, I have come to see you because you have a good reputation as a heart doctor, and I think I need a heart transplant.' The doctor asks the patient to describe his symptoms and says, 'I agree that it sounds like you need a heart transplant,' takes a knife out of his drawer and cuts into the patient's chest. After he withdraws the knife from the chest cavity, the doctor sends the patient home with the instruction to come back next week for follow-up and to call if there are any problems in between appointments. The therapist who agrees to do intrusive exploration of the client's psyche without appropriate preparation will likely produce similar consequences.

The first issues that need to be addressed if the psychotherapy is to be well-grounded are those that relate most directly to basic well-being. For many individuals severely traumatized in early childhood, this means issues relating to their own safety, such as suicidality, involvement in abusive relationships, disabling addictions, extremely disordered eating patterns, dangerous self-mutilation or, in some cases, issues relating to the safety of others, such as child abuse or pressing homicidal impulses. It is crucial that the therapist elicit as much information as possible about these issues in the first sessions. To do so it may be necessary to ask about them in a straightforward manner. It may not be obvious to the client that her six admissions to the hospital for overdoses in the past year are relevant to a therapy process in which she expects to deal with her past, or she may not mention them out of shame or fear that the therapist will not wish to work with her if she is aware of her suicidality.

Some severely dissociative individuals who do not engage in extreme levels of self-destructive behaviour have, nevertheless, defensive patterns to focus on in the early stage of the therapy process. For example, periodic binging and purging, drinking too much when under stress, engaging impulsively in unsafe sex, getting involved with people who are destructive, compulsive and extreme patterns of exercise – all of these are relatively socially sanctioned behaviours. They are quite common and are not immediately perceived as dangerous. However, it is important for both the therapist and the client to deal with them at the beginning of a therapy process, because they illustrate the ways in which the individual will be likely to cope under stress.

An individual's problems may not be extreme in the early stage of therapy, but it would be a mistake to ignore them and move immediately into trauma work without helping her to understand her characteristic ways of coping with stress and beginning the process of developing new and more creative coping strategies. Drinking that is only occasionally out of control, for example, can become a full-fledged and more entrenched addiction when an individual is beginning to deal directly with memories of trauma and the associated feelings and has not learned other ways of titrating emotion than through the use of alcohol. Long-term, in-depth therapy for trauma survivors is a grueling and stressful project, and it is the therapist's responsibility to ensure that the client is engaged in developing the strengths that she will need to make substantial changes in her life.

Focusing on present-day issues and helping people make changes in the areas of their lives that are currently problematic creates a safety net to ensure that the therapy process is helpful rather than harmful. This intervention also alters an emotional dynamic that keeps trauma memories inaccessible in a more natural way than digging around specifically to unearth these memories.

This is how it works. Experiences that are too traumatic to be integrated into an individual's general memory system become stored in consciousness in a compartmentalized fashion. Though these experiences appear to be forgotten, they are just as present as memories that are more accessible to general consciousness, and they affect an individual's way of thinking, feeling, and behaving at least as much as, and sometimes more than, experiences of which the individual is consciously aware.

Although Western thought privileges linear, conscious self-awareness and assumes perception, memory, and identity – the combination of which we experience as the self – to be unitary, both contemporary science and philosophy challenge this notion. Subjectively, most of us have a compelling sense of a unified self. In fact, many relatively independent systems and subsystems operate simultaneously to produce what we experience as affect, cognition, motor activity, and behaviour, and we are only consciously aware of a small percentage of what is going on at any given time.

· This systems view of mental functioning, whether framed in neuroscientific terms as modularity, psychological terms as polypsychism or 'states' theory, or philosophical terms as poststructuralism, necessarily yields contradictory contents and/or controls – dissociation. Generally, most people are not aware of the plethora of systems and subsystems that are operating as an effect of our ongoing day-to-day functioning. When the self-system is in disharmony, however, the multiplicity of self-systems tends to be more obvious (Erdelyi, 1994).

Memory is no more unitary than any other aspect of mental functioning. There are experiences that are completely erased and cannot be retrieved. Much of what we call 'forgetting,' however, is an attentional shift due to neglect or defence rather than an erasure. An experience may also be actively operational in an individual's present-day life without that individual being able to make a cognitive connection to the original experience. Declarative memory, in which a linear representation of a part event is preserved, is different from procedural memory, a dramatization of that event that is dissociated from the individual's conscious awareness (Bornstein & Pitnam, 1992; Erdelyi, 1993; Lewandowsky, Dunn & Krisner, 1989).

A person who has been abused as a child may not remember, may remember only partially, or may remember the details but be out of touch with the affective component of the memory. The abuse experiences are still influential on how that person processes her present-day life. This influence exerts itself on a number of levels: biologically, cognitively, affectively, and behaviourally.

A survivor of severe abuse may well have an exaggerated startle response when tapped on the shoulder. She may also have difficulty distinguishing between relationships that are respectful and those that are abusive, being generally mistrustful in her relationships with people, always expecting to be betrayed, and, paradoxically, often becoming intimately involved with abusive partners. She may become furious at relatively minor or even imagined slights, or terrified in situations that most people would not find particularly frightening, and then numb and distant in situations that are emotionally laden. She may find herself behaving in a repetitious and compulsive fashion, doing things she consciously does not wish to do and finding it impossible to control her behaviour with any degree of consistency. Her physiological responses, her thoughts, feelings, and behaviour seem to her – and often to others – unexplainable, illogical, and perverse. She often calls herself 'crazy' or 'bad.' Mental health professionals may well label her 'borderline personality disorder,' which is often spoken in a tone that connotes a combination of crazy and bad.

Her thoughts, feelings, behaviour, and sensations are not illogical. They simply look that way because the survivor does not understand she is responding to her early experiences as they have been incorporated into her biology and her psychology. If, for example, I am swimming in the ocean and I feel a burning sensation on my leg, my knowledge of the ocean may well influence how I understand my reaction. If I have no idea what has happened I may jump out of the water and stand on the beach, rubbing my leg, alternately jumping up and down and yelling, and then, when I look at my leg and see nothing much, trying to keep quiet until I can't stand it anymore, and I start jumping up and down yelling again.

If I don't know what has happened and no one around me knows either, other people are likely to respond in ways that may be well-meaning – or may not be – but are unlikely to be helpful. They may be embarrassed that I am making such a fuss over what appears to be nothing and ignore me or walk away. They may rub my leg and exacerbate the irritation, so that rather than the pain easing off in a short period of time, it spreads in both location and duration. If I am very expressive, they may call an ambulance or the police, and I may be taken to a psych ward where I have to talk my way out of a situation that I do not understand.

If, on the other hand, I am aware that large jellyfish with long tentacles live in the ocean; that it is possible to swim into one of the tentacles without seeing the creature; that the sting of the jellyfish is extremely painful, even when there is hardly any external sign of the poison that has been injected; and that the worst thing you can do is rub the affected area, then I can feel free to jump up and down and yell, making it clear to everyone who is listening to me that I have been stung by a jellyfish. I know that, bad as it is, the acutely uncomfortable stinging sensation will be gone in fifteen or twenty minutes. In this context, my screams will not only allow me to bear the sting without doing anything counterproductive, such as rubbing my leg, but they will also warn other swimmers that there is a large jellyfish in the area. This gives other people the opportunity to protect themselves by getting out of the ocean until someone finds the creature and removes it from the swimming area with a net.

Most people who have been severely abused as young children are more like the individual who is suffering from the jellyfish sting and does not know exactly what happened or what to do about it. Unfortunately, there are not likely to be other people around who immediately recognize the signs of the trauma and know how to respond appropriately. A child who is being abused, particularly when the abuse is sexual, does not have the capacity to comprehend the situation and to act in the most effective way in the interests of her own self-protection. The younger the child, the less able she is to understand what is going on, but even adolescents are often extremely naive in analysing an adult's actions and motivations. This makes the child vulnerable to the manipulations of the abuser, and he is usually able to control not only her actions (ensuring that she put up with the abuse) but also her thoughts, feelings, and sensations.

The circumstances may be very different from one situation to the next. One child may have no contact with protective adults, and no matter what she says or does, no one acts as her advocate. Another child may be surrounded by caring adults, but the offender or offenders manipulate her thought processes in such a way that she is not able to reach out for the help that could potentially have been available.

In any case, the child is badly hurt, and no one intercedes on her behalf. She learns to defend against these injuries in the best way she knows how, by relying on her own mental resources.

The younger the child, the more likely her first line of defense will be a global form of denial, what we see as pervasive dissociative coping strategies. Dissociation is a defense that can seem magical to the hurt child. One child said to me, when I asked her how she felt just after her classmate in kindergarten pushed her down on the playground, 'It didn't hurt me at all. I just put my eyes up here (pointing to her eyelids) and I forget about it.'

The immediate solution, however, becomes an ongoing problem. The child manages to escape from the traumatogenic reality, but she does not learn to understand the situation and develop age-appropriate coping skills to deal with it. The simple dissociative mechanism gets locked in, as do the interpretations, feelings, and sensations connected to the trauma. This eventually leads to the circumstances in which the adult survivor finds herself. She is haunted by the effects of the trauma in her daily life while at the same time doing everything she can to avoid anything that reminds her of the abuse.

Generally, this scenario plays itself out in self-defeating or self-destructive behaviour of some sort. The little girl on the playground, for example, had been severely abused in her family. Though she found it very difficult to remember the physical and sexual abuse that was eventually documented by the child protective authorities who removed her from her home, those experiences did not disappear simply because she was able to compartmentalize them in her mind.

In school, she re-enacted various aspects of the original abuse situation she endured at the hands of a number of male relatives (who were also her only caretakers, her mother having died when the girl was born). She was alternatively timid – expressing the terror she had felt – and aggressive – venting the rage at her abusers, and their incorporated rage as well, on her less threatening classmates in ways that were similar to some of the acts that had been perpetrated on her. She took very little interest in playing with other girls and was constantly attempting to play with the oldest and roughest boys on the playground, who did not take kindly to the intrusions of this strange little girl. When they would eventually lash out at her physically, she would dissociate from the experience, and during the next recess, she would frantically try to get them to play with her once again.

This child's behaviour was frustrating to her teachers, who alternately framed it as crazy and bad, always implying that it was irrational and perverse. In fact, the child was doing her best to both express and deflect the scenario that had been etched into her consciousness from her earliest days. Males take care of you, males hurt you. You need them to survive, and therefore you must disconnect from the hurtful things they do to you. The child continued to use the radical dissociative defences that protected her in the original abuse situation, in which there was no escape, as protective mechanisms in her present life, and in doing so, was not able to engage in a more complex process of figuring out the current situation and coming up with solutions that served her better.

By the time an abuse survivor reaches adulthood, her patterns of simultaneously expressing and deflecting her traumatic experiences are likely to be more complex and more entrenched. Childhood abuse has been called, ironically, 'the gift that keeps on giving,' because the lessons it teaches, the themes it sets down that must be replayed again and again, even many of the physiological effects, are reinscribed at each developmental level. A volatile four-year-old may become an introverted eight-year-old, who may become a provocative adolescent, who may become a young adult who uses drugs and alcohol, and so on. Each new developmental stage incorporates new coping mechanisms, layered over and often intertwined with the previous ones in a way that can make an individual's behaviour patterns seem perverse indeed, not only to others, but to herself as well.

The core of an effective treatment process is interference in this dynamic of simultaneously expressing and avoiding painful material. The survivor needs help to change in her present-day life the patterns of re-enactment that have enabled her to leak out some of the affective energy connected to the early abuse experiences and, paradoxically but effectively, keep the intensity of the traumatic material at a distance.

Focusing on present-day life and making as many positive changes in this arena as possible provides a solid basis for engaging in the difficult and sometimes destabilizing process of remembering, reliving, and reprocessing the individual's trauma history. Making changes in the present so that it is not a re-enactment of the traumatic past is also the best way to encourage any buried material that might be influential to emerge at a pace that leads to the maximum degree of resolution with the minimum degree of disruption. I do not assume that such material is always there, or, if there, that such material is always related to experiences of child abuse. I have no preconceptions about what a given individual will come to understand as influential in her life history. It is my responsibility as a therapist to be open to hearing my client's story as she understands it and to help her create the changes she wants in her life.

In the early 1970s, long before abuse became a popular topic in the media and an acceptable focus in mental health circles, I found in my therapy practice that a significant number of unhappy people did have histories of child abuse of various kinds, which they remembered to varying degrees before entering into the therapy process. I also found that many unhappy people did not experience abuse as children; there were other sources for their dissatisfaction with life, either in their childhood experiences or in their adult lives. There are many ways of getting hurt in our society, both as a child and as an adult. Women (and males who are not white, middle-class, able-bodied, stereotypically masculine, or are in some way different from the norm) are systematically subjected to many forms of oppression and victimization in a capitalist patriarchal culture. These experiences often have profound effects, damaging their self-worth and creating severe and ongoing personal and social problems.

I do not privilege a childhood history of abuse as a traumatogenic agent over other ways in which people come to feel disturbed, depressed, or depleted. Individuals experience oppression of all sorts that does not divide itself into neat categories but rather is idiosyncratically combined in the ongoing creation of their lives. One woman says she suffered more as a girl than as a girl with brown skin as she was sexually assaulted by the male members of her family. Another woman remembers the constant taunts of her classmates and the contemptuous racist treatment by her teachers as the most painful and diminishing experiences of her childhood; the unpleasant sexual touching by her brother was much less traumatic than the shaming she suffered outside the family setting. Another woman found the constant pressure in her teen years to conform to heterosexual norms and her compliance with the abusive treatment by male peers during that time in her life to be the source of her most severe difficulties with self-acceptance and her ongoing struggle with suicidality. Many individuals experience multiple oppressions as they negotiate their lives from a one-down power position along a number of lines: gender, sexuality, race, class, religion, physical or mental ability, and so on.

The ways in which people are hurt and in which they transcend the diminishment that can be the result of oppression is the raw material of the healing process. To simplify it (to engage in some form of reductionistic 'abuse therapy') is to do another level of violence to people who have usually already suffered more than their share of interpersonal violence. From the beginning I try to create an atmosphere in which my focus is on the individual's strengths, her desire to have more than she does at present.

When I first began engaging in psychotherapy with people who were severely dissociative, they spoke to me in terms of 'getting the abuse out of my system,' 'throwing it up,' 'getting out all the garbage he put into me.' I listened to them, and that experience resonated in me, countertransferentially I now think. It made sense in a visceral way and satisfied my need to find a relatively hasty solution to these extremely painful problems. Without considering it too critically, I operated for a while within the framework of what I have since come to call 'the vomit theory of psychotherapy.' Horrible stuff was fed to the survivor, and it is the therapist's job to help her throw it up, as quickly and thoroughly as possible.

I have come to understand that the vomit metaphor is inadequate for the complex and multi-levelled process of in-depth therapy. It is not difficult for a therapist to facilitate a regurgitation of a great deal of volatile and painful affect in combination with images that may or may not represent an individual's historical experience of reality, especially when working with a highly trance-prone person. As part of the therapy, this kind of cathartic work can be an important part of the healing. When it is the central part of the treatment process, it almost always represents a re-enactment – the imposition of something developmentally inappropriate and over-whelming – rather than a resolution of the original trauma. It is a form of revictim-ization.

This is not something that the survivor can easily tell the therapist. Clichés and half-truths such as 'you will feel worse before you feel better' make it appear to the survivor that, although her life appears to be going down the tubes as her symptoms escalate and she can concentrate on nothing but abuse, all of this is a sign that she is indeed getting better. Also, there can be a tremendous relief in the immediate release of pressure that results from catharsis. The endorphine rush that often follows cathartic work can become as addictive a tension release as heroin, self-mutilation, or bulimia. Abreaction of trauma, although painful and frightening, may feel like a healing process. However, without the appropriate context, it can be simply one more self-destructive coping mechanism that gets the survivor through the day but never leads to any deep and satisfying resolution.

I have become convinced that effective therapy works in a dialectical pattern. Marsha Linehan (1993) uses the term 'dialectical behavioural therapy' to describe the comprehensive program she has developed to treat individuals with borderline personality disorder. I was unfamiliar with her prior – and somewhat different – use of the term when I first began to theorize the process of therapy this way. The concept of dialectic, as originally proposed by the nineteenth century philosopher, Georg Hegel, refers to the passage of thought from less comprehensive forms to increasingly more comprehensive ones through a process of contradiction. Catego-ries compete with one another, and out of this interaction emerges a category richer and clearer in spirit than either. A thesis is challenged by a counter-thesis or antithesis. These conflicting and seemingly contradictory concepts are then reconciled and integrated into a higher-level cognition (synthesis). This synthesis serves as another, more complex thesis for the development of further progression. Hegel posited an analogous process vis-à-vis the unfolding of the process of history and the evolution of the material world (1937).

I find this a useful way of conceptualizing the therapeutic process. Focus on day-do-day problems ('I want to stop my problem drinking' – thesis) sometimes enables the individual to make some immediate changes in her life. Occasionally this can occur through fairly simple problem-solving, cognitive restructuring, suggestion, and encouragement. However, this is often not enough. The thesis turns out to be too simple to represent reality for the individual, and then a more complex look at the present – and often the past as well – is needed to make room for change ('In order to survive this degree of fear and pain, I must numb myself. Drinking, from the time I was a teenager, has always been a sure way to do so. Therefore, drinking is not a problem for me, it is a solution' – antithesis). The struggle becomes incorporating the seemingly contradictory realities of the sincere desire to stop drinking and the desperate need of drinking to survive into a synthesis that works in the creation of concrete behavioural change. Such a synthesis might look something like this: 'I shall try some other ways, besides drinking, of creating enough distance from those surges of unbearable feeling that make it so difficult for me to function, and I shall find a social setting in which other people are trying to do the same thing so that I can get some support while trying to make these difficult changes.'

Sometimes issues regarding the past must be touched on in order for there to be any room for change in the present. For example, one individual may be able to change her addictive drinking by attendance at AA meetings at the suggestion of the therapist, who tells her that there is little likelihood of making any significant progress in therapy while her life is in the grip of a full-fledged addiction. Another person may need to process the ways in which alcohol was a part of her upbringing or her abuse experiences, or learn hypnotic distancing techniques to defend against destabilizing flashbacks before she is able to take the step of actually giving up drinking.

In any case, the emphasis is on creating change in the individual's present-day life rather than dealing with past experiences. Only as much work on the past is facilitated as is necessary to enable the individual to make such changes. It is tempting for both therapists and survivors to get excited when they begin to get in touch with experiences and feelings that are clearly important and meaningful; if a little bit of work makes such a difference in terms of changing dysfunctional behaviour patterns, then surely more focus on the past, more intense remembering and reliving of hurtful early experiences, should make more change happen – and faster. This completely understandable desire for quick results can be the source of serious problems as the therapy process proceeds.

Many issues might appropriately be the therapeutic focus in the early stage of the treatment. Often individuals, particularly highly dissociative abuse survivors, seek treatment when they are in crisis in their present-day life. For example, they may have functioned adequately or even excelled in their career throughout most of their adult life, but they have recently found themselves unable to cope in that setting. As part of socializing my clients to therapy, I encourage them to maintain as high a level of personal and professional functioning as possible throughout the therapy. In my experience, this has more than one advantage. The most obvious is that they get to have a life as well as a healing process.

Initially this may not be to everyone's liking. Creating and maintaining a responsible day-to-day life is difficult for anyone, and particularly difficult if you are being flooded with unpleasant posttraumatic stress symptoms, if your interpersonal problems make it hard for you to have satisfying personal or professional relationships, or if you were forced into inappropriate responsibility as a child and experience adult demands as a repeat of this experience. Some individuals give up the mundane struggles around family, employment, or schooling, when they start to get really involved in their therapy process; they make healing their full-time job. This may be a relief at first, but it can have devastating consequences in the long run. It is not only not good for the client to have finished a six-year therapy project and found she has lost her home, her career, and her children, but disengaging from the responsibilities of daily life in the present is likely to deprive her of the ballast she needs for her healing process.

I encourage my clients to attempt to keep functioning in the workplace or school (and to maintain as much equality as possible in their intimate relationships and friendships rather than becoming ensconced in the role of 'sick one who needs all the care and support') as well as they can manage. I often find myself doing a great deal of work immediately with people about their lives in the present – their jobs, their intimate relationships, how they relate to their children, how they manage anger, manage money, eat, exercise ... the things anyone talks about in therapy.

With clients who are severely dissociative, this mundane kind of therapy some-times looks just like any other kind of therapy. Sometimes it doesn't. Talking about something as basic as eating, for example, may necessitate accessing half a dozen altered states of consciousness before any clarity emerges about why, as the client reports deadpan, 'Ten pounds have been lost in the past week. That makes thirty this month.'

Generally, I think the principles that apply to minor problems also apply to life-threatening ones and that the basic strategies that work with less dissociative clients work with more talented dissociators. It is central to the effectiveness of anyone's psychotherapy process that the therapist create an atmosphere in which the client can communicate as much information as is necessary, so that the problem can be addressed as fully as possible. With people who dissociate, this may mean encour-aging a few alters to emerge and talk about the situation directly, or it may mean helping the presenting part of the person to get in touch with parts of herself that have previously been inaccessible. It is then up to the therapist to find ways to focus on the aspects of the situation that are amenable to change and to help the client facilitate that change.

The dissociative individual may need to express herself in a childlike state in which she conflates eating with being forced to perform oral sex. She may speak the language of an adolescent who is obsessed with being thin, as a punitive adult who declares that they deserve to be punished by being deprived of food, and as a compliant, helpless adult, who says, 'I tried to do the things you suggested last week, but every time food is in front of me I gag for some reason and, even if I do manage to get some food down, I usually throw up shortly afterwards.

The binge type of anorexia nervosa is (with bulima) associated more with a history of trauma than some other eating disorders. It is easy to hypothesize that the problem in this case is overdetermined. Some of the information that emerges from the client may relate to abuse and cognitive distortions that confuse eating with coercive sex. Profound and pervasive social messages that are communicated to all women in a patriarchal society prescribing a correlation between extreme thinness, sexual desirability, and basic worth appear to be operative as well. These are all usually cognitively embedded and deeply felt confusions, and they cannot be dealt with quickly.

This does not mean that the individual cannot be helped to stop starving herself. However, behavioural programs that do not consider the ways in which the client perceives her eating pattern as a solution rather than a problem are not effective; they replicate the authoritarian atmosphere of the individual's childhood in a central and sensitive area, basic sustenance, and consequently reinforce her defences. Although the therapist does not have to know everything about why her client cannot eat, she must understand enough for her interventions to be credible and therefore effective.

Often, in the early stages of therapy, it is enough to communicate to the part of the person who thinks she is three and is being orally raped, that you do not think anyone should do that to a child and then to help her create a self-hypnotically-induced safe place where she can hide whenever she is scared. More mature parts of the mind can be engaged to facilitate this protection of the child, particularly at mealtimes. Brief empathic negotiations about levels of weight gain can often alleviate the anxiety of the teenage state who is convinced that consuming one apple will cause her to gain fifty pounds, resulting in at least enough leeway to allow some eating. The self-punitive part of the self can often be engaged as a helper in the project of negotiating and enacting behavioural change, keeping control with the individual and thus avoiding a fruitless power struggle between the client – who knows she has to stay thin and get thinner to survive – and the therapist – who is just as convinced that the client must change her eating habits, or die.

Behavioural interventions do not get to the bottom of eating disorders as a manifestation of personal experiences of sexual assault or part of a more general socialization as a woman to patriarchal norms. It is rarely possible to deal with all that in the early stages of therapy. However, helpful, concrete cognitive/behavioural interventions – in combination with an indication that the therapist is aware of the complexity of the issues – give the client the message that the therapist is not simply attempting an end run around defenses that were constructed with good reason. On the other hand, the therapist presents herself, not only as sensitive to the deep and compelling need her client has to starve herself, but as a sensible person who is thoroughly grounded in the present. From that perspective she is reaching out with practical strategies and firm support to help her client make the behavioural changes necessary if she is going to live to engage in the process of truly resolving the problem.

The therapist who gets lost in the elaboration of the abuse history while her client is in immediate danger in the present cannot be of much help. Indeed, she may make things worse, as will the therapist who tries to impose an overlay of feminist ideology on a teenage alter who *knows* she must be thin to have any worth at all. Therapists who cannot let their clients know that they begin to understand and are compassionate, but simply try to legislate change ('You must eat or you will die' or 'The biological changes that accompany starvation are making it impossible for you to think clearly. Gain weight – and then we can work on your problem') from an experience-distant position of power are not likely to create enough of a connection with their clients to facilitate any but the most superficial and temporary type of change at best, or provoke reactive exacerbation of the symptoms at worse.

Incremental change is much more likely to be stable over the long haul than sudden, dramatic turn-arounds. A woman who has eaten nothing but black coffee and crackers for a week has made a great gain by adding milk to her coffee and a few slices of fruit to her diet. Trying to persuade her to eat more without acknowledging the initial efforts and without helping her to communicate what she went through making the first change will simply reverse the process. Each change in the present and the sense of accomplishment that such change evokes builds the support for more challenge and more change in the present. It also builds the strength to face the past without getting mired in it.

Therapists who frantically push their clients to eat full meals because they are afraid the client will die if she does not gain a lot a weight in a hurry, are guaranteed to fail in helping their clients to change from not eating enough to survive to being able to do so. The therapist's anxiety can only interfere with the process of change, and unless the therapist is able to deal effectively with her or his own need to see change faster than a client can produce it, she or he will do more harm than good.

This is not only true about life-threatening issues such as anorexia or suicide, although the tendency to push for change that the client cannot make is greater in situations in which the consequences of not changing are so extreme. If the therapist has a personal stake in producing any kind of changes in the client's life at a rate only the therapist finds acceptable, that dynamic is bound to block the client from doing the work she needs to make the changes she wants and can accomplish.

There are situations in which it is the therapist's responsibility, as a member of society, to take coercive measures if it is perceived that the client's life is in immediate danger, that the client is an immediate danger to someone else, or if the client has abused a child. These exceptions to the usual framework of confidentiality and respect for the centrality of the client's perspective to the therapy process should be stated clearly to the client as part of the socialization to treatment.

In some cases, an action such as hospitalizing a client is seen by the client as a protective intervention, and it does not interfere with the treatment process (likewise for reporting homicidal intentions or child abuse). In other cases, the client's anger at having her autonomy pre-empted in this fashion can destroy the therapy process. In any case, the therapist engaging in these coercive measures is saying, 'I have not been able to find any way, within the boundaries of my role as your therapist, to help you keep yourself or other people safe in a way that is demanded socially. Therefore I must step out of my role as your therapist and engage in my responsibility as an agent of the state.'

It is important to be clear about one's responsibilities as a mental health or social service professional in this regard. This clarity offers protection to both the client and the therapist. For the client, it provides a bottom line. For the therapist, it makes it clear that, as a therapist, we are not responsible for making our clients change, for making them do anything. However, in certain circumstances, we are responsible to declare the limitations of our role as therapist, both to the client and to the legally mandated representative of society (the psychiatrist on duty at the hospital in cases of suicidality and maybe the police if the person must be incarcerated forcibly, the children's aid society in cases of child abuse, and the police in cases of homicidality).

It may seem like splitting hairs to distinguish these roles – therapist and agent of the state – from each other. However, being clear – both with our clients and particularly with ourselves – about these different roles can make a great deal of difference to our ability to function clearly and cleanly as therapist. It is not our responsibility to legislate change, but simply to be as creative as possible in helping our client dismantle her defense system, layer by layer, so that she can make the changes she wants in her life.

Experience makes a great deal of difference to how often a therapist must invoke these bottom lines. I have never – yet – had a client forcibly incarcerated in a hospital or had to report a client to the police or to the children's aid society. I have always been able – based on our original agreement about these issues and our ongoing relationship – to persuade individuals to take the actions that were necessary to protect themselves and others. Making the limits of my role clear early in the therapy process makes a considerable difference in how often my clients present me with an emergency that forces me to invoke my role as agent of the state.

In the first five years of my work with severely dissociative abuse survivors, my practice was located in a sexual abuse treatment program that was part of a child welfare agency. Doing therapy in this setting is somewhat like learning emergency medicine at Bellevue Hospital in New York City. You see a wide range of cases, and you learn a lot about the bottom line. I carried a card around that said I had the right to apprehend children from their caretakers. My clients knew this, and it often came up for discussion.

Many of these individuals had had unpleasant experiences with child welfare authorities, and my location in that agency was a source of conflict for some of them. I let it be known that I did not see the power to act as an agent of the state to enforce community standards of child protection as undermining my role as psychotherapist. I was clear that I would much prefer never to have to use that power directly, but I would have no hesitation in doing so if I believed it was the only way to protect a child from immediate and serious harm. When the conversation was theoretical – as it always was as part of the socialization to therapy – my clients agreed with me that children ought to be protected and that if every avenue of keeping them safe with the voluntary help of their caretakers has been exhausted, then it is an unfortunate necessity for state authority to be invoked.

Learning to accept that level of responsibility and to be clear with my clients about it has been helpful in keeping these responsibilities and the distinction between my role as therapist and my role as agent of the state in the foreground in the therapy process of people in which the issues play themselves out more subtly, at least initially. At the earliest emergence of an issue like suicidality, which invokes both my roles, I make it clear that I am not in charge of whether a person lives or dies, just as I am not in charge of whether a person kills someone or abuses a child. My focus is on creating a structure that the individual can invoke herself, so that she is responsible for her own safety or the safety others, if that is the issue. This sometimes involves making contracts with the client; there may be times when this sort of concrete intervention is necessary and helpful. At other times, it is not necessary, appropriate, or even polite, as it implies a less sophisticated ability to function on her own behalf than may be the reality.

One of my clients told me a story recently that illustrated this point. She was talking about a close relative who was always threatening suicide and how the family, time and time again, became enmeshed in the hopeless dynamic of trying to save him from himself. As she was complaining about this situation, she suddenly grinned and said, 'You know I used to be just like that.' I said I had never had that kind of experience with her since I had known her, and she replied,

Yes, sure you did. At the beginning, when I was first coming to see you, I left one session feeling bad. When I came back the next week, I said to you that I had been strongly tempted to commit suicide, and I wondered what you would have felt if I had gone out after a session and killed myself. You said, quite kindly, that that would have been very unfortunate (my killing myself, that is). When I left that session I was stomping around saying to myself, 'Unfortunate! Unfortunate! I would be dead, and she says that's unfortunate.' But I never tried that on you again, and, in fact, I mostly stopped doing it with other people as well. I just kept thinking, 'Unfortunate!' and I felt stupid trying to make it other people's fault that I feel so bad sometimes that I don't know whether I want to live.

People who have had a history of not being properly cared for as children are often looking for the boundaries that were missing when they were children, and their parents were not able to ensure their safety. Having experienced frequent intrusion on their autonomy in combination with neglect of their welfare, however, they resent the imposition of rules from the therapist, while at the same time they create situations in which the therapist will be provoked to impose her own will on the reluctant client.

This is a basic dynamic in many therapeutic relationships, particularly those with trauma survivors whose early socialization plays itself out repeatedly in the present in double-binding relationships. Their internal ambivalence and conflicted confusion is externalized and re-enacted, creating havoc in their day-to-day lives, but relieving the pressure of facing and working through their deepest difficulties. This re-enactment is often particularly prevalent and intense in relationships with medical and mental health professionals. It represents the double bind which pervaded their childhood, and it needs to be addressed again and again, in a variety of ways, throughout the therapy process. If, however, it is being continually acted out, it will never be worked through. As Dawson and MacMillan (1993) stress '[H]elpful therapy cannot be conducted in an atmosphere of acting badly, acting out, chaos, regression, and repetitious distorting of interpersonal negotiations' (p. 56).

Therapy conducted in this sort of atmosphere can be a continual replay of, 'I am going to do something dangerous; see if you can stop me. I am going to neglect to care for myself (or my children) in very basic ways; see if you can make me.' If this dynamic becomes entrenched in the therapeutic relationship, not only will no significant therapeutic work be accomplished, but a need for escalating levels of dangerous behaviour may be created in order to fuel the process in the same way that increasingly higher doses of some drugs are needed over time to get the same high. Therapy (or mental health interventions of any kind, including crisis line interactions and emergency room communications) in these circumstances reinforce the legitimacy of suicidal threats or acts of self-harm as negotiating currency, and the risk of successful suicide or increasingly dangerous self-mutilation are increased by the interventions that are supposed to be preventing them.

Working with trauma survivors means facing the reality that one is working with a population who do pose a risk of suicide. There are a number of studies documenting the reality that a significant sub-group of these people successfully complete suicide (Stone et al., 1987a, 1987b, 1990; Paris et al., 1987, 1989; Fryer et al., 1988; Gunderson & Zanarini, 1987; Kullgren, 1988; McGlashan, 1986). The data also show that many individuals who commit suicide do so while in hospital – or shortly after discharge. It is possible to argue that hospitalizing a person of this sort – especially repeatedly – amounts to taking someone from a moderate-risk group and placing her in a high-risk group (Dawson & MacMillan, 1993).

One of the best ways of avoiding this trap – all our training to the contrary – is not to ask trauma survivors repeatedly about suicidal ideation. When a client raises the issue of suicide herself, I often respond with a reflection of how distressed she must be to be considering taking her own life. If pushed to take control, I sometimes say something along the lines of, 'I know you often feel like killing yourself, and I also know that if you really decided to do so, I probably could not stop you. Is that right?' The individual almost always agrees, sometimes with an edge of defiance. I continue, 'But for now, painful as it is, you are alive, so how can I help you under these circumstances?'

Sometimes this leads to a healing conversation about the anguish she is currently experiencing or about how exhausting it is always having to struggle to find a reason to stay alive. Sometimes it leads to productive strategizing regarding ways to avoid life-threatening actions. Sometimes the answer to the question of how can I help is, 'There is no way you can help,' or 'I don't know how you can help.' We are now in a position of accurate communication. We can agree that there may not be anything immediate and concrete I can do to help and that I truly wish to be of help if possible.

It can usually be taken as a given that most severely dissociative trauma survivors who have acknowledged their profound ambivalence about living and their pressing impulses to die will respond positively when pressed about whether they are suicidal. By continually bringing up the subject, when we do so for the sake of easing our own anxiety, mental health professionals are acting as past caretakers did – creating a context that is supposed to be nurturing for the client, but is, in fact, simply self-protective for the professional.

Consider a few scenarios among many of the ways such conversations play themselves out. If the person says she is not presently suicidal, a conversation that was unnecessary for the client's welfare has been initiated for the sake of reassuring the professional, and, in fact, thoughts of suicide are much more likely to be in the foreground after such a conversation. 'She is my therapist. She is probably aware of something that I am out of touch with. Come to think of it, she's right. I am acutely suicidal today, and I have just been in denial.'

If the person says she is thinking about committing suicide, the professional can suggest hospital – thus fostering regressive dependency and intervening in a way that is known to be unhelpful in the majority of cases. If the individual refuses to go into the hospital – even though she has strong and vivid suicidal impulses and cannot promise not to act on them – the professional can either certify her, thus declaring her literally incompetent, or can agree to allow her to leave, even though she has stated clearly for all to hear that she will most likely be dead before the night is out. The professional may even insist on hearing about suicidal ideation and then refuse adamantly to hospitalize the individual because, the professional declares in a smug and irritated manner, she is just manipulating him with her constant threats of suicide.

How are any of these possible conversations helpful to the suffering person, who just does not know what to do with floods of intense dysphoric affect? We often exacerbate people's already almost unbearable difficulties when we behave in self-protective ways without thinking them through.

This is not to replace one unhelpful overly-general rule with another: 'Always ask about suicide plans, dwell on details, and hospitalize if the person has pressing impulses and clear plans.' should not become 'Never ask anyone about suicide and never hospitalize for suicide under any circumstance.' There are people and groups of people for whom these guidelines do not apply. There are also many occasions for productive therapeutic conversations about suicide with trauma survivors. On the whole, however, with the population of depressed and distressed trauma survivors, continually pleading with them, cheerleading them, and acting on them to prevent suicide is not only ineffective but can be very dangerous.

A clear awareness on the part of the therapist of the degree to which she is helpless in imposing her agenda on her client is the most effective prophylactic against becoming engaged in these unproductive power struggles. Only an acknowledgment of our inability to make circumstances or people conform to our need to have them be a certain way allows us to operate cleanly and efficiently within the realm of our genuine power. If I have to incarcerate a client in the hospital against her will because I cannot find any other way to keep her alive in the short run, it is important for me to recognize that I have not facilitated her safety as I would have if we had found a way together to help her contain her self-destructive impulses. What I have done is protect myself by being a responsible agent of the state and invoking the bottom line when I could not find any way as a therapist to help.

This intervention may or may not end up being helpful to my client. She is more in control of that than I am. If she chooses, she may kill herself in the hospital or when she gets out of the hospital, and I have no control over that. She may also find within her a desire to live and leave the hospital ready to engage more actively in the therapy process. The power and the choice is all hers.

When this kind of a scenario is played out in relation to a person the therapist has a complex mixture of feelings about– in this type of situation there is usually at least the combination of attachment, compassion, and frustration – it can be very difficult for therapists to maintain consistent contact with the realization that they are basically powerless to make the client do what they want her to do. However, therapists who are able to bear the reality that their power is limited and to use what power they do have clearly and consistently are much more likely to stay out of the destructive and often spiralling trap of, 'Make me stay alive if you care about me. Don't you dare intrude on me if you respect me.'

If at all possible, in circumstances in which hospital admission – voluntary or not – is necessary for crisis management, it is usually preferable for the admitting professional to be someone other than the primary therapist. Also, therapy should be suspended while the person is hospitalized. Many people break the pattern of frequent and counterproductive hospital admissions when they become involved in a therapy relationship in which they feel both validated and challenged, and in which there are absolutely no secondary gains to be derived from the therapist as a result of self-destructive behaviour.

Basically, the healing process, when it is most effective, moves in a spiralling motion. Day-to-day safety and constructive living patterns are focused on and established so that the difference between the past and the present becomes emotionally evident. This may cause an emergence of feelings, reactions, or memories from the past that are then accessible to therapeutic intervention. Working with this material causes further disruption in daily life, and these issues must be attended to in a conscientious and thorough fashion, which creates further psychosocial change, which then triggers further reactivity, and so on.

The client often wants the work to go faster and pushes the therapist to go deeper quickly, with the idea that the faster they work the sooner the process will be over. It is crucial that therapists be thoroughly grounded in the clinical experience that teaches us solid change can only be made on a secure foundation. Trauma work, memory processing, experiential engagement with volatile feelings like rage and grief – all of these important therapeutic tasks can be extremely harmful if an individual has not built the supports in her daily life and the intrapsychic structures that enable her to do such work constructively.

As each new level of present-day safety and, eventually, life satisfaction, is established, another level of contact with the pain and abuses of childhood can be unearthed with new resources and increased personal strength to explore and heal old wounds. The healing process often seems like circling back to the same place and struggling with the same issues at deeper and deeper levels. Each engagement with the past leads to an increased ability to build a new life in the present not driven by the dynamics of childhood survival patterns. Each new level of present-day growth and achievement stirs up memories, feelings, and griefs, and provides the grounding for further cognitive restructuring and deeper, more secure psychosocial change.

Eventually the momentum of the spiral slows down. The survivor finds that she can live and celebrate the present without constantly being drawn into the past. She owns her history. Her history no longer owns her.

When therapy is seen as a dialectical process, assessing the success of the therapeutic process is not measured by goals that focus on the dissociation per se, such as the integration of personalities ('I had forty personalities and now I have four; I am getting close to the end of my therapy'). The goals of therapy are framed in terms of the increase in capacity to function in a developmentally mature fashion. I keep an eye on four basic issues throughout the therapy process as a way of measuring progress. Though dissociative strategies play a part in all of these areas as they manifest themselves in an individual's life, only one of them relates specifically to changes in dysfunctional or immature levels of dissociation.

The Development of the Capacity for Positive Attachment

Peter Barach (1991) defines multiple personality as an attachment disorder complicated by the sequelae of physical and/or sexual abuse. Pervasive anxiety regarding close relationships, defensive detachment, patterns of abusive attachments, compulsive caretaking – and a variety of other attachment patterns that are re-enactments of preoccupied, neglectful, or actively harmful early caretaking relationships in which the child learned how to survive vis-à-vis other people – are key areas that should be dealt with in therapy and monitored for change.

Communication patterns are part of developing and maintaining attachment. An infant who learns that her cries will be responded to in a way that meets her needs is a child who is learning to communicate actively and directly. Passive-aggressive communication patterns, in which an individual attempts to coerce other people into responding in a particular way, pervasive assumptions that one is communicating one's needs accurately and other people are simply willfully withholding what is desperately needed, and the inability to interpret accurately other people's feelings and responses are all characteristic communication distortions that trauma survivors exhibit in attachment situations. These issues must be addressed for treatment to be successful, and new communication skills developed to replace the maladaptive ones.

The Ability to Tolerate Affect

Abused and neglected children are mistreated as objects rather than respected as sentient creatures, and they must comply in the process of their own destruction for the sake of survival. Through many repetitions of these experiences, they learn that feelings are futile and, in fact, dangerous. They cut off their feelings when they can; they explode when they have to. They do not know how to tolerate – much less benefit from or enjoy – intense affective states. Therapy is a context in which an individual can develop the capacity to bear feeling, gradually, incrementally, a little bit at a time.

Most survivors of severe trauma exhibit a profound and chronic depression. The vital expression of emotion has a tonic effect on the person as a whole – physically, mentally, and spiritually. When affect is blunted, an individual slows down, and there is often an alienation in life-preserving functions, such as immune responses. An accumulating body of evidence suggests that depression and despair create a significant pre-disposition for illness. Many survivors of the World War II death camps, for example, found themselves unable to face – and therefore to mourn –

their catastrophic losses. They suppressed their feelings as best they could in their efforts to put the past behind them. Many were successful in creating new families and new lives for these families. Unable to grieve thoroughly, however, they themselves became depressed, physically ill, and died early (Krystal, 1995).

The degree of depression that trauma survivors experience usually correlates with the intensity of all of the emotions that they need to experience if they are to heal – fear, anger, and particularly, perhaps, grief. Their inability to tolerate affect, however, precludes them from being able to handle even ordinary day-to-day emotion easily, much less face and feel the powerful emotions that are a normal consequence of their traumas and losses. Marsha Linehan's (1993) elegantly articulated *Cognitive Behavioral Treatment of Borderline Personality Disorder* places central importance on the evolution of the capacity to tolerate affect. She describes people with these kinds of problems as the psychological equivalent of third-degree burn patients. They have no emotional skin. As any response is torture, they must constrict their movements to avoid unendurable suffering – alternately flailing about in agony when circumstances force them to move. Until they learn to tolerate, understand, and express emotion, they have little room to grow and often little motivation to live.

Some individuals are aided by an appropriate medication regimen to ease their depression. For trauma survivors intent on liberating themselves from chronic depression, however, medication is only the beginning of creating a calmer internal context within which to feel what needs to be felt. Many trauma survivors, who have had numerous unsuccessful medication trials, have finally learned to tolerate feeling enough to process their painful past and present situations with the intense emotion appropriate to them, and have then gone on to live depression-free and medication-free lives.

The Ability to Modulate State Transition

It becomes clear, as this list evolves, that the items are not independent. One of the least conscious yet most important tasks of parenting a young child is the teaching of state transition. Newborns are more dissociative than multiples. They experience discrete psychophysiological states, and are not cognitively capable of making connections between these states (Wolff, 1987). When a week-old infant wakes up hungry, she is utterly engulfed in the state of unmet need for food. When she is appropriately fed, she becomes completely blissful. The next time she wakes up hungry, she cannot say to herself, 'Oh, I remember this. It wasn't very long before that beautiful fed feeling came over me.' She is again engulfed in unmet need.

An attentive caretaker is empathically connected to the inability of the child to tolerate any space of time between the perception of hunger and the meeting of her need to eat. That same caretaker also teaches the child to develop the ability to connect one state to another, to learn from past experiences and therefore to be able to bear increasingly intense affect without panic, and to move more gradually from one state to another – from hunger to satiety, for example. The newborn who screamed when she was hungry becomes a one- or two-month-old baby who can hear her mother's voice saying, 'I'm coming, honey,' and be soothed by the remembrance of the other times in which that voice meant a state of fulfilment.

Therapy is a milieu in which individuals can learn to be their own empathic parent through the modelling of the therapist and the incorporation of the therapist's attitudes of soothing, affirming, and challenging. As the ability to tolerate and modulate affective states develops, the need for rigid barriers between dissociative self-states gradually decreases. An individual can learn to experience and acknowledge a state of anger that then turned to pain (or anger mixed with pain) rather than having to say, 'First Jim came out, and he almost belted the guy. Then suddenly Sally was there – I don't know why or how – but she was just sobbing and sobbing.'

The Development of a Mature Sense of Responsibility

Many adults who are abused and/or neglected as children never grow from the very young developmental state of understanding themselves as responsible for all kinds of things they have no control over (or even have nothing to do with) in combination with denying utterly responsibility for their own actions. One of the most significant signposts of treatment progress is the increasingly consistent ability to assign appropriate responsibility for actions and in relationships. This indicates a developmentally more sophisticated ability to tolerate the existential helplessness implied in acknowledging that one is not and cannot be responsible for everything and everyone and the concurrent capacity to take responsibility for what one does indeed have some control over.

The development of maturity and responsibility can be seen in the ability to distinguish thoughts and feelings from actions, a capacity often stunted in survivors of severe childhood trauma, who can be cognitively and emotionally arrested to some degree at the developmental stage in which magical thinking predominates and to think something is to make it happen. Learning to think a variety of thoughts and feel a range of feelings and still behave responsibly is a landmark of treatment success.

Each of these issues, which can also be framed as a basic treatment goal, is dealt within the context of the therapist/client relationship (sometimes in the foreground, more often in the background) and also in terms of the client's present-day life.

Insights about past hurts and consequent deficits and distortions in these areas are always milked for everything they can offer towards the goal of creating steady incremental change in present-day circumstances and relationships.

Treatment as a dialectical process vis-à-vis therapeutic focus on the client's present-day life and her past, particularly her most basically formative childhood experiences, is one way to look at the structure of the treatment process. Another perspective is to ask what it is about therapy that creates change. What is mutative, what generates healing, or, as Heinz Kohut (1984) entitled his last, posthumously published book, *How Does Analysis Cure?*

What is it about therapy that enables a person to make substantial changes in her life? Many things may happen as part of therapy that contribute to change – problem-solving, the development of insight, catharsis, skill-building, cognitive restructuring, behaviour modification. They are all important, but not basic. None of these are therapy-specific effects. Insight can evolve through reading a book that is relevant to one's own situation; problem-solving happens in many situations; screaming one's head off while driving through the car wash may create a cathartic release. Although all of these experiences, when activated within the treatment process, may be helpful, individually or together they are not the same as therapy.

What is basic is the therapeutic relationship, the instrument through which all of the interventions and the experiences of the enterprise we call therapy are initiated and maintained. There are many types of therapeutic relationships. A parent who accompanies a foster child to a play therapist's office for an assessment and spends five minutes with the therapist supplying demographic data is a client of that therapist. So is the individual who sees that same therapist four times a week for six years in psychoanalysis. Obviously, there are significant differences in terms of the depth and character of the therapeutic connection that each of these people would develop with the therapist.

As well, there are different characteristics of therapists, as well as a wide range of therapeutic modalities practiced and styles within which they are practised that make a difference to the character and depth of the therapeutic relationship. A one-shot assessment session with a relationally skilled and empathic practitioner may create a therapeutic connection that remains alive internally for years in a transformative way within a client who experiences little connection to her regular therapist, who is distant in manner.

I am stressing this point because, although I take the position that it is the therapeutic relationship that enables therapy to mediate change in a significantly different way from reading self-help books, spending time with supportive friends, attending AA meetings, or practising yoga, I am not assuming that all therapy relationships partake of the qualities that create deep change.

I find the self psychology literature the most helpful in addressing the issue of the therapeutic relationship, and much of the way that I think and talk about it can be found in its basic texts, especially recent formulations that stress the very postmodern axiom that psychological phenomena cannot be understood outside the contexts in which they are shaped (Stolorow & Atwood, 1995; Mitchell, 1993; Stolorow et al., 1987). The emphasis in self-psychological treatment (usually termed 'analysis') is on the therapeutic relationship, the psychological field created by the interplay between client and therapist, as the only reliable and relevant source of information therapists can garner in terms of their role of facilitating personal change for the client.

Self psychology – taken to its logical conclusion, as its more recent theorists tend to do (Brothers, 1995; Mitchell, 1993; Stolorow & Atwood, 1995) – is essentially social. There is no such thing as the individual outside of her context, and the self is envisioned as the interactional configuration of the self in relation to others. Knowledge is understood as narrative, as a context-dependent creation of meaning, in a way that is singularly postmodern.

Although context is important in a radical way in recent self psychology, its meaning is limited to the intersubjective field (usually seen as a dyad) created between therapist and client or caregiver and child. The interplay of larger social forces on these radically related dyads is not emphasized – or usually even noted. Self psychology has certainly been influenced in its evolution from Kohut's challenge to Freudian mechanistic metapsychology (Kohut, 1971, 1977, 1984) by the climate of postmodern thinking that understands the notion of the isolated individual mind as a modern fiction. However, self psychology, including 'intersubjectivity,' which claims for itself post-self psychology status (Stolorow & Atwood, 1995), remains, first and foremost, a variant of psychoanalysis. Its focus is always on the complexities of the narrowest units of interaction – in early development, the child/caregiver 'system of mutual reciprocal influence' (Beebe & Lachmann, 1988); in the therapeutic process, the client/therapist system of mutual reciprocal influence. This is both the strength and the limitation of psychoanalytic theory.

The self psychology description of the way therapy creates change for the individual is its most widely useful contribution. My own basic training was psychoanalytically based, and, long before I ever happened upon the self psychology literature, I always viewed the therapeutic relationship as the key to the healing properties of psychotherapy. I am therefore going to talk about it without using the self psychology jargon, which I find exceptionally irritating. I do, however, wish to acknowledge the richness that can be found in many of the major writings in the contemporary psychoanalytic literature. A more thorough discussion of the issues I shall only touch upon can be found in the works of such writers as Stolorow, Brandchaft, and Atwood (1987), Mitchell (1993), and Wolf (1988), all of whom offer an overview of the many theories that have evolved as psychoanalytic theory and practice has been radically transformed over the course of the twentieth century.

Empathy, the therapist's capacity to allow an individual's experience to resonate within her or him such that the experience can be processed and understood from a radically experience-near vantage point, is the basic tool of the therapy project. Sometimes referred to as 'vicarious introspection,' empathy is not sympathy (in which the sympathizer shares the other's feelings), identification (in which the feelings are appropriated as one's own), or observation from the outside inwards. Empathy is a neutral activity. The therapist, when in clear empathic connection with the client, does not suffer or enjoy with her.

This does not mean the empathic therapist cannot be friendly, take the client's side at times, be irritated with the client occasionally, or feel surges of rage at the abusiveness of her perpetrators. Such reactions are not empathy, however. Data obtained from the empathic connection with the client can and should be combined with other data, such as observation, clinical records, reports from the client about important life events, clinical experience, and so on, but all of this information must be subjected to the empathic field of communication before it yields reliable data for use in the healing process.

Empathy is not only the way in which therapists know what they know so that they can be helpful to their clients. The experience of empathy also constructs the basic healing matrix for the client. A person's sense of self is enhanced by the awareness that another person is focusing on her with a high degree of absorption, accurately understands her inner experience, and is responding with positive affect. The quality and intensity of that focus is not very different from the focus of the nurturing primary caretaker(s) on the infant. Within the ambience of the responsiveness of the caretaker the child develops a vigorous, cohesive, and harmonious sense of self. Once therapists understand that their responsiveness can be experienced as a vital and transformative component of the client's self-organization, they will never again listen to their clients in the same way (Stolorow et al., 1987).

Healing takes place in the therapeutic relationship through the transformation of the client's mental schemata through which she organizes and gives meaning to her life. Unassimilated memories – and the cognitions and affects associated with them – are activated in a charged transference toward the therapist. Healing occurs as the interactions are reworked, this time with a different outcome. As a result the client's way of understanding herself and the world – her basic meaning schemata – are re-transcribed (Modell, 1990). Some of this change is noticed and consciously analysed; much takes place outside of conscious awareness – incrementally, very slowly, but often with dramatic, long-term, stable effects.

A consistent attitude of sustained empathic inquiry on the part of the therapist promotes the unhampered unfolding of patterns of experience, including disturbances in the structural properties of a person's sense of self. This unfolding may occur in a variety of ways. The transference relationship with the therapist, in which all kinds of intense feelings are experienced, is one of the most obvious, but there are usually many other ways in which the individual engaging in therapy finds herself in the midst of an upsurge of reactions that are not particularly grounded in the realities of the present.

This needs to be understood, particularly by the therapist, as an achievement rather than as pathology. Only within this context can early developmental derailment, thwarted developmental strivings, and the resulting psychological distortions and constrictions be accessed and healed. However, understanding that an upsurge of uncontrollable feeling and distorted thinking are the sine qua non of a therapy process powerful enough to be effective is a very different thing from encouraging licence in acting out these patterns.

When individuals who become intensely involved in an in-depth therapy project act out the impulses that are being stirred up, it can result in harm for the client, for other people in the client's life, and for the therapy process itself. For example, an individual who has defended against her severely damaged sense of self by working hard to build a career and a family life that is visibly successful will, sometime in the course of psychotherapy, most likely become flooded with the perception that everything she has worked so hard to build is a sham. She may, as well, experience intense resentment towards the responsibilities that have accrued from the course her life has taken.

I do not care about the business anymore. Why should I work so hard building it up for the sake of my employees and to keep up a lifestyle I no longer care about? If I had known what I know now I would probably never have had children, much less trained them to expect the level of care from me that they do now. Nobody ever cared for me. Why am I breaking my neck taking care of other people?

To some degree, this may represent a genuine rebellion against a pattern of engaging in inappropriate caretaking behaviour that has served as a way of covering up an individual's own needs for nurturance; to the extent that this is what it represents, change can be made in the way she conducts her life that will enhance it. However, it is very likely that at least some of what is being demanded is a regression to a state in which she does not have to behave like a responsible adult but wishes to be cared for like the child should have been whose cries are now resonating through her being. In this case, if she is to maintain her self-respect, she must continue to behave in ways that are socially responsible, even though this behaviour no longer serves the defensive function of covering up the pain of her unmet needs.

It is not easy for the client herself to distinguish between a genuine need to make healthy change and a defensive need to act out regressively. The therapist is responsible for maintaining as much clarity as possible in this area or a great deal of damage can be done very quickly. Careers can be destroyed and already fragile relationships with spouses, children, and other important people in the individual's life can be permanently wrecked if the therapist is not able to guide the powerful process of therapy constructively, so that it does not become yet another harmful experience in the individual's life.

Individuals suffering from multiple personality can express these impulses to disrupt their lives when they start to get in touch with the intensity of their deeper feelings in ways that make a difficult situation even more complex and confusing. The following would be a typical example of this:

I know we need to keep on working so that the mortgage can be paid. It's just that Damien keeps coming out and putting sand from the parking lot in the machine so that no one in the whole place can work. He thinks it's pretty funny to watch the boss trying to figure out what happened, but I worry that someone is going to get hurt one of these days.

It would be easy for a therapist to encourage a quick termination of employment under such circumstances or circumstances that are even more obviously dangerous. However, that solution could quite possibly set into motion a pattern of behaviour that would make it difficult for the person ever to return to the work world. If issues of entitlement, which need to be addressed therapeutically, are acted out and no responsibility is taken for the dynamic – 'We can't work, even though we want to earn our own way, because Damien keeps wrecking things' – both life and therapy can easily land on the rocks.

The key to creating a constructive process is engaging with all of the parts of the person who have any stake or interest in the situation to find ways in which the impulses can be expressed rather than acted out. The therapist must consistently communicate the message that is central to the development of maturity – that feelings can be extremely powerful, but they are still just that, feelings. Pain is just pain. Grief is just grief. Anger is just anger. Sexual feelings are just sexual feelings. When they are converted into action, however, they have many effects that must be responsibly considered. When a person is in the early stages, or even a difficult middle stage of an intense therapy process, it is wise to encourage her to be extremely conservative about acting on unclear impulses.

Basically, therapy is about building a relationship within which pre-empted developmental processes are revitalized. The configurations mobilized by the therapeutic process are not pathological, but rather developmental strivings that have been thwarted and arrested on a personal level in the individual's life and by the power of many other social forces as well. The therapist's consistent empathic attunement and acceptance of the client's feelings and needs reinstates processes that had been arrested, distorted, or aborted – at earlier stages of the client's life, certainly, but also last week – in personal encounters and through exposure to myriad cultural experiences that diminish an individual's robust connection to herself and to other people.

Depending on how deeply divided an individual is, the therapy process may evolve differently. Some people are able to communicate largely through the adult aspect of themselves – speaking for all parts of themselves to the therapist. Other people need to speak from their compartmentalized selves, and in these cases, each personality develops a relationship with the therapist. In these cases, the relationship with the therapist may become a point of reference for the personality states to communicate with each other. Complaints about favouritism, rivalry over the amount of time spent with the therapist in sessions, and problems with the behaviour of other personalities outside the sessions should be referred back to the self-system for consideration, and all points of view should be respected. Within this context, longings, pain, rage, and grief can be felt, expressed, heard, and understood in a way that is unique to the therapy situation. The appropriate response of the therapist to the expression of these feelings reactivates the development of a harmonious, resilient, and joyful sense of self that was arrested in the past.

The more deeply parts of the individual connect with the therapist, the more important it is for the therapist to remember that the client is one person and to facilitate communication among the various parts of the person. As the therapist does this, the individual aspects of the system or personalities will gradually transform. They will not be as stuck in rigid and repetitive patterns, and the early stages of a fluid, responsive self will begin to emerge.

The client becomes deeply attached to the therapist as this process unfolds. This is inevitable and entirely appropriate. Deep healing in therapy does not take place without deep attachment. How the therapist manages this attachment will determine whether the relationship evolves into a healthy bond that empowers the individual or one of unhealthy and regressive dependency. Early socialization to what therapy is and what it is not makes the former the more likely outcome.

The therapeutic relationship may well be one of the strongest and most transformative relationships a person ever has. It is also just therapy. By that I mean it is a relationship that is essentially disposable. When clients are encouraged to use their therapist as their main support person, creating all of their important connections with that person, it is very likely that the good that the connection effects will be undermined by the degree of dependency. This actual dependency on the support of the therapist outside the contracted therapy time not only discourages an individual from learning to build supportive relationships that are equal in nature, and therefore keeps her in a one-down position in terms of getting her needs met, it also eventually restricts the scope of the therapy process. If a client is desperately dependent on her therapist to answer daily telephone calls, she is not as free as she should be to acknowledge and work with her deeply felt rage at the therapist for not providing her with everything she needs, or if she feels free to rail at the therapist in calls that increase in length and frequency, a sado/masochistic relational dynamic will build between the two that will eventually make effective therapy impossible.

Emergency phone calls once in a while are part of many solid therapy relationships. Therapists cannot be their clients' support system, however, if they are to function effectively as their therapist. The client who is learning to maintain her own life and to build on it while developing a bond with her therapist in which she is affirmed, soothed, nurtured, and challenged is the client who is also developing her own capacities for self-affirmation, self-soothing, self-nurturing, and self-challenge.

This is the way a healthy parent/child relationship is supposed to evolve, as the child becomes the loving, capable, independent person her parents encourage her to be. It is also the path of healing for a person who started in therapy with an extremely depleted sense of self and substantially impaired capacities for self-care and self-fulfilment. It is a process that enables her to discard the defensive armouring built to protect the fragile self against the effects of serious emotional injury and to maintain a modicum of cohesiveness and functioning.

This framework for understanding the healing properties of the therapy process can be applied to a wide range of issues. Gonsiorek & Rudolph (1991) have applied self psychology concepts to gay and lesbian youth in relation to their coming to awareness about their sexuality. The sexuality of the heterosexual child may well be anticipated and responded to positively by the caring authority figures in the child's life. This is rarely the case, even for lesbian and gay children and adolescents whose parents are generally nurturing and accepting. A wound is, therefore, created that, even though it occurs later in life than the kind of injuries to the self that self psychology emphasizes, can be significantly painful and damaging. The lesbian or gay adolescent whose self-esteem has been chronically injured throughout childhood may well be less able to withstand the threats that accompany coming out as gay or lesbian. The stress – both social and psychological – with which these young people must grapple results in a greater likelihood of their developing serious problems, such as substance abuse and suicidality, than their heterosexual peers (Gonsiorek, 1991). Gay and lesbian youth who find adults and peers who serve an affirming function in their lives – accepting, admiring, supporting, and inspiring them – have the opportunity to heal the wounds created by the rejection of such an important aspect of themselves, or prevent such wounding altogether.

It is important to recognize that the type of relatively complete therapy process that is being described here is not the only treatment of value. For a wide variety of reasons, individual clients and client/therapist dyads never manage to work through all of the issues that need to be dealt with if the abuse survivor is to be able to have the happy, productive life she desires. Treatment that is not entirely successful and complete in this way can still be enormously helpful for the client. Demonstrable change for the better in specific areas of the client's functioning is the signpost of a therapy process that may not be perfect or complete but still must be considered a success in terms of meeting some of its goals.

Many clients structure their treatment in increments, both for practical reasons and because they cannot handle the intensity of the therapy process without taking significant breaks to replenish their strength and rekindle their motivation. The therapist must be open to allowing the client to pace her own treatment and set goals that are meaningful to her at a given time, rather than assuming that the therapist knows best, and, from that vantage point, attempting to persuade the client to complete a treatment process according to the therapist's norms of success.

Successful psychotherapy obviously has great advantages in repairing damage and enhancing capacity. Good therapy can have profound effects; it is, however, no panacea. A successful therapy process does not ensure a life without difficulties, pain, or contradictions. Many people who have freed themselves from the preoccupation with their struggles for basic survival and have come to embrace their own power move to a level of consciousness about personal, social, and political issues for which they did not previously have the energy. An ongoing and uncomfortable awareness of the inequities and injustices that are endemic to life within the confines of a capitalist patriarchal culture – as it plays itself out in the minutiae of everyday life as well as on a global scale – is one of the more common outcomes of a therapy process informed by a feminist analysis. This kind of therapy prescribes resistance rather than conformity to many prevailing social norms. It fosters openness to the reality that all living things are in a state of interdependence and none of us is free until we are all free. That sometimes opens individuals up to experiences of transpersonal anguish that are less likely to be personally disabling than the individual's previous suffering, but can be very uncomfortable nonetheless.

Therapy does not replace old discourses, full of cumbersome contradictions, with unproblematic ones. A successful healing process does not give women unlimited choices or free them from the necessity of engaging in the ongoing construction of their own subjectivity within the context of a culture that denies them. It does not spare women from feeling their own pain and the pain of those they love. Above all, therapy does not create of the world a sacred space in which all creatures live in a state of mutual respect and nurturance, a world in which the powerless are no longer exploited by the powerful. Therapy does not create justice.

But therapy can be a vehicle through which people whose capacity for justice-seeking was stunted and distorted can come to find their place in the struggle to create a different world from the one in which they were harmed as children. It can foster the growth of that personal still centre from which the individual can make whatever contribution generates most naturally and most passionately from the self she continues to create for the rest of her life.

6

Boundaries in Psychotherapy

There are two or three things I know for sure but never the same things and I'm never as sure as I'd like.

Dorothy Allison (1994)

All psychotherapy occurs within the framework of the therapeutic relationship. There are many aspects of the recovery process that can take place without involving ongoing personal interaction between a therapist and client, such as reading self-help books or attending twelve-step groups. There are probably recovery computer programs for all I know; if there are, there is no reason why they should not be helpful. None of these resources and activities, however, are psychotherapy.

The therapeutic relationship, the central vehicle through which therapy takes place, is a relationship like others in some ways and unique in other ways. It is a business relationship in that it involves a contract. The therapist provides services and usually gets paid for doing so, either by the client directly or by a third party. It is a nurturing relationship of unequal power, like the parent/child relationship. It is usually a relationship of positive affect, in which the participants appreciate each other, like a friendship. Yet, it is not strictly business; nor is it a friendship, or a parent/child relationship.

The idea that the relationship between psychotherapist and client has some special elements is hardly new. Freud (1912/1958) introduced the term 'transference' in 1912 to describe the phenomenon in which feelings from the client's formative relationships are felt with intensity toward the therapist, whether or not these feelings have much to do with the reality of the present-day therapy situation. It was Freud's belief that the ability to re-experience these emotions in the analytic context was one of the key features that made therapy instrumental in creating deep psychological change. The analytic concept of the therapist being a 'blank screen' upon which the client can project his or her own conflicts, feelings, and distortions is the basis upon which some strict analysts will not even answer questions like, 'Are you married?' 'How long have you been in practice?' and so on, except with the traditional, 'Why do you ask?'

The discipline involved in maintaining this posture of distance is immeasurably difficult. Freud himself did not consistently enact a strict psychoanalytic stance in his own practice. He helped certain patients financially, gave them gifts, and talked to them about the details of his family life. However, though it is difficult for even the most convinced and fully trained classical analyst to maintain the strict relational limits that early psychoanalysis demanded, the therapeutic model proposed by Freud, in which the analyst uncovers the secrets of the mind and cures the patient through rational interpretations, places the therapist in the position of the person who learns by virtue of her or his objectivity, a scientist uncovering facts. From this vantage point, these limits make theoretical sense. Relational closeness would equal contamination of the field in which this authoritative and curative rational understanding is sown. Such an analytic relationship would logically be characterized by abstinence and emotional distance on the part of the analyst.

Over the course of the growth and development of the psychoanalytic model, there has been a shift from the notion of the insight of the analyst as curative to an emphasis on the active engagement of two people in the project of a collaborative therapeutic relationship as the source of the healing. Jokes about the interminability of classical analysis – defined by Woody Allen as 'whining on the couch' – and its ineffectiveness are legion – 'I have been in analysis for fifteen years; I am going to give it another year and then I am going to Lourdes' (*Annie Hall*). Contemporary therapists are much more likely to believe that change is created by the therapeutic interaction rather than by the incorporation of insight discovered by the therapist and imparted to the client.

This radical change in perspective occurred within psychoanalysis as part of a paradigm shift taking place in the culture at large. Scientists, scholars, and artists in many disciplines were challenging the belief that rational thinking offers us singular, unmediated access to nature, to reality. From a contemporary point of view – very different from the scientific perspective of Freud's Victorian and Edwardian social context – knowledge is embedded in the context it surveys and is therefore pluralistic, constructed, and ever-changing. This makes a great deal of difference in how the therapeutic relationship is understood. Rather than the therapist uncovering, in an unambiguous fashion, the truth about the client's experience, the truth is created within the framework of the communication between client and therapist. This puts today's therapist in a very different position from the scientist/analyst of Freud's day.

By the 1960s in North America, the challenge to traditional therapy as represented by psychoanalysis was in full swing, and the classical psychoanalytic framework for understanding the therapy relationship, and all of the hierarchical structure that went with it, was challenged in almost every new therapy that grew up at this time.

The women's liberation movement has been one of the most fertile grounds for the growth of new therapy models. Leaderless consciousness-raising groups, settings in which women gathered to talk about their personal experience and to help each other understand these experiences politically, were the first structures within the most recent wave of feminism created to implement that basic feminist principle 'the personal is political.'

Consciousness-raising groups never replaced professional therapy as a resource for the many troubled women looking for psychological help, and gradually, throughout the 1980s, the energy and insights generated in these settings were channelled into the development of models of professional psychotherapy based on feminist principles. Some of the earliest (Wyckoff, 1980) challenged all the existing structures and practices of the medical model as it relates to women's mental health, and they operated outside the boundaries of mainstream mental health settings. Group therapy was the main and often only treatment modality offered, and an egalitarian therapeutic relationship between group facilitator and participants, with frequent self-disclosure on the part of the therapist, was prescribed. Based on the assumption that women's personal difficulties are a function, not of individual intrapsychic dynamics but of cultural expectations within a social context in which women hold a subordinate economic and social position, radical political activism on the part of the therapist was usually her key qualification and political activity on the part of the group members was encouraged as an important part of the solution to individual problems.

At the same time as the 'radical psychiatry' movement (Wyckoff, 1977) was promoting groups led by women whose training was in the area of feminist activism rather than clinical psychotherapy, there was also an emerging critical voice from within the mental health professions, decrying the sexist nature of most therapy processes and relationships. Psychological frameworks for understanding women were developed that took into consideration women's socialization within a patri-archal culture and focused on women's differences, strengths, and capacity for evolutionary change rather than promoting an adaptation to male standards of achievement and behaviour (Baker-Miller, 1976; Chodorow, 1978; Gilligan, 1982). Scepticism about diagnostic categories was pervasive, and women were encouraged to name their own experience. A self-defined feminist therapy literature tried to integrate some of the challenges of radical feminist therapy, the principles of liberal feminism with its emphasis on sex roles and their discriminatory ascription, and the new psychologies of women in order to offer an alternative model of therapy practice to feminists (Lerman, 1976; Carter & Rawlings, 1977; Sturdivant, 1980; Greenspan, 1983; Ballou & Gabalac, 1985; Rosewater & Walker, 1985).

When the limits of the therapy process were even considered within these frameworks, the emphasis tended to be on posing a radical challenge to the hierarchal model of traditional psychotherapy. Therapists were encouraged to create equal relationships between themselves and their clients, and notions like transference were frequently debunked as an unnecessary outgrowth of a patriarchal therapeutic structure.

There has been a lot of movement in the thinking about the issue of boundaries in therapy in the past ten years. Feminist therapists have been increasingly aware that some of the rebellion against traditional therapy structures in the name of egalitarian principles involved ignoring many of the complexities of power that are inherent to the therapy relationship in which, by definition, one individual is framed as the helper and the other as the one asking for and presumably needing help. It has become clear that a cavalier abandonment of concepts such as transference and therapeutic boundaries does not do away with the power differential in the therapeutic relationship. It simply places it out of sight, where it is less likely to be monitored and therefore more easily exploited.

The struggles among different racial, class, and cultural groups in the women's movement to gain recognition for both the specificity of their experience and its frequent erasure by white middle-class feminism has informed the contemporary feminist therapy movement. Power issues are less frequently ignored by feminist therapists today than they were in the early feminist therapy movement.

In fact, there has been a complete reversal in the ideology of some of the earlier practitioners who labelled themselves 'feminist therapists.' Hogie Wyckoff's guidelines for leader self-disclosure in facilitating group therapy – 'I struggle with the members of my groups the same way in which I struggle with friends or lovers' (Wyckoff, 1980) – would be endorsed by only a small minority of contemporary feminist therapists. On the contrary, it is now common for feminist therapists to create very strict guidelines differentiating the relationship between client and therapist that is not strictly therapeutic. Laura Brown (1994) introduces such guidelines into her relationship with her clients in the initial session and asks them to sign a contract that states explicitly what will be expected of both client and therapist. One of the expectations is that the relationship will be strictly a professional and therapeutic one and that it will not evolve into any other kind of relationship, even after the termination of the psychotherapy.

These strict definitions about the limits of the therapy relationship are a reaction to the thousands of abuses of power that have been perpetrated by so-called helping professionals that have come to light in the past decade (Bouhoutous et al., 1983; Gartrell et al., 1986; Pope & Bouhoutous, 1986; Herman et al., 1987). Sexual exploitation has become the focus of the most concern as both the popular press and research studies report high levels of sexual abuse of children and adults in relationships of trust – abuse by parents, teachers, clergy, coaches, physicians, and many other authority figures, including psychotherapists.

The response to this increasing awareness that many vulnerable individuals are being exploited in the very places where they seek help and sanctuary has tended to run to extremes. The False Memory Syndrome Foundation, focusing on adult children's allegations of sexual abuse by caretakers, particularly fathers, during childhood, denies the scope of the problem. Its members point to aggressive therapeutic techniques as responsible for what they claim are the 'false memories' of thousands of women that they were subjected to sexual assault in childhood. The media have been quick to pick up on stories about loving parents being tormented by their children, who, under the influence of ambitious and self-serving therapists, are destroying devoted families with inexplicable accusations. Some people, including mental health professionals, have embraced this perspective with relief.

In general, however, the widespread reporting of sexual abuse in all relationships of authority has become a fact of life, and the recognition that the exploitation of vulnerable individuals is a very real aspect of a substantial minority of these relationships has become a serious and abiding concern for most responsible professionals. The recognition that such abuses of power are not only endemic in family relationships but in all relationships in which there is an imbalance of power, including psychotherapy relationships, has been one of the factors that has most powerfully influenced some mental health practitioners to address the issue of the power imbalance in the therapeutic relationship, emphasizing the interpersonal guidelines that make therapy relationships different from others, such as friendship or sexual relationships. One of the core questions raised as part of this challenge concerns the limits of the psythotherapy process. If therapists are not archaeologists digging for transparent truth, if they are not friends, parents, or lovers, then what are they? What is therapy, and what is it not?

This is what the notion of boundaries is all about. Boundaries are one of the most important building materials for structuring the therapy, for creating a framework that distinguishes the therapy relationship from all of the other relationships in which people participate. The boundaries of any relationship are an essential part of what makes the relationship function effectively in terms of its own goals.

It is interesting that the word 'boundary' as it relates to the therapeutic relationship has now come to have one particular connotation – it almost always refers to a limit, a delineation of appropriate barriers or walls between the therapist and client that enable the therapist to fulfil her fiduciary duty to the client without exploiting the therapeutic relationship to meet her needs at the client's expense. In fact, the concept of boundaries in the clinical context is much broader and more subtle than we would be led to believe by this common conflation of the word 'boundaries' with appropriate limits (or, as in 'boundary violation' or 'boundary crossing,' clinical or ethical misconduct relating to inappropriately tearing down limits in a way that is harmful to the client).

The therapeutic relationship is as much about walls that are let down in ways that are idiosyncratic to the clinical context as it is about walls created around the treatment relationship defining its framework. Empathy, or vicarious introspection, is basic to both the process of data collection – how we know what we know – in the in-depth therapy encounter and to its healing effect. We are capable of creating an empathic connection with another person only to the degree that we can allow ourselves to loosen the boundaries that distinguish one individual from another.

Frequently, people tell me things in my meetings with them that they have not only never told anyone else, but also never consciously decided to tell me. I often ask people questions in a therapy session that I would never think of broaching in a social or business setting. This does not occur because I am more brash in a therapeutic communication than I usually am; on the contrary, I am much more aware of and respectful of people's sensitivities when I am relating to them as therapist than I tend to be in other social, professional, or personal situations. This erosion of the limits on what people consider appropriate or safe to talk about takes place because the empathic connection that develops – sometimes slowly, other times almost immediately – between client and therapist is constructed by the process of the dissolution of certain of the interpersonal barriers widely experienced as necessary in other social settings.

As therapist, I sometimes feel my client's feelings transiently as if they were my own and thus am able to understand what my client is feeling, even when she has little awareness of those feelings herself. This temporary release of my affective field for use by the client makes it possible for me to take a stance of sustained empathic enquiry in a fashion that is experienced, in balance, as more nurturing than threatening.

I consciously (and also not so consciously) allow myself to be open to my clients in a way that I am usually not in other social or business relationships. This is not the kind of openness that results in self-disclosure for the satisfaction of my own needs; it is an openness that I deliberately structure for use as a vehicle for therapeutic intervention. It is the vulnerability of the therapeutic relationship in this particular way – in which the usual barriers to interpersonal communication are regularly dissolved – that makes it so important that proper therapeutic boundaries (in the current use of the word) be responsibly constructed as a basic part of creating a safe healing space for the client.

Boundaries are not context-free rules; in fact, they do not exist at all outside their context. Boundaries have as much to do with attitudes as with actions. I do not see myself as a scientist who has to stay out of the affective field of my relationship with my clients in order to maintain some kind of pure objectivity. I do, however, see myself as needing a type of clarity with my clients that I do not pretend to be able to maintain consistently with other people in my life, to whom I look to get my personal needs met – colleagues, friends, family, and intimates. The central difference between a therapeutic relationship and other relationships between adults is that the contract between therapist and client explicitly or implicitly states that the central purpose of the relationship is directed toward the needs of the client.

This does not mean that it is not a relationship, that is, that the therapist does not engage with personal feeling or that some of the therapist's needs are not met. The expression of the therapist's feelings and the meeting of the therapist's needs, however, are not the purpose of the relationship. When the expression of feeling on the part of the therapist enhances the client's participation in her own healing process, then that communication is appropriate and constructive within the context of the therapy project.

When I offer an empathic response, for example, to my perception of a client's pain, and she snaps back a hostile rejoinder, it may well be (it also may not be) that I experience a personal affective response. If I am engaging in the therapy along the line of its basic contract – that the therapy be structured to facilitate her healing process rather than being a relationship that provides nurturance and healing for both of us – what I do with that response depends on the needs of the client. One client in one moment may be best served by my quiet presence, and she may experience any comment on her reaction as judgmental and emotionally assaultive, or as a cry on my part for her to stop expressing herself in particular ways so as to take care of my emotional needs for affirmation. Another individual – or the same individual in another moment – may find it facilitative of her self-awareness and respectful of her desire to communicate with me and with others in an open way, to know that I experienced her reaction as harsh and dismissive.

I do not choose my response by how likely I think it is that an individual will accept a confrontation compliantly or gratefully. A desperately eager agreement may be a sign of an interaction that has hindered growth, and some people feel obliged to rebel furiously against input to cover over the vulnerability they feel while processing it. There is no set of rules that enables the therapist to figure out – quickly and certainly – how to choose from a range of possible responses. It is up to individual therapists to formulate their own decisions, and to engage continuously in the personal struggle to be clear about the effects of their actions in each particular situation with each individual with whom they work.

The issue of therapist self-disclosure – whether telling stories about one's life to illustrate or amplify relevant issues, or letting the client know how she is affecting her therapist, or protecting the privacy of my personal life – is emblematic of the process of creating therapeutic boundaries in general. The boundaries I set in any given therapy situation are ones that enable me to develop a clarity of communication with a particular client that facilitates her healing process.

I do not perceive my clients as needing to be completely and utterly unaware of who I am as an individual in order to be able to project freely and fully onto me within the therapeutic context. In fact, I have a public persona that is not particularly impersonal. I teach in a lot of places and have been known to illustrate theoretical or clinical points through anecdotes about my background, my experiences of childrearing or of being a child, egregious clinical mistakes I have made, and other revelations that I think might enhance the learning process of my students. One of my children attends a nursery school that is located on the grounds of the hospital in which I work, and day hospital patients sometimes pick up their children at the same time as I pick up mine. Members of my family have accompanied me to hospital functions that are attended by patients as well as staff. As well, some of clients – through their own personal or professional sources – know a great deal about me before I meet them, even if we have had no direct connection with one another.

I know how much it meant to me when I discovered that my graduate school adviser, Jeri Wine, was a lesbian who did not feel the need to hide her sexual orientation to be professionally successful, and I am open about being a lesbian whenever it seems to be appropriate and relevant. My sexuality is not a personal issue that I feel the need to be circumspect about. I am no more private about the fact that my partner is a woman and that we raise children together than most heterosexual therapists are about their family circumstances. I have family pictures in my office; I occasionally have had to change appointments because of childcare foul-ups. I do not think that my stance is unusual. Except for those who are rigidly analytic in their training and their stance, it seems to me that most therapists are not completely guarded about the basic circumstances of their lives, although there can be grounds to take that position with some clients or in certain settings.

Most clients are not particularly interested in the details of my life when they come to my office to talk about their problems, and, in the majority of cases, the issue does not come up. If it does, however, I am as comfortable telling clients that I am a lesbian as I would be – in fact, was, at one time – telling them I was married. Now – as then – there might also be times when, rather than answering a question with the information requested, I would say, 'Why does that interest you at this moment?' Such a decision not to answer personal questions would reflect my clinical judgment about the response that would advance the individual's healing process, rather than my politics or my personal need for openness or for privacy.

This professional stance of relative openness about my life has consequences – just as the practice of utter separation and privacy would have – both for me and for my clients. Effectively managed, it does not need to present a problem to creating and maintaining clear and clean therapeutic relationships.

I do think, however, it is much more difficult for an effective therapy process to take place with people with whom I already have another role, or if I develop roles and relationships other than the therapeutic one with clients in ongoing therapy. This is a basic therapeutic boundary that works for me – the prohibition against dual relationships. Even this rule, which I think of as basic to my current therapy practice, is enforced to different degrees with different clients, depending on my perception of their needs and our relationship.

If I am engaged to give a training seminar to a large group of employees at a client's workplace, do I ask my client to absent herself, or do I refuse the invitation because I have a client who works there? Maybe I do the one, maybe the other, and maybe I decide that there would be little harm in acting as my client's teacher for one day. Again, it depends on my perception of my client's needs and her perception of her needs. In any case, my decision is based on my value that her treatment comes first, so if I do think there is a significant chance that this transitory dual relationship would undermine her therapy process, and my client could not absent herself without adverse consequences for her, even if it is clear that the organization needs this training and I am the best person to offer it, I act accordingly and decline to teach in that situation.

Acting in the role of therapist for a significant other (partner, sister, good friend) of a current client is also a dual relationship, although we do not tend to think of it that way. I have a relationship with my partner's therapist and she with me, even though I have only met her once when we bumped into each other at a bank machine and were introduced by my partner. I have an impression of her and she of me, I am sure – all mediated through my partner. And that is how it should be; that is how it is with the partners (or siblings, friends, parents, and so on) of most of my clients. I often find myself saying to clients, 'My reflections about this relationship (about this person) are a result of what you tell me. I do not have any independent knowledge about it outside of what you communicate to me.' My ability to say this can make all the difference in facilitating my client's ability to listen less defensively to interpretations that may be threatening to her.

It has been my practice for a long time not to accept into my practice partners, close friends, or relatives of current clients, and sometimes even former clients. This has been one of the luxuries of practising in a large urban area, and I do not think that it can or should translate into a rule with universal application. However, having said that, my recent experience of practising in a small town in a rural area with few mental health services has made me even more aware of the potential for serious and sometimes insurmountable problems that can arise in attempting to engage in an in-depth therapy process with two or more individuals who are intimately or closely involved with each other.

The therapeutic relationship is an intensely personal experience, and a client needs a great deal of room to be able to feel the array of responses to the therapist without outside influences that threaten her sense of security in the relationship. 'My therapist thinks that I should start standing up for myself when we fight and not always let you get your own way,' is the kind of occasional strategy to which most therapy clients, even those who try not to do so, resort under pressure. An upsurge of anger at the therapist brought into the relationship in this way is inevitable, and this is not usually a big deal.

However, the effect can be quite different if the therapist so referenced is the therapist of the partner as well. No matter how rational a client tries to be, no matter how many times she says to herself, 'I am only hearing my partner's (or sister's or mother's) point of view,' it will be a hurtful experience. It will ripple into many areas of the individual's consciousness and may well do significant damage to the therapeutic relationship.

Even communications that are not adversarial – a client talks enthusiastically about how much her therapist recognizes her strengths in a particular area, for example, and how affirming that is – can be extremely unsettling. They can have unintended meaning for an individual who may be struggling that week – or even that year, or throughout her entire therapy process – with her own insecurity about whether her therapist thinks well of her, or for an individual who may need to project her sense of worthlessness onto her therapist and truly believe for a while that her therapist does not appreciate her strengths, in order to wrestle with her own damaged self-esteem. A client engaged in this aspect of her therapy process may need to hear nothing about how her therapist appreciates anyone but her.

Sometimes it proves very helpful to see a client's partner or children – anyone with whom the client wishes assistance in communicating – in an occasional joint session, but the effects of doing so on the primary therapy relationship should be considered by the therapist – and discussed with the client – before assuming that such an intervention will be helpful. Even if marital or family counselling is clearly indicated in a particular situation, the couple can engage a professional who is not the primary therapist of either of them, and there are times when this is the appropriate route to take. There are some people who are not adversely affected by having couple or family sessions with their personal therapist and, in fact, such sessions enrich their personal therapy process as well as dealing with issues directly related to their intimate or parental relationships. But there are also people who, in such a situation, would feel impossibly divided, jealous, intimidated, invaded – or a variety of other reactions that could undermine the primary therapy relationship, as well as make it difficult to focus effectively on the relevant relationship or family issues.

Individuals who are severely dissociated may initially be able to divide their perceptions into separate mental compartments in a way that enables them to say honestly, 'It does not bother me to talk about therapy with my partner; it feels fine that she is seeing you too. In fact, I am glad she is seeing someone I know is competent.' However, as an increasingly integrated consciousness develops, hurts and misunderstandings often emerge full-blown and well-established, and issues that might possibly have been resolved had they been dealt with immediately can become intractable.

Just as it is not possible to enact an absolutist stance about some other dual relationship prohibitions, it is sometimes impossible to avoid seeing people who are significantly connected with each other. In fact, sometimes therapists will not even be aware that they are doing so until both treatments have progressed beyond the point where the therapist and/or the clients feel able to terminate either. There may be no easy answers that enable a therapist to avoid these situations under all circumstances. It is still important to know that – awareness of the potential pitfalls and good intentions on the part of everyone involved nonwithstanding – in-depth psychodynamic therapy relationships can become impossibly compromised when a therapist is treating two or more clients who are engaged in significant relationships with each other.

Carrying principles about dual relationships to an extreme makes it clear why discretion is always involved when following general rules. If I discovered, for example, that I frequented the same bank as a client in the small town I practise in, what would I do? Although this could only be construed as a dual relationship by the most stringent of standards, there might be situations in which I would take my business elsewhere. If my client was closely related to the bank manager, for instance, and she showed up a few times to pick him up for a lunch date and waited outside the manager's office (which, in my bank, is none too private) while I was doing personal business, and I also found myself in frequent contact with her and her children while I was waiting on line for a teller, I might feel enough of a sense of boundary violation that I would switch banks. In a large city, this would not present much of a problem. In a small town, services being limited, I would consider the question much longer, and my tolerance for some degree of boundary blurring would be greater. In an isolated rural area or village, I may well have no choice but to both think about and handle the question of boundaries and privacy differently.

I find it helpful in my practice to create fairly rigid guidelines about dual relationships with clients in therapy with me, but this does not absolve me from the necessity of considering every situation on its own merits. I would have no trouble declining a client's offer to type for me in any situation I can think of, but would I automatically refuse to go to an art exhibit to view a client's paintings? It would depend on the situation whether I would see that as an extension of my mandate as therapist or as a boundary violation.

I am the co-director of a personality disorders service in a psychiatric hospital. I am not the primary therapist of the patients on the inpatient unit or involved in the day hospital program, but I do see many of them, for a while, in private sessions, as well as in a group therapy context, as part of their participation in the hospital programs. My role with these clients is – in some ways – more multileveled and complicated than my role with my private clients, whom I serve as primary therapist, often for half a dozen years. The intensity of our relationship is also titrated by our mutual group participation and the reality that several other program staff serve a therapeutic function for them as well.

Each therapeutic context and each relationship presents different challenges. Because each client and each therapist is unique in both strengths and vulnerabilities, and because each therapeutic relationship and the context in which it takes place is unique, somewhat different limits work well in different therapeutic relationships and in different contexts. The purpose of the creation of the boundaries, however, is always the same – to facilitate the therapy process and both the therapist's and the client's effective participation in it.

The degree of attachment and dependency that often accompanies an in-depth therapy process can be both the driving force behind the healing process and its downfall. Boundaries – that address the issue of what can be expected from the therapy and the therapist and what cannot – are central to a stable therapy that does not overwhelm either client or therapist.

When I have my initial interview with a prospective client – or even someone who is inquiring about therapy by phone – I make it clear that the type of therapy I offer is only appropriate for people who can build their own support systems. I do not guarantee that I will answer calls right away, and I do not provide an ongoing support service by telephone. There are a number of reasons for this. One has to do with my needs, resources, and availability. I travel all over the province of Ontario in the course of a week. I travel to other places in Canada and the United States one week out of every month, sometimes more. I am simply not in a position, literally, to provide the consistent backup that people who are going through an intense and sometimes destabilizing treatment need.

However, my schedule is only part of the picture. I used to extend myself a lot further for clients in crisis than I do now, and my experience has been that, whereas the sense of being cared for that can be generated by a therapist putting herself out in extraordinary ways for a client can be a powerful therapeutic motivator, in balance, the disadvantages for the client, in terms of regressive dependency, outweigh the advantages.

Creating a context in which I can be fresh and enthusiastic about my work is part of my responsibility to both my clients and to myself. I am at a point in my life when I would burn out very quickly if I did not have considerable time in which to focus on other professional endeavours than the facilitation of the therapy process of my clients in individual psychotherapy.

At this point, I consider it part of the task of socializing people to the process of therapy to help them learn how to construct their own support systems. I make it clear that I am in no position to give them all the help they will need, and I encourage them to use the sessions to talk about their struggles and successes in building friendships, and sometimes other professional relationships, and in finding creative ways of using these resources to keep them on track between therapy sessions.

I try to teach clients who may not have done this before to manage their peer relationships so that they are as equal as possible, rather than structuring them strictly around their own needs. This can be difficult for people when they are acutely anxious and disturbed. The struggle to offer time, energy, and attention to people who have been generous with them, however, tends to give these relationships a multidimensional quality that makes them satisfying to both parties in a healthy manner and therefore more likely to outlast the crises in the client's life. This ongoing effort to develop reciprocal relationships easily repays the work involved – in enhanced self-respect, in a sense of being able to get one's own needs met without compromising one's integrity, and in a sense of balance to the therapeutic relationship.

Engaging in a healing process within the context of a web of supportive relationships also increases the likelihood that the therapeutic relationship can be fully mobilized in the service of the tasks of therapy, rather than being a catch-all. If most of a person's important emotional needs are being met in the therapy – or if both therapist and client are colluding in the illusion that this can happen – some of the most important tasks of treatment will be difficult to accomplish. The therapeutic relationship, if it is to be the powerful vehicle for change for which it has the potential, must be the container for all of the longings, rage, disappointment, grief – all of those emotions that got dampened, distorted, or derailed in some way at an earlier point in the client's life.

If clients get in the habit of needing to hear their therapist's voice on the telephone each day to remain basically stabilized, come to experience themselves as being in serious danger of death if they cannot talk directly to their therapist each time they feel suicidal, or come to rely on their therapist for up-to-the-minute advice about all the daily decisions of life, there is little room for dealing with these issues in their intensity or working them through maturely. Only two choices will emerge, and neither will lead to the completion of an effective healing process. The client can suppress a great deal of the material key to healing in order to maintain a level of compliance that makes the day-to-day enactment of the neediness and the caretaking demanded bearable for the therapist. She also has the choice to act out her powerful feelings over and over again as part of negotiating ever-expanding access to the therapist, which will inevitably never be satisfied. Such a relationship will eventually make any therapist feel overwhelmed and abused, and it will eventually make any client feel undernurtured and abused.

A consistent attitude that says, 'I care about you too much to damage your self-respect by treating you in your relationship with me as less of an adult than you are – no matter how galling it may be to the client at times – is the basic boundary of the therapeutic relationship, and it eventually comes to be appreciated and counted on. Deep and pervading feelings of childlike dependency or tantrumous rage will still be felt and expressed. The impossible demands and the rageful disappointments that follow will be contained, however, to be explored in the therapy sessions and eventually resolved rather than leaked out in extra-therapy interactions. That is the challenge of the adult psychotherapy participant, to take those infantile feelings and transform their energy into the fuel for running a productive present-day life, rather than acting them out to the detriment of present-day relationships and responsibilities.

This is not something that most clients know how to do when they enter therapy. If they did, they would be able to manage their own treatment. Unless the therapy is short-term and fairly superficial, clients will come up against the key personal defenses that protect them from mental and emotional material that had to be kept under some control if they were to develop a cohesive sense of self and some ability to care for themselves practically in the midst of chaotic experience. Those defenses combine suppression and expression in a style unique to each individual, and it is an important element of the effectiveness of the defense system that its operations remain, in a large measure, out of the individual's conscious awareness. Therapy has to be structured in such a way that it has the capacity both to contain and to work with these feelings, and the balancing of the containing and the expressing aspects of the process is the art of pacing. The process of therapy must loosen the defense structure enough to allow for change, and do it slowly and gradually enough to allow the client to maintain basic stability.

Boundaries, as the word implies, are an element of this structuring process. Since each individual client's set of defenses – and each therapist's for that matter – is different, the structure that will work well for each client/therapist dyad will be different. Therapists should not create therapeutic boundaries in order to exercise control over their clients. We do so because, without boundaries, neither the therapist nor the client would be able to bear this long-term and often grueling enterprise.

Judith Herman (1992) quotes Patricia Ziegler, an experienced therapist who declares, 'Patients have to agree not to drive me crazy ... I tell them they owe me the respect not to scare the daylights out of me.' This is a boundary that make some sense, but it does not create clear-cut rules and regulations. What drives me crazy and scares the daylights out of me may be very different from what will disturb another therapist, or even me in another context. For example, if I were working in the context of an inpatient hospital program, an individual's hurling herself headfirst against the cement wall of the unit would not drive me crazy or scare the daylights out of me. I would expect that level of self-destructiveness occasionally from hospital inpatients, and the facility will presumably have the resources to contain the individual's explosive actions until she can find another way to express herself without doing serious damage to her body.

If, however, a client periodically uses my waiting room or treatment room as a venue for physical self-harm, that behaviour would scare the daylights out of me and drive me crazy. Because I do not have the resources to contain the damage that such behaviours can create – both to the individual perpetrating them and to other clients in the setting – I would question seriously whether an individual who engaged in self-injurious actions in my waiting room was an appropriate client for my outpatient therapy practice.

I therefore create a boundary that declares that clients are not allowed to injure themselves on the premises of my office. This does not mean I can control my clients' actions, or even that I think that they can necessarily control their own actions. What it does mean is that the consequence of their behaviour – if together we cannot find a way to get it under control – is that I may be unable to continue to provide therapeutic services to them in my outpatient practice.

The particular boundary of calls between sessions is an issue that seems to come up frequently in the therapy process of highly dissociative trauma survivors. I have not found it necessary so far to create hard and fast rules about phone calls between sessions. Most of my clients understand – from the way in which we talk about constructing support systems to meet their needs between sessions and their responsibility for their own safety – that I am not able or willing to be a crisis line. It is very seldom anymore that a client calls me for anything except making instrumental changes in appointment times. The occasional emergency call I do get is usually brief and appropriate.

However, if the stimulation of the therapy process proves to be too much for a particular individual, and she becomes overwhelmed with her needs or her anger in such a way that – rather than building and relying on a supportive network to maintain her stability – she cannot resist calling me frequently between sessions, then for both her sake and mine, I am likely to construct particular limits on her therapy process like, 'No phone calls except to make or change session times.' Though that may initially seem harsh and be interpreted as a lack of caring involvement, I have found that it creates a structure in which the sessions are valued and used productively. The individual is not constantly tempted to undermine her life by creating crises so that she can access direct contact with me.

Since I am clear about the way I work before I agree to initiate a treatment process with someone, my clients may not like this kind of limit, but they do not leave therapy in a state of outraged abandonment. If they truly decide that they need a therapist who will offer freer access between sessions, then I am completely supportive of their need to transfer to a professional who works differently from me.

Boundaries that would be appropriately firm in one situation would be abusively rigid in another. Limits that empower under certain circumstances stifle under others, and the boundaries that I create in a therapy process depend on both my needs and the needs of each client I see. This is true of one-shot assessment sessions as well as long-term therapy.

I make it clear, while contracting to do most assessments, that they are not a prelude for accepting clients into my practice. This is not an issue that is non-negotiable and unethical in itself, like some others (for example, no sexual contact with clients, the most obvious non-negotiable limit). However, in the vast majority of cases, my role as assessor and consultant to the primary therapist would be undermined by an awareness on the part of the client and the therapist that once they connect with me, supposedly for the purpose of assessment and consultation, there is a good chance that the client could be transferred. Under the guise of working on enhancing the ongoing therapy situation, they would be working at issues of termination.

That is a general policy. In each assessment, I institute other limits that are idiosyncratic to its particular circumstances. For example, one woman was referred to me for assessment because of ongoing difficulties in her relationship with her primary therapist. The therapist had both the qualifications and the experience to determine her client's degree of dissociation; she was just having a hard time managing the therapy process.

I attempted to establish some communication about this client's relationship with her therapist and her view of how her therapy was progressing. Each time I opened the subject, the client would begin to tell me about the details of her abusive childhood. I finally declared that, although I understood that the way she was hurt as a child was an extremely important issue, in this session, with the limitations on time and its particular focus, abuses from childhood were not an appropriate topic. I knew I was on the right track when she looked at me with unbelieving eyes and said, 'You mean you don't want to know about how my father killed my puppy?'

When I said that, indeed, that is what I meant, she muttered sullenly that she was being abused in her therapy too; was she allowed to talk about that? When I agreed that that would be fine, she went on to say that her doctor had promised her that she would be fully supportive if she decided to work with her, and to begin with she had seemed wonderfully present and nurturing. But now, she seemed to be changing – withdrawing from her just like everyone else. She had been seeing her every weekday, and the doctor had always accepted her emergency telephone calls in the evenings and on weekends. Recently, however, the doctor had said that she could only see her three times a week and would accept only five telephone calls each week outside of office hours. The client went on to say that she could not possibly open herself up if she were not supported more fully, and that she thought that her doctor was behaving unethically by withdrawing in this way and reneging on her promise. After she had spoken vehemently about this for some time, I asked her if she wanted to know what I thought, since she and her therapist had both requested this consultation. She nodded, and I said that, if her therapy were to have a good chance of success, I thought that three times a week was quite likely too often for her to be seen on a regular basis and that she should immediately start learning to use the local crisis services constructively, so that she would not have to call her doctor at all after office hours. She heard me loud and clear. She glared at me and said, 'Don't you dare tell *her* that.' I replied that my written agreement, signed by her, directed me to see her and then offer an opinion to her doctor as to the results of the assessment. She got out of her chair, towered over me and said, 'Well I have changed my mind. If you say one word to her, I will see you in court.'

I have never before or since told anyone presenting for assessment that the rule of the session was no talking about childhood abuse. Usually people do not want to do so anyway, and when they do, it is relevant to the assessment process. In this case, my setting down what on the surface seemed like an odd guideline immediately opened up the core of the issue that needed to be looked at for the assessment to be useful – the distortions in this client's sense of entitlement and the counterproductive compliance of her therapist that were engulfing the therapy. Once she was unable to deflect from this main theme into the atrocities of her childhood (the details of which presumably would distract me as well as her), she could not avoid talking about what was really upsetting her in the present.

This was not a pleasant session, but it accomplished its goal – to assess what was the problem in the therapy. This is the way limits should work – making it possible for the therapy to do what it is supposed to do. The requirement that the therapist be both consistent and flexible – and, above all, creative in understanding what particular limits mean for individuals – can make the ongoing process of setting, negotiating, re-setting, and re-negotiating boundaries one of the most challenging aspects of the art of psychotherapy.

Difficulties in dealing with boundary issues are one of the most frequent reasons therapists request consultation. Therapists who are new at offering treatment to individuals with dissociative conditions can find themselves floundering in deep water without a life-jacket if they 'go by the gut' or 'fly by the seat of their pants' and then find themselves engaging in practices with this group of people that they would never think of doing with other clients. The need for creativity and flexibility can be greater in the treatment of highly dissociative clients, but the need for a therapy based on sound theoretical principles and accurate assessment of what is going on is commensurably as great.

When in doubt, therapists should delay doing things they feel pressured to do but uneasy about and run – not walk – to a consultation with a trusted colleague with more experience in the area of the treatment of dissociative conditions. By catching countertherapeutic dynamics before they become entrenched, timely and helpful consultation can save a great deal of headache and heartache for both client and therapist.

Appropriate boundaries are the building blocks of an effective psychotherapy treatment, and the evolution of a set of guidelines that creates a helpful container for the powerful feelings evoked over the course of the therapy process is an ongoing matter. Judith Herman (1992) quotes a client as defining boundaries in this way: 'What my psychiatrist calls rules and I call moving targets.'

In the past thirty years, the professional community of clinical psychotherapists has moved from the position that professional distance is the hallmark of the therapeutic relationship, to the breaking down of that distance and of many of the professional conventions that went with it, to a return to a reliance on strict rules to make therapy safe and workable. Much of this movement is an historically inevitable and generally useful dialectical challenge. Sometimes, however, as the wheel turns, one place it stops looks much the same as the previous one.

I see some of the more rigid positions about the boundaries of the therapeutic relationship as no more useful than the previous 'if it seems to work, do it; anything goes' framework, and almost as likely to cover up rather than illuminate abuses of power in the therapy relationship. One example of this type of rigidity is a guideline that is increasingly commonly proclaimed in codes of ethics: 'once a therapist, always a therapist.'

Frankly, that seems like nonsense to me. I understand that in many cases – maybe even in the majority of cases – in which individuals engage in a long-term, in-depth therapy process, the emotional reality of the situation will be 'once a therapist, always a therapist.' To a substantial degree at any rate – enough to make the evolution of a friendship or a business or collegial relationship or sexual partnership complicated and inadvisable and, indeed, unethical under some circumstances – many clients continue to experience themselves in a one-down power position vis-à-vis their former therapists. Some clients also want and need to keep open the possibility of returning to therapy with the same therapist after termination. For that to be a reasonable expectation, the boundaries of the therapeutic relationship must remain intact.

Creating a hard and fast rule that forbids any such relationships once the therapy contract is terminated, however, belies the wide variety of therapeutic relationships and limits the evolution of relationships in ways that might well be perfectly healthy and ethical in particular situations. Even, in my opinion, offering a specific time limit, like 'no friendships, business, or sex with ex-clients until two years after termination' – although it offers the advantage of encouraging professionals to consider the complexities of ongoing post-termination relationships with ex-clients and avoid acting impulsively – is a compromise that solves neither aspect of the problem. If it is indeed impossible to create an extra-therapy relationship with certain clients that is as equal as any relationship can be in a patriarchal society, then it is not going to be a whole lot more likely that all of the factors that made it a relationship of significant power imbalance will fade away in the course of two years of non-contact.

Carter Heyward's (1993) book, *When Boundaries Betray Us*, looks at this issue from the point of view of a client who was a confident professional who had been in therapy a number of times before and who brought her troubles with exhaustion and burn-out to a feminist psychiatrist. It is a first-person account by the author, a lesbian feminist Episcopal priest and theologian, of her experience of being profoundly affected by a therapy process that initially excited and empowered her, but eventually shattered her.

I read this account as text. It is a story created by the author, the client in the situation she describes and analyses. The author not only creates her own character, she also creates the character of the therapist. When commenting on the therapeutic dynamic, I am commenting on the dynamic as described in the book, in no way assuming some sort of transparent reality that stands outside the text itself. I am offering a reading of the story of the therapy relationship, not commenting on the way a particular therapist (whose identity I do not know) conducts her practice. I do not offer this caveat because I have any concerns about the veridicality of this particular account. It is my belief that this is the only responsible way to approach any piece of writing.

When Boundaries Betray Us draws a compelling picture of a serious empathic failure on the part of a therapist who used her professional power, including the power to play with the limits of the therapeutic relationship, to cover over a profound countertransference that eventually destroyed the therapy and left the client in a state of emotion devastation.

The relationship between the client and the therapist had many difficulties, as I read it. It was a relationship between a bright and engaging therapist who very quickly developed a raft of non-therapeutic feelings towards her bright and engaging client, didn't recognize this, and didn't take appropriate action. My reading of the client's increasingly insistent request that she and the therapist become friends after the therapy ended was that this was the only way the client could name the reality that what was going on between them was not a clear and clean therapeutic relationship structured to meet the needs of the client, but something much more like a friendship with an erotic element.

The therapist in this account did not meet her basic responsibility to create an ambience of accurate empathy. As noted previously, empathy is vicarious introspection, what Freud called *einfuehlung* (to feel oneself into another), to open oneself up such that the emotional experience of the other can resonate within us and then to pay attention to that experience as a source of awareness about the other.

The therapy described in *When Boundaries Betray Us* is a painful story of a 'promise of empathy' and a 'failure of empathy' (Lewinberg, 1994). The therapeutic relationship began with excitement on both sides. The therapist and client sat on the floor of the office with a candle between them, and they discussed issues of interest to them both – women's spirituality, for example, and the oppression of women, lesbians, and gays within the institutional church. The client opened up. She felt accepted and understood, and she became vulnerable to the therapist in a way she probably would not have become open to the same person had she not been her therapist. The therapist also enjoyed the sessions, until the client began to question the context.

The account then becomes a story of rampant, unprocessed countertransference. The client was opened up by the ambience of empathic resonance originally created by the therapist, and that openness was used against her when the therapist's fears and needs began to get in the way, and the therapist could, consequently, no longer maintain a stance of sustained empathic inquiry. The therapist alternated between being cold and distant and angry and hurtful, in response to the client's questions about why the two of them could not be friends after therapy. Sometimes the therapist said no; sometimes she said maybe, she was giving it serious consideration. Always the therapist appeared in the account to be talking about her own needs and feelings, without any acknowledgment of this.

I do not say this because that is the analysis offered in the book; it isn't actually. The clarity in the book vis-à-vis the therapeutic relationship derives from the descriptions of concrete incidents, vignettes, and snatches of dialogue. Sometimes when the author is theorizing as client about her relationship with her therapist, there is a confusing combination of inchoate rage and desperate defensiveness on behalf of the therapist, her motives, and her character, that is evocative of a battered wife who has not quite yet disentangled herself from the abusive relationship. This tone is very different from that of the theologian who speaks – sometimes on the same page – so clearly and powerfully about this painful passage as a spiritual journey.

The story, as I read it, was about a therapist whose own needs for intense, sympathetic communication got in the way of her ability to structure a therapy process centred on her client's healing. This problem has nothing to do with what topics are discussed or whether client and therapist sit on the floor or on chairs. The same dynamic could occur in the most conservative of settings under fluorescent lighting.

It is also no crime for a therapist to get countertransferentially entangled with a client. Some degree of countertransference is inevitable in in-depth therapy relationships. There are a couple of things a therapist could do if she found herself in that position, either of which I think would have been more ethical than continuing to misrepresent the situation (presumably to herself as well as to her client). She could tell her client she liked her a lot and would be happy to continue their discussions on a more informal basis but couldn't continue to take her money for what was a non-therapeutic relationship. Some therapists would consider this a violation of their personal frame of no extra-therapy relationships with ex-clients, so it is a solution that would not work for them.

The therapist could acknowledge her own feelings and – probably with the help of a clinical consultant and possibly a therapist of her own – realign the relationship so that she could act responsibly in the role of therapist. This would enable her to bracket the issue of the evolution of their relationship when the therapy was completed ('Whether or not we will become friends is just not something I can know during the course of the therapy.') or present her practice of 'no extra-therapy relationships with ex-clients' straightforwardly and tactfully and be able to listen and explore openly all of her client's feelings, including any feelings that the client had about a post-termination personal relationship.

Instead, as I read the encounter, the therapist in *When Boundaries Betray Us* alternately got her own needs met in the relationship and then pulled back into the power of the profession when her client started to ask to have the reality of the situation acknowledged. I do not think that the issue in that relationship was whether or not clients and therapists should be friends or lovers after therapy ends; it was a problem of emotional dishonesty on the part of the therapist.

This is not the way the book has been taken up in the vast majority of professional contexts. In both reviews of the book and in discussions that I have been a part of, this book has been almost invariably framed as a dangerous challenge to the obvious need for boundaries in the therapy process.

Many therapists seem to identify with the character of the therapist that the author has created, and I have heard clinicians and students rage about difficult clients, like the author, who want their own way and won't take no for an answer. Sometimes, in book reviews (Hunt, 1994; Fortune, 1994) and collegial discussions, passing mention is made of therapist error ('She could have been more consistent about her limits'), but the focus is almost always on this irritating client (called clinical names like 'narcissistic' or 'borderline') who created so many unnecessary problems for herself and her therapist by not shutting up and accepting her therapist's word as law.

Ironically, under the guise of an emphasis on the importance of therapeutic boundaries for the protection of the client, there seems to be very little awareness that this was a therapeutic relationship that provoked powerful feelings in a client through an aggressively personalized stance on the part of the therapist, and then double-bound the client in an emotionally abusive way by alternately stimulating her feelings and then discounting her responses to the situation. Most discussions of the book see it as a story of a powerful, demanding client who overwhelmed a therapist who was just trying to make the client obey the rules for her own good.

The relative power of the client and the therapist within the context of the therapeutic relationship is thus turned upside down, and the client is framed as the villain who is assaulting one of our most revered, newly developed social structures – the therapy relationship. The very nature of the therapy process to stir up powerful feelings in the client and the responsibility of the therapist to ensure that this intensity is grounded and helpful rather than largely destabilizing to the client – the very reason for clear therapeutic boundaries – seems to be ignored.

This self-righteous imposition of overly generalized and rigid rules in combination with no appreciable sensitivity to the issues of what therapy is, how powerful a tool the therapeutic relationship can be, and what the most basic responsibilities of the therapist are to ensure that the client is helped more than she is hurt in the relationship, does not speak well for the way in which we are currently engaging in the struggle to develop ethical standards in our professions.

As therapists, we should be consciously developing an ever-increasing level of comfort with an awareness of our countertransference responses to our clients. If we have not worn away our narcissistic sensitivities against knowing we are imperfect, significantly flawed human beings by the time we are relatively experienced therapists, this is a dangerous business to be in. When I come up against a therapeutic impasse, I routinely examine my participation in the relationship for countertransferential distortions that might be the source of the problem. If I cannot uncover anything of the sort in myself and the problem persists, I take it to a colleague whom I trust to help me see what I might be blind to on my own.

If, even under these circumstances, I can find no evidence of problems of my own that might be blocking the process, this does not make me particularly happy. Problems of my own I have some control over; what I create I am quite likely to be able to change. If the impasse does not originate or is not being sustained by my countertransferential blindness, then it is likely that what I have on my hands is a difficult situation which time, patience, and trying as many new things as I can think of may or may not be able to ameliorate. I much prefer dealing with my own problems to recognizing the reality that I may not have the power to help people make the kind of changes in their lives that I would like to see them make.

There are destructive individuals who are abusive to their psychotherapists in obvious ways (Comstock & Vicery, 1992), and others whose demands and distortions make it impossible for even the most rigorous and conscientious therapist to satisfy them. Not everyone who requests therapy wants to take on the responsibility of facing and dealing with themselves openly and honestly.

Not all clients respond positively to an empathic therapist. For example, a sociopath might sever a therapeutic relationship upon discovering that his therapist was empathically attuned to him, and many other people have less clear-cut but profoundly ambivalent responses to the experience of being accurately understood. But that is the choice and the struggle of the client in the therapy relationship, just as it is the adolescent's choice and need to ignore, reject, or mock sensible parental care as part of the struggle for independence and the creation of a mature self. Whether accepted or rejected – or, more often, some complicated combination of both – it is the therapist's responsibility to create an atmosphere of empathic connection within which the client can grow and change.

I find it disquieting that so many therapists identify with the psychiatrist in *When Boundaries Betray Us*, not in terms of a cautionary tale about what could happen to any of us if we are not emotionally honest in our work, but as a righteous professional who was abused by a pushy client who would not do therapy the way she was supposed to. It seems to me to be a particularly 1990s response. We have indeed come a long way in the past decade or so in understanding the importance of clean and clear therapeutic boundaries in creating an effective healing process. We are well aware of the problems that derive from ignoring the issue of power differential in the therapeutic relationship. But the solutions we have come up with are still, by and large, primitive. In many situations we have tried to place simple and not very workable rules over the complicated process of in-depth interpersonal therapy, and then mislabeled this inadequate response to a very real issue as 'boundaries.'

Along the same lines, we seem increasingly to count on large professional regulating organizations and courts of law to monitor a process that demands a high level of accountability to the most vulnerable in our midst and a sophisticated ability to look at complex issues responsibly, which have never been the strengths of large professional bodies or the legal system. Professional bodies should hold their members accountable for ethical violations, and there should be a place for judicial redress for malpractice or ethical misconduct. But these are just the beginning.

We have been taking some of the most obvious first steps. We need to continue unlearning, relearning, and reshaping our communities so that we can be truly accountable to one another and to our clients. Expending too much of our energy in trying to ensure quality of care through simple all-embracing legal or professional standards enforced in contexts historically constructed to protect the powerful will only divert that energy from the difficult process of creating more effective community support and accountability.

My dismay at the direction in which the professional community is moving in solving complex problems with simplistic rule-making does not mean that it is my style to be particularly casual about boundaries. I have become acutely aware of how extra-therapy contact with people can take the edge off the therapeutic project, and I am inclined to be conservative about any social or professional contact with clients for that reason. I try to avoid social gatherings (or business occasions, teaching, or consulting situations) where my clients are present because I have found that in many cases our therapeutic relationship limits the client's freedom to relax socially, conduct business objectively, or learn freely – and limits me in these respects as well.

I have also found that, more often than not, the struggle to engage in the dual relationship greatly dilutes the therapy process, and I do not get much satisfaction conducting half-baked therapy.

In some cases, I might well try to avoid such extra-therapy situations forever with particular ex-clients, if I perceive that the therapist-client affective intensity and power differential remain alive and strong in our interactions. I do not make such a choice because I consider my clients to remain my clients forever, but because the relationship that evolves with certain ex-clients, as with other people who have never been clients, is not conducive to an ongoing relationship that is useful for me or for them. This, however, is not a rule that I make; it is a practice about which I have a right and a responsibility to use my discretion.

What troubles me about what I see as an increasing tendency to legislate boundaries – again except those dealing with the sexual, financial, or professional exploitation of clients currently in therapy – is that it creates an *in loco parentis* responsibility on the part of the therapist to a degree that is insulting in a relationship between adults. It is critical to acknowledge the dimensions of power in the structure of the therapeutic relationship. It is just as important not to become locked into a deterministic analysis in which dominant groups appear to be the only ones who can have individual agency and subordinate groups are seen to be totally and forever trapped in structures of oppression. A useful feminist critique demands the recognition of structures and agency on both sides of the equation in order to allow for resistance and change and to present the complexities of the sources of power and weakness in women's lives (Gordon, 1986).

Therapists should still be aware of the potential for exploitation in post-termination relationships of a social, business, or sexual nature. Clients or ex-clients are also not precluded from taking appropriate action against a therapist if it is their perception that they have been exploited either during therapy or after therapy was terminated.

There are many clients with whom I would not develop a friendship after they completed their therapy process because I would not experience it as a relationship of equals. It is my responsibility to be as rigorous as I have it in my power to be in my exploration of the possible consequences of developing a friendship or a collegial or business relationship with an ex-client. However, with little collegial discussion and no convincing empirical evidence, to declare by fiat that an everlasting and unalterable power differential is part of the essence of the therapist-client relationship is disrespectful to the relationship and both of its participants.

Reducing the therapy relationship to one of transference/countertransference in this way disallows one of the most important and transformative aspects (or at least possibilities) of the therapy dynamic: the evolution from a relationship of unequal power in which transference is an important tool in facilitating the client's regression and consequent exploration and growth to a relationship of relative freedom from transference limitations. Jean Baker-Miller (1976) talked about therapy as a relationship of 'temporary inequality' at a time when most feminist therapists were denying the depth and complexity of the therapeutic power differential. I think this is still a good way of thinking about it. In fact, a particular therapy relationship may not play itself out this way, but it makes more sense to me to keep the door open for that kind of transformation than, under the guise of protecting the client, order unchanging and unchangeable hierarchical power relations between therapist and client.

Sanctions like 'once a client, always a client' are hegemonic, and they are created in the service of protecting the profession rather than protecting the client. They imply that the balance of power between client and therapist is, if not completely static, at least capable of very limited movement for the rest of each of their lives. Thus, they patronize and infantilize individuals who contract for a relationship in which we are the helper, the wiser, the clearer, for a specific time period only, not for eternity.

If a therapist genuinely needs the degree of personal boundaries and insurance of safety that these sanctions purport to offer, surely it is basic to any form of ethical negotiation to spell out the conditions and the limitations of the contract before the relationship is underway and the client is unable extricate herself from being a client forever in a way she may believe is against her best interests. However, although I know many therapists who say they personally subscribe to the value that it is unethical to develop post-termination relationships of any sort with ex-clients, I do not know of many therapists who routinely include in their introductory conversation, in which they and the client decide whether they wish to contract for treatment, a clear statement that one of their policies is to have no extra-therapeutic relationship with clients or ex-clients *in perpetuum*. I think therapists have a right to decide that making clear and unambiguous rules about post-therapy involvement of any sort with ex-clients is the best policy for them to follow, but I think that, if they need that degree of separation between their professional and personal lives – or if it is their belief that all their clients need that boundary – then it should be part of the initial contract.

There are a number of people I have declined to see in treatment because I wanted to have the opportunity of developing a personal or professional relationship with them. Clients should be made aware that they are also making those kind of choices and that when they contract to do therapy with a particular individual, this precludes developing other types of relationships during the course of the treatment, and, in some instances, forever.

Many professionals, who do not take the prohibition of extra-therapeutic relationships and associations with all ex-clients as an absolute, make an exception in the case of sexual relationships. They would acknowledge that there are many areas in which discretion should be used. Sexual contact, however, is removed from the realm of issues professionals can use their judgment about and is prohibited absolutely, forever, and under all circumstances.

It is important to emphasize that there are many – probably most – counselling relationships in which post-termination sexual contact would be unethical. For example, because of the nature and intensity of the long-term relationship that a highly dissociative trauma survivor usually has with her psychotherapist and the degree to which sexual abuse survivors are particularly vulnerable to revictimization, sexual contact with a client who has been treated for a severe dissociative condition – even long after the therapy was over – would likely be exploitive and therefore unethical (Barach, 1994).

The therapist must be aware of the possible dangers involved in post-termination relationships with ex-clients, and especially sexual relationships. However, I think that this severing of sex from the notion of the possibility of a growing and changing relationship is a manifestation of the growing sex panic of some groups in the radical feminist movement and in the feminist and humanist therapy movements, aligning them with the radical right in terms of sex negativity and misplaced scale (Rubin, 1993). It represents a disconcerting and dangerous degree of comfort with defining, interpreting, and legislating fit forms of desire and sexual behaviour. In the context of the feminist therapy community and the lesbian therapy community, a set of strictures functions with the authority of the symbolic 'law of the Mother' (Creet, 1991) – the morality that an abstract or reified contemporary feminist or lesbian community (externally or internally) legislates for contemporary women.

Rigid rules and regulations construct the comforting illusion of a guarantee of 'no harm' in times when therapy is a very risky business. They create an anonymous, automatic morality for which no one must accept responsibility. Therapists can sidestep facing, theorizing about, and struggling with the issue of power in the therapy relationship – who has it? what is its use? what happens when it is misused? Rigid rules create an atmosphere in which sloganizing and name-calling replace reasoned dialogue about difficult clinical, ethical, and political issues and where professionals are afraid to think important issues through for themselves or in communication with their colleagues for fear of being labeled 'unethical.' An ideological structure is imposed on clinical work that stifles its creative possibilities and privileges conformity to the rules of the group over the individual therapist's responsibility to engage in thoughtful exploration of the therapeutic process and relationship in all its complexity.

What global sanctions regarding post-termination relationships with clients do *not* do is deter sexual predators who are professionals from exploiting their clients or ex-clients nor do they deter professionals who, without conscience, exploit their clients or ex-clients, financially, professionally, or in a variety of other ways. They also fail to create an atmosphere in which confused and vulnerable (but not socio-pathic) professionals who engage in sex (or other dual relationships) to the detriment of a client (either during the professional relationship or after its termination) would be able to communicate their feelings, impulses, and intentions to colleagues or supervisors and expect to find a non-judgmental forum in which to wrestle with the issue and possibly avoid acting in harmful ways.

Imposing overly general rules about the boundaries of professional relationships creates an atmosphere that stifles therapists' exploration of countertransference and other personal issues. Professional doctrine or legal strictures become an escape valve that frees the therapist from that difficult bottom-line responsibility. Ideology under the guise of ethics hides the discomfitting reality that any relationship, including a therapeutic relationship, is a balance of the good it does for the people involved and the harm it does, and that there is no possibility of doing 'no harm' ever, despite the inspiring and useful direction of the Hypocratic oath *'Primum non nocere.'*

If a rigid, or even the relatively conservative application of the 'no dual relation-ships' proscription that I have been espousing is absolutely essential to effective psychodynamic therapy, it would be impossible to treat clients in small, isolated communities in which there is an inevitable overlap of roles, or at least the results would be substantially compromised. The only study I know of that addresses this issue indicates that this not the case (Beskind, Bartels, & Brooks, 1993). Certainly before we assume it to be so, we need to do a great deal more research. As Charcot is quoted by his student, Sigmund Freud (1893/1962), 'La theorie, c'est bon, mais ça n'empeche pas d'exister' ('Theory is good, but it doesn't prevent things from existing').

Cultural traditions in which the healers in a community are a part of the social fabric of that community must be respected (as well as challenged and explored when they are seen as problematic by members of the community) rather than swept aside by professionals outside the community who feel confident that their standards of ethics have universal application. When I acted as a consultant to a Native Canadian social service agency that provided therapeutic services to an urban Abo-riginal population, one of the most complex issues was the development of bound-aries protecting the therapy process that respected both traditional values of the integration of the healer within the community and the contemporary urban sen-sibilities of the workers, who had been trained in mainstream mental health practice as well as through traditional Native teaching. Rigid rules about the practice of therapy that ignored the cultural complexity that was the experience of these workers and their client community would have been criminally insensitive to the goal of this agency and its workers – to develop culturally appropriate and creative services that combined traditional healing with mainstream mental health practices.

The solution of exempting different racial or cultural groups from complying with strictures that are framed as mandatory for everyone else seems both patronizing and a case of sloppy thinking. The workers in this urban Native organization had to struggle to create a set of practice guidelines that made it possible for them to accomplish their particular goals with their particular group of clients. In that they share a struggle with every other responsible professional – the struggle to create structures that empower rather than diminish both the healer and those who seek healing by honouring the customs and values of both and being willing to offer challenge to those customs and those values, both to themselves and to their clients, when necessary.

This is a time when the professional pendulum has swung from deconstructing the boundaries of the therapeutic relationship to reconstructing them, sometimes in a rigid fashion that subverts the collaborative struggle at the heart of an in-depth therapy process. The issue of the boundaries of the therapeutic relationship is one of the most difficult and complex of clinical and ethical issues. The bottom line in making a value judgment about whether a particular boundary in any relationship is useful, respectful, and ethical is its power to facilitate our capacity to reach out to other human beings, including our clients, in a grounded, passionate, and genuinely moral way. In order to do that we need to be rigorous in examining the complexities of our relationships – including their shadows and their depths. If we do so we will find, in this area as in so many others, that simple solutions are no solutions at all.

7

Abuse and Memory in the 1990s

The Delphic injunction 'Know thyself?' did not refer to memory. It required that we know our character, our limits, our needs, our propensities for self-deception. It required that we know our souls. Only with the advent of memoro-politics did memory become a surrogate for the soul.

Ian Hacking (1995)

The issues of memory has become central to the issue of trauma, particularly childhood sexual abuse. The ways in which we now think and talk about memory as it relates to trauma evolved from the late nineteenth century, when the word 'trauma' acquired a new meaning. Although it had always been in the medical lexicon as meaning lesion or wound, at this point in history the word acquired the meaning most common today: 'a psychological hurt, a spiritual lesion, a wound to the soul' (Hacking, 1995, p. 4).

In the past fifteen years, we have seen the issue of memory and trauma expand from the domain of the psychological sciences and its treatment venues, in which the lesions of early childhood trauma were examined with the goal of healing the individual so wounded, to the more public realm of the legal system, in which some of the perpetrators of the harm were – for the first time in history in any great numbers – held accountable for the damage they had inflicted on the children in their care.

Psychotherapy services delivered to abuse survivors are profoundly influenced by their social context. The shift of emphasis from thinking about child abuse, and particularly child sexual abuse, as a personal psychospiritual issue for the individuals who have been harmed in this way (when it was acknowledged as a reality at all) to framing it as a crime against society, has had many consequences for the ways in which we respond to abuse survivors in therapeutic practice. The clinical community is just beginning to recognize and deal with some of the complications that have evolved from this expanding of the social context in which psychotherapy is conducted.

I was trained as a therapist in a psychoanalytically-oriented community organization in the 1960s and early 1970s. Everyone who was in training as a psychotherapist was also engaged in an intensive personal therapy process as well. We were not taught to think about our clients as a different class of people with a different set of problems from ourselves. Most people had psychological problems, it was assumed. The differences in terms of prognosis were seen to derive from the willingness and the ability of individuals to acknowledge their own troubled areas and to wrestle with them honestly.

We used hypnotic techniques to enhance our ability to focus on past events and related emotional reactions that, presumably, were causing turmoil in the present. Within this context, many people recollected being abused in one way or another in childhood. This was not considered particularly unusual, and those of us who were not subjected to physical or sexual abuse generally thought of ourselves as having been poorly treated in some ways and to some degree. Hence the personal problems that led us to seek therapy.

As a group, we also thought of the maltreatment of children – or at least the insensitive treatment of children, leading to psychological damage – as fairly universal in a society we saw as repressive and oppressive.

We not only thought that most of our parents, relatives, teachers, and so on – all those adults who were influential in our upbringing, – had treated us somewhere on the continuum from not so well to very badly, we considered ourselves quite likely to be engaging in some of the same damaging childrearing practices ourselves, and we consciously struggled to open our eyes and change our behaviour towards our own children.

The climate around the issue of child abuse has changed considerably since then, and many of the changes are for the better. Short of the most egregious examples of life-threatening abuse, no one went to the police to protect children. Looking at maltreatment on a continuum as completely as we did tended to lead to conflating rape with fuzziness around boundaries – 'emotional incest' – and they are not the same. In general, we now think that crimes against children belong in the public realm. Very few therapists would now say with the conviction of the psychoanalytically trained therapist of twenty or more years ago, 'It doesn't matter whether these things you picture in your mind actually happened or not. What is important is their psychological meaning for you.'

It clearly does matter whether particular events actually happened. It is worth creating some categories to distinguish these areas from one another, in order to facilitate appropriate and just action. For example, if I start having images or dreams about a particular individual sexually abusing me as a child, and I am not certain whether or not these experiences represent historical reality or not, this would necessarily affect my actions under certain circumstances. If I were planning to send my child to his household for childcare, I would rethink my arrangements. Whether or not this individual abused me or is likely to abuse anyone else, my first responsibility would be to ensure the safety of the child. In such a situation, I would reason that, although I do not know what my images mean, at the very least they mean that I am not comfortable with the babysitting arrangements I have set up, and I would take my misgivings seriously. If I were considering hiring this person for a job that involved contact with children, I, personally, would also feel bound to act conservatively – although, if challenged, I should probably have some good reasons for not selecting him for the position, other than my mental images of him as an abuser.

What would such images mean for my relationship with that person? I consider that I have more flexibility when it is my own welfare at stake. I can decide that I wish to continue spending time with this person, knowing that he may have abused me in childhood, because I like him, because I am not sure what the facts of the situation are, or because I want to use our proximity to explore the issue. I also have a right to decide that I do not wish to be in his company, and it is my right to act on this wish, whatever the reason.

If my relationship with him allows me to question him about whether or not he perpetrated the acts I am picturing, I also have a right to do so. However, accusations about acts of child abuse, based on images or feelings that are not clear memories, can be incredibly hurtful, and generally, I think that we are obliged ethically to be cautious about the harm we inflict on others. What this ethical guideline means is that we are ought to weigh the good an action will accomplish against the harm that is likely to accrue before we act in a way that is likely to hurt another person. How we decide to act will then depend on all the circumstances of the situation. How certain am I that my mental images represent historical reality, and on what is my conviction based? Is there any benefit to be derived from my speaking out. To me? Regarding the protection of others? What are the risks involved?

Making such an accusation in the public realm – such as a court of law – demands even more rigour regarding the veridicality of the abuse memories. We have seen vast changes in the past fifteen years as to the type of evidence that a judge will take seriously – stories of sexual abuse told by children as young as four and five, for example. Credibility is now accorded to many individuals who would never have seen the inside of a court as complainants not long ago. This is positive change, and with it has come some important responsibilities. One of these is to distinguish between a courtroom and a treatment room.

The evidence needed to bring a perpetrator to accountability in a judicial context is different from the evidence necessary to persuade a psychotherapy client that she has suffered personal harm in childhood. And so it should be. It is not unusual for people to act impulsively when they are in the emotionally charged situation of beginning to suspect someone of abuse. Actions such as confrontations, civil suits, and police reports can have far-reaching consequences for everyone involved, including the person who initiates them, and they should be seriously weighed.

Psychotherapists working with individuals who are considering taking such steps have a responsibility to help them look at the situation from the broadest viewpoint possible, if they are given any opportunity to do so. Taking a hands-off stance, or even worse, offering countertransferentially-based encouragement ('Good for you. Let's get some of these buggers') without helping the client explore the possible ramifications of her actions, is an abrogation of the therapist's professional responsibility.

Many clients, for example, when they begin to become aware that they were a part of activities that were harmful to others – as well as being abused themselves – become so agitated with guilt that they attempt to initiate police action against their perpetrators. Sometimes this is necessary and appropriate, such as in situations in which it is truly known that children are presently being abused or in which the perpetrators are stalking the client in the present. The few such investigations that I am aware of that have been fruitful in this regard have been cases of intra-familial sexual abuse, and in most of those cases, a guilty plea was entered by the perpetrator. In other similar cases, and in all of the more complicated cases involving multiple perpetrators, I know many individuals who were revictimized as they attempted to bring to justice individuals who had abused them many years before. Quite often, their own healing process had to be put on hold for months – or even years – as they were able to concentrate on nothing but the judicial process or the confrontational personal interactions that created, in the present, an atmosphere of threat and invalidation that closely resembled the abusive childhood milieu.

Many trauma survivors believe that not to be a continually angry and obviously suffering witness amounts to silence and submission. Yael Danielli tells the story of her patient who refused to take the medications that – after years of sleepless nights – finally allowed her some relief because, as she said, 'My nightmares are the only connection I maintain with those people close to me who were exterminated in the death camps.' A Vietnam veteran is quoted in a similar vein, 'I do not want to take drugs for my nightmares, because I must remain a memorial to my dead friends' (Caruth, 1995, p. vii). For sexual abuse survivors, 'I have to tell the authorities about these atrocities,' may represent some version of this cognitive frame that 'if I do not speak they will have won.' If accurately understood, the wait to speak until one can do so productively can be reframed as the development of an outraged and effective witness who can thwart her perpetrators, first of all by her own healing and success, and then by bringing a steady and credible voice to any challenge she may decide to throw out.

Many trauma survivors, especially those suffering from severe dissociation, are not able to communicate with the police or in a courtroom setting in a way that is likely to make them believable witnesses, according to the standards that apply in these contexts. Perpetrators and their supporters are usually in a much better position to play their part in the social drama of a criminal investigation and trial than a severely dissociative survivor of childhood abuse. I encourage people who want to lay charges against their perpetrators – or file a civil suit, or even, in some, though certainly not all cases, confront individuals personally – to wait until they can be stronger witnesses on their own behalf, and on behalf of the other children they hope to protect. An individual charged with an offense and found 'not guilty' cannot be charged with the same offense again. Putting off bringing issues of past abuse into the legal arena can make sense, even for an individual who is completely convinced that she will not be free of the influence of the perpetrator until he is held publicly accountable for his actions.

As well as the ethical and the practical dimensions of public accusations of sexual abuse, it is important for an individual to explore her own motivations. Asking some key questions can be helpful in this regard. What are the emotional dynamics involved in my wanting to accuse a person when I am not at all certain, when I am fairly certain – when I am completely certain, for that matter? What am I hoping to gain from making such an accusation, and are my hopes realistic? Am I imagining a flight into health? (Once he is shamed, I will regain my self-esteem and the sense of integrity he robbed from me.) Am I hoping that my mother will leave him and show a protectiveness and loyalty to me that I have never felt from her before? Am I hoping that the pain that I always experience when I am with her will be alleviated when she is, at last, given the opportunity to be the mother I have always wanted her to be? Do I imagine that the money I am hoping for as a result of the civil suit will enable me to find peace? Will my anger be satisfied when he is embarrassed publicly by my accusations?

From a legal standpoint, the motivations of the complainant do not – or should not – matter. Why should an abuse survivor not be rageful, not want revenge, not want her mother to love and protect her, not want her perpetrator to pay emotionally, financially, or any way at all? Within the context of the survivor's healing process, however, her hopes, dreams, and motivations matter a great deal. When people act on their first impulses, without seriously considering the emotional, practical, and ethical dimensions of their actions (or without having the information to take such things into consideration), they are often the ones to suffer.

Therapists must discourage their clients from going public with accusations the client is not certain about – or does not have the grounds to be certain about. A dream or some dissociated mental images should not turn into a court case with few or even no intermediate steps that make them more properly termed '*memory*.' Such experiences can be understood in many ways, and it is the responsibility of the qualified therapist to ensure that premature certainty does not replace the thorough exploration and processing of such material. This is a critical part of conducting effective treatment. It is also our responsibility as citizens as well as a psychotherapists.

Frightening as the thought is, much of our social safety depends on the judicial system. It is a truism to say that when we undermine the civil rights of one member of society, we undermine the civil rights of us all. It is a cliché, however, worth taking very seriously in times in which the courts are being used as a weapon in many personal and political disputes.

Professionals are much more likely to be cavalier about the issue of mistaken, false, and even malicious allegations of sexual abuse until they encounter such a situation personally. Although I have thus far escaped being the object of such an accusation, I have known more than one professional who was accused of such acts in circumstances that persuaded me to a certainty that they were not guilty. In the cases with which I am personally familiar, the allegations were the result of a combination of confusion and malice.

Fortunately, in those cases, there were factors that led the investigating authorities to come to the conclusion that the accusations were not grounded in fact. However, it did not have to go that way. We are well aware that the structure of the judicial process does not ensure that the guilty will be punished. We may be less aware of legal situations – possibly because there are many fewer of them – in which the innocent are not exonerated. And even when practitioners are cleared of criminal charges or complaints to professional regulating bodies deriving from mistaken or malicious allegations, the process is usually extremely frightening, painful, and disillusioning to the individuals involved, despite the outcome.

We are naive if we think that this could not happen to us. It is especially important for professionals working with adult survivors of severe trauma to be realistic about the propensity that some individuals – who have been badly hurt in their formative years and have been socialized, in many cases, by sociopaths – for easing their own torment by hurting others. They can do this deliberately, by mistake, or by some complicated combination of both. The psychotherapist, who is the repository of all the client's projections, including being seen as an abuser at times, can be one of the most likely objects for revenge attempts, under certain circumstances. Those individuals who tend to present this danger to their therapists combine the tendencies to distort reality and to repeat malevolent patterns imposed on them as children. They are more inclined to act out than to work through upsetting material.

Abuse survivors can also be induced into attacking their therapists by important people in the client's life who are threatened by the effects that therapy is beginning to have on an individual who was once malleable and susceptible to total control. False accusations, which almost always lead to discontinuation of treatment, are an effective way of undermining the power of a therapist who is presenting this sort of danger.

Comstock and Vickery's (1992) article entitled *The Therapist as Victim: A Prelim-*

inary Discussion notes that there have been increasing reports of severely dissociative adults victimizing their therapists, including filing frivolous complaints and lawsuits, harassing other clients of the therapist, spreading untrue rumors about the therapist, invading the therapist's personal space, harassing family members, killing pets, and destroying property. Such behaviours may sometimes be in response to therapeutic error or inappropriate behaviour on the part of the therapist, but they also occur in situations in which the therapist has been entirely professional and competent.

Attacks of this sort serve a purpose for the distressed individual, such as discharging intense and unbearable affect. Causing pain or instilling fear in the therapist – often perceived to be maddeningly powerful and invulnerable, like the abusers of old – can provide a cathartic release for individuals who have a tremendously difficult time containing their feelings. The adversarial transactions and the hateful emotion that accompanies them can restore the equilibrium of an individual who is feeling unbalanced.

Distorted attachment behaviour can be expressed in such malicious attacks. A robust vendetta against a therapist can offer a sense of identity and purpose to a person who is both extremely agitated and extremely empty, and who does not have any idea of how to develop healthy relationships in the present that fulfil her need for connection and nurturance. People who combine severe dissociative symptoms with aggressive behaviour and extreme self-centredness can become enmeshed 'in a magic circle of seeking new and devaluing exhausted sources of gratification in a series of idealizations and dissatisfactions and internal restlessness' (Svrakic, 1985).

Abuse survivors do not make false allegations against their therapists – or anyone else – very often. But because this occurs in only a very small minority of cases does not mean we can be complacent in our assumptions that it never happens – or that, if we behave in an ethical and professional manner, it will never happen to us. Such wishful thinking can rebound in a way that is dangerous for both survivor and therapist. We can miss signals that should tell us that the need to relieve the stress of intense feelings is far outpacing the survivor's ability to process those feelings constructively. The survivor can be abandoned in a morass of powerful and destructive emotions that she cannot acknowledge or work through with a starry-eyed therapist who has a need to idealize her clients.

It is important for any therapist working with trauma survivors to be able to understand and encompass hateful emotion and the immature cognitions that often accompany such feelings. All or nothing thinking is normal in young children. At early stages of brain development, children do not have the neurological capacity to experience ambivalence (Fisher, 1995). When a loving and securely attached toddler says 'I hate you,' she does not mean, 'I am angry at this moment, but I am aware that you are very dear to me as well.' At that moment, anger is all she is able to feel. This inability to contain contradictory notions or feelings is often not outgrown in adults who were severely traumatized at an early developmental stage. Very intelligent individuals can have utterly distorted cognitions when it comes to key concepts about themselves. One of the most common is the notion that if I am not totally good, I am bad. Often the most difficult part of taking reasonable responsibility for one's actions – rather than global blame for everything – stems from this way of looking at things.

This type of primitive thinking has sometimes characterized advocacy for abuse survivors. The notion that women or children never lie – or even more preposterously, that women and children never have faulty powers of recollection and that everything they say they remember must, necessarily, be taken at face value – is clearly undemonstrable. Why should survivors of severe interpersonal abuse or neglect in childhood be less prey to the limitations of all human beings?

Historically, of course, these propositions were made to balance the more pervasive cultural belief, supported with particular vigour by mental health professionals, that allegations of childhood sexual abuse were always the product of the fevered imaginations of hysterical women or lying children. However necessary and understandable this swing was, no cause is served by sloppy thinking and slogans that do not hold up in the light of logic. Although we are now immersed in a political climate in which moderate thinking feels like a terribly mild and unsatisfying weapon against the histrionic attacks that seem to be mounted with increasing frequency, reasoning that parallels the dichotomous conceptualizations of young children – and adults who have not had the opportunity to grow out of the developmental periods in which they were traumatized – merely discredits us.

The reality is that memory is a complicated affair. Much of what we remember in the broadest sense of the term never translates into narrative truth. Our stomach knots when we hear a certain sound. Our limbs become paralysed when we are in the presence of a certain person. Our mind goes blank when we are addressed in a certain way. We are more profoundly influenced by the limbic system than by the frontal cortex, and a powerful and effective therapy process is usually as much about dealing with and healing from this type of enactive memory that it is about uncovering all the facts of a situation.

Memories of severe trauma are rarely laid down in a narrative fashion, and they are only partly healed within a narrative frame of reference. Bessel van der Kolk (1995) describes the job of psychotherapy as helping suffering people transform wordless, emotion-laden, right-hemisphere information into empowering autobiographical narrative. That is certainly part of the task. However, an equally powerful part of the healing process takes place at a much more primitive level than the level of language, insight, and figuring things out. We are beginning to know a little bit about what happens in the brain as this process takes place.

Nobel prize-winning neuropsychologist Karl Pribram declares that neuroscience is always trying to document what philosophers and clinicians know from a different frame of reference. Although the processes of brain functioning are extremely complex, and there is a great deal about even basic brain functioning that science has not yet understood, relatively recent scientific technology has enabled neuroscientists to examine the relationships among consciousness, emotion, and the brain directly in a way that was previously impossible. Sensitive electrodes can be inserted into the brains of test animals, allowing a researcher to see clearly the effects of various stimuli on different parts of the brain. Magnetic resonance imaging (MRI) and positron emission tomography (PET) provide a window onto the topography of the human brain. For example, scientists can now watch the amygdala – a knot of nerve cells located close to the brain stem – become active in the brain of a person who suddenly becomes frightened.

Researchers are examining the brain for more clues about the processes by which memories are acquired, stored, and retrieved. The role of the hypocampus in the coordination of the retrieval of memories of concrete facts and events and the role of the amygdala in the activation of emotion-laden enactive memories (particularly memories involving a high level of fearful affect) are of great interest to clinicians treating trauma survivors, whose memory processes are deeply connected to their suffering, and to their healing.

For the past two years (1995 and 1996), a conference has been held in Alexandria, Virginia, entitled *Trauma, Loss and Dissociation: Foundations of 21st Century Traumatology*. This now annual event is organized to bring together neuroscientists, researchers who specialize in animal behaviour, child developmentalists, and clinicians specializing in the treatment of traumatized individuals with the ambitious goal of bridging the gap between research, theory, and practice. Over the course of the four stimulating days of these conferences, so many new facts and ideas are presented that I – and many others as well who are stretching to comprehend even the basics of the neuroscience – do not have the capacity to make memories out of much that I listen to. But I do come away from the sessions with renewed conviction that the issue of memory is far more complex than would be imagined if all one were exposed to were the recent, rather simple, ideologically-driven debates. Those of us who are trying to do effective and responsible clinical work long before the data are accumulated and understood in hard scientific terms must use what research we can find – and comprehend – and then combine it with our basic clinical common sense.

This common sense tells us that most of what we are fairly certain happened to us will be true in its general details, and that we will get some of the specifics wrong. Abuse survivors are not more likely than the rest of us to have perfect memories, uninfluenced by time, emotional reactivity, and a variety of other factors. This does not mean that survivors of all sorts may not have many memories of trauma that have always been accessible, just as anyone else can have many memories of childhood experiences. Although survivors may have paid little attention to these experiences – dismissing them as unimportant, reframing them as their fault, or discounting and distancing in a variety of ways – these are memories that are no more or less likely to be based on reality than anyone else's memories.

However, a minority of clients who use therapy to deal with childhood abuse – 12 to 28 per cent according to a recent research summary (Bowman, 1995) – enter treatment for other psychological problems and report almost total amnesia for childhood abuse until they are engaged in a therapeutic process in which they are encouraged to explore their thoughts, feelings, and sensations in a milieu they experience as relatively safe. Within this context, they begin to see images and experience sensations that they come to understand as relating to historical abuse encounters. This is an experience that is contraintuitive for most people who have not been traumatized in this way. We all have faulty memories, but most of us remember the most significant events in our lives, at least in a general way, once we get past our first few years. How is it that some people can completely forget hideous acts perpetrated against them day after day for years?

The answer is we do not really know how it can happen – that is, how the brain sequesters information that is powerful and important (such as memories of repeated acts of child abuse) and renders it inaccessible either for a period of time or for all time. There is enough research going on to encourage speculation, but we are nowhere near certainty as to the mechanisms that are operating in a process we loosely call forgetting. We do know, however, that such a phenomenon – forgetting experiences of abuse and then, sometimes, remembering them at a later time – happens, and not infrequently.

A number of studies shed light on different aspects of this phenomenon. Although some apologists for the point of view that the uncovering of widespread child sexual abuse in our society is a witch-hunt without foundation in reality declare that there is no evidence that a child would forget a truly traumatic experience unless the event occurred before age of three (Wakefield & Underwager, 1992), the research shows that such forgetting is common. Briere and Conte (1993) found that a majority (59 per cent) of individuals in therapy dealing with issues related to childhood sexual abuse had forgotten the abuse experiences for some period of time before the age of eighteen. Herman and Schatzow (1987) found that 28 per cent of the women in their study had "severe memory deficits" for their abuse experiences, and 64 per cent reported some inability to remember. Loftus, Polonsky, and Fullilove (1994) report that 31 per cent of their sample of sexually abused women had incomplete memory for their abuse, and 19 per cent reported previous periods of total lack of recall of the abuse. Kristiansen et al. (1996) reported 51 per cent of the participants in their study had experienced some disruption in their memory of childhood abuse.

This wide range of results from retrospective studies suggests that more research needs to be done before we can say with confidence how common forgetting experiences of child sexual abuse is. Even the lowest percentages, however, indicate that such forgetting is by no means uncommon.

When systematic attempts are made to verify abuse memories, as many as 80 per cent of the reports can be corroborated through physical evidence, perpetrator confession, or eyewitness testimony (Bagley & King, 1990). Coons (1986) was able to obtain independent verification of abuse memories in 85 per cent of a sample of twenty individuals suffering from severe dissociative conditions. Seventy-six per cent of Herman and Schatzow's clients in group therapy found independent evidence for their abuse memories (1987). Seventy-three per cent of the subjects in the Ottawa survivors' study of recovered memories of child abuse (Kristiansen et al., 1996) found corroboration for memories of abuse experiences.

A prospective study (Williams, 1994) also fills in some of the gaps in the retrospective research. One hundred and twenty-nine women who had been forensically examined and medically treated for sexual assault (some single incidents; some multiple incidents of abuse by the same perpetrator) as children in an American inner-city hospital in the early 1970s were interviewed seventeen years later. They were not informed of their victimization history and were told only that this was a follow-up study of the lives and health of women who, as children, had received medical care at the hospital. Over one-third (38 per cent) did not report the sexual abuse that had been documented in hospital records; nor did they report any other abuse by the same perpetrator. Additional findings, such as their willingness to report sexual assaults at other times in their lives, suggest that most of these women actually did not remember the abuse, rather than simply chose not to speak about it.

Although some who did not remember the abuse were very young at the time, others just as young remembered their experiences. In fact, most of the girls were at least seven years old at the time of the abuse, and nearly one-third of those abused between the ages of seven and ten and over one-quarter of those abused between the ages of eleven and twelve did not recall the abuse. These findings suggest that having no memory of child sexual abuse experiences is common, not only among white middle-class adults in therapy (Briere & Conte, 1993), but among a community group of primarily poor, African-American women.

Exactly what happens in the brain when people forget traumatic events in this way is·not yet clear. It may well be quite a while before neuroscience catches up with clinical observation. Although there is much we do not know about the coping mechanisms (whether we label them 'repression,' 'amnesia,' 'dissociation,' or just plain forgetting) that render the memories of some traumatic events inaccessible to consciousness for a while, and then, in some cases, accessible again, we need to theorize about the process in order to do our work. We must also be aware that our theories are bound to be challenged and enriched in time. Obviously, more research is needed to test specific hypotheses concerning the psychological mechanisms through which abuse memories are laid down, are lost, and are recovered (Williams, 1994).

One way to conceptualize this phenomenon of forgetting significant, traumatic events is to use a different way of thinking about forgetting and remembering. According to this concept, some of what we call forgetting is actually dissociation – that is, the partitioned assimilation of information and experience. Memory is the returning to the compartment into which the information was assimilated (Crabtree, 1993). State-dependent knowledge, in which one learns something in one state of consciousness and then cannot recall it in another, altered state of consciousness is a well-known phenomenon. For example, if an individual learns innumerable verses of a bawdy song when drunk, it is quite likely that the song will not be recalled in any detail the next morning. However, if the same level of intoxication is reached the following evening, or even the next month, the song may well be remembered in full.

This appears to be what is sometimes happening in the therapy process when information that seems to have been entirely forgotten is retrieved in altered states of consciousness. In fact, the notion of 'forgetting' is misleading in this context. It is more a matter of shifting states of consciousness rendering previously inaccessible material accessible.

Memory of traumatic experiences can be quite different from the memory of everyday events that are not particularly noteworthy. Generally, information processing consists of making mental models and trying to fit new experiences into the schemata already developed. These cognitive models determine the extent to which new information is absorbed and how it is understood and integrated. Thus, memories of particular events can become inaccurate when new information and old are mixed together in the development of flexible mental schemata that allow an individual to use the information in an adaptive fashion (van der Kolk & van der Hart, 1995).

For example, when I was a young, inexperienced, and intensely perfectionistic mother in the 1960s, I spent a fair bit of time with a neighbour who had a couple of children the age of my own and who was also a university student. We had these important things in common, as well as a need for company and support, but we were very different in our approach to childrearing. She was more or less reproducing, according to her, the conventional and satisfactory way she was raised in the 1940s and 1950s, and I was trying to do it all differently. In this context, I loaned her A.S. Neil's treatise on permissive education and childrearing practice, *Summerhill*, and another book along the same lines, *The Free Family*, by two disciples of Wilhelm

Reich, about their adventures raising their five small girls. When she returned the books, I asked her what she thought of them. She replied that she hadn't seen much new in them, and that she was basically raising her children to be self-reliant, just as the books recommended.

I do not think I said anything, but I can remember being flabbergasted that she could incorporate ideas that were so different from hers into her frame of reference, without even noticing the differences. It was not that there was anything wrong with her childrearing practices. Her children were well loved and probably did grow up to be self-reliant. But her ideas and the ways in which she carried them out were, as I saw them, very different from those the books proposed. She made the books work for her, however, and though the accuracy of her interpretation is highly questionable, it was undoubtedly adaptive. Integrating them as she did into her mental model of what it was to be a competent mother was very sensible at a time in our lives when we needed all the support we could get for our fledging efforts as parents.

The memories that are made from this kind of adaptive reworking process – and all the other reworkings that go on further down the line as the impression of an experience is bent to match a later experience, which gets connected to another experience, and another, and so on, in the creation of the cognitive framework that shows us how to understand the world – are malleable through this constant reworking. Traumatic memory, however, is sometimes much more fixed, much less malleable – and therefore much more reliable as to detail – than less charged memories, for the very reason that such memories are more difficult to integrate into a general cognitive schema. Van der Kolk and van der Hart (1995) note that it is ironic that some abuse survivors most desperately need what is falsely claimed about them. They need the same kind of normal bad memory that most of us have – malleable, flexible memory that does not have such a vise grip on the present.

Many individuals encode their experiences in a way that is not distorted. Vivid and detailed recollections of traumatic events are often retrieved from dissociated states of consciousness, where previously they had been inaccessible to the individual's day-to-day consciousness. The notion of state-dependent memory, in which dissociated memories that were encoded under conditions of great stress are brought into focused awareness – that is, remembered – in another situation similar enough to the original to cause the brain stimuli to travel down the same neural pathways, thus activating the original memory, is one familiar to clinicians working with trauma survivors.

In child welfare settings, for example, mothers are frequently triggered to remember their own abuse histories – or to become upset about them if they never dissociated them off from their general awareness – when their children disclose sexual abuse. Again, this is not an unusual experience. It is not uncommon for people to block the memory of unpleasant events and then recover them suddenly in a context that stimulates their conscious recollection. The reason for the compartmentalization of the memory of such experiences is the same as for the abuse survivor: to enable the individual to concentrate on the tasks of daily living rather than be continually focused on the traumatic, upsetting, or even simply disagreeable event.

This is not to imply that all memories of traumatic experiences are fixed and reliable. Assessing the accuracy of memory retrieved from altered states of consciousness involves exploring the degree of distortion inflicted on the individual's perception in the original state, as well as the influences that are later brought to bear. Contexts in which children are subjected to the extreme forms of bizarre and sadistic treatment are contexts in which deliberate 'gaslighting' is a common occurrence. Children appear to be brainwashed into a twisted view of reality that serves the interests of the abusers in a variety of ways. This can make the task of understanding what actually happened in a given experience being remembered particularly difficult, and sometimes impossible.

Fortunately, although we may often find ourselves holding an opinion or an impression about the veridicality of our clients' reports of their experiences, it is not the therapists' responsibility to determine the accuracy of our clients' memories of trauma. It is the role of the therapist to facilitate the healing process. Part of that healing process for the survivor of childhood abuse is often to come to some understanding of the events of her life – what happened to her and how it affected her. It is up to her to create a meaningful autobiographical narrative. Therapists who usurp the role of their clients in the slow and difficult process of putting together the pieces of their life's puzzle are not doing their clients any service, no matter how much their clients may implore them to supply the final paragraph of the story for them.

'Believe the survivor' was a basic principle of early abuse survivor counselling. It evolved as a reaction against almost a century of denying, discounting, and reinterpreting, by mental health professionals, the reality of child sexual abuse experiences as lies, fantasies, or wishful thinking. This tenet was never meant to provide a shortcut through the complicated and difficult process of developing self-knowledge and personal wisdom.

The command to believe those who spoke about their histories of childhood assaults was also not meant to defy common sense. Members of the clinical community have always been aware that everyone remembers some events quite accurately, some events partially (perhaps mixing up some of the details with some other events and forgetting some details altogether), some events in only the fuzziest way, and some events, which are witnessed by others, not at all. No one who has considered the subject holds the view that anyone's memory is perfect and complete.

It also makes no sense to claim that one group of people has a completely unique cognitive or moral capacities. Therefore, to declare that women are credible when they report childhood abuse merely means that there are no conditions per se that preclude them from competently testifying to their own experience (Campbell, 1995). It is not a claim, as some of the False Memory Syndrome Foundation's spokespersons maintain, that 'absolute belief in the accuracy and truthfulness of all charges is the only appropriate stance' (Ofshe and Watters, 1994, p. 5), or that 'memories are always true' (McHugh, 1993, p. 18).

The False Memory Syndrome Foundation is an advocacy group for parents who are accused of sexually abusing their children. It was created in 1992 by Pamela Freyd, whose daughter Jennifer accused her father of incest. Although no one can state this with certainty, some of its members have probably been mistakenly or falsely accused, and some of its members probably did abuse their children; certainly some of them have been convicted in a court of law of sexually abusing their children. As well as parents and other relatives of people claiming to have been sexually abused in childhood, the FMSF has drawn a number of influential academics – psychiatrists, psychologists and sociologists – as members and/or advisors.

This is a relatively wealthy organization, with a large public relations budget, and one of the main solutions to their perception of the problem of so-called false memories is to bankroll lawsuits against psychotherapists who work with abuse survivors, with the long-range goal, according to their newsletter, of shutting down the business of sexual abuse treatment altogether. Their attacks on individual therapists are often scurrilous and irresponsible, and although they pay lip service to the reality of child sexual abuse as a social problem, they do not advocate education to remedy what they see as therapeutic mistakes and excesses. Rather, they support the destruction of the community of psychotherapists in the courts and in the media, the court of public opinion.

The False Memory Syndrome Foundation's professional proponents' most common tactic is to attribute to clinicians a view of memory – the video recorder view – that is not held by many, if any, therapists. McHugh says that therapists who attempt to recover hidden memories are committed to the belief that 'memories are always true' (1993, p. 18). Lindsay and Read declare that such clinicians 'think of memory as a sort of video library of their personal histories, and of remembering as akin to replaying a video of the past ... that memory is perfect and complete, requiring only the proper cues to allow people to retrieve accurate records of past experiences' (1994, p. 284). Ofshe and Watters claim that 'Recovered memory therapy's conception of how memory functions assumes that the *human* mind records and stores everything perceived' (1994, p. 5). They all set up a 'straw man' – the credulous psychotherapist who does not have the wits to realize that every ostensible memory retrieved in therapy may not be accurate and infallible.

Stephen Braude, examining the subject of multiple personality from the point of view of a philosopher rather than a clinician, notes that the attacks directed against mental health profession by these FMSF advocates are either utterly naive and ignorant about the professional literature on dissociation and memory, or they are intellectually dishonest. He concludes that, disheartening as the latter conjecture (a tactic of deliberate dishonesty) may be, it is a great deal more credible than the possibility that these intellectual luminaries could unknowingly resort to 'transparently fallacious arguments and shoddy dialectical tactics that they presumably would not employ in other contexts, or whose defects they would be quick to spot if they had been the target of that criticism' (Braude, 1995, p. 254).

Elizabeth Loftus, one of the most voluble FMSF advocates, is a psychologist with a distinguished twenty-year career in the area of memory research. Her work indeed shows that individuals can be suggestible enough to be persuaded to describe unpleasant events that never happened but were suggested to them by a researcher. Her research also shows that when people do remember things, their memories are often faulty about some of the details, particularly the peripheral details, and that, in fact, memory experiences are always subjected to some degree of cognitive distortion (Loftus, 1994, 1993, 1979). None of this is surprising; nor does it in any way undermine the credibility of a sound psychotherapy that involves the recovery of some memories that were inaccessible to the client before the therapy process was initiated, as Loftus seems to assume in recent publications and public addresses on the topic. In fact, as Richard Kluft (1995a) noted, some of Loftus' most famous studies attesting to human suggestibility – for example, the scenario in which a boy was persuaded that he experienced an unpleasant event that had never happened (getting lost in a mall) – are more convincing as an explanation of the retraction syndrome, in which relatives (who have a clear stake in effecting the suggestion) persuade abuse survivors to believe that their abuses never happened.

In attempting to alter the legal and social climate that has enabled increasing numbers of sexual abuse claims to be heard openly, the False Memory Syndrome Foundation has taken up the issue of memory contestation (just how reliable are our so-called memories, really?) but has limited its focus to one group of citizens – women who declare that they were sexually abused in childhood. This is a flagrantly political strategy, and it poses a threat to the credibility of any marginalized group that would make a public claim about harm done to them in the past (Campbell, 1995).

Research on memories of all ages and genders of people in all sorts of situations (except, ironically, the relevant one of severe, early trauma) is used to indict the memories of one group of people, women claiming to have been abused in childhood. In challenging the credibility of this one group, a special discourse has been created to serve the political purposes of the attack. In this discourse, all manner of ways of reporting events with more or less accuracy – mistakes, screen memories, lies, confabulations, partial memories, basically accurate memories with a few details wrong – become 'false memories.'

The FMSF proponents and their like are creating a double standard for credibility in offering personal testimony. Most of us are assumed to be reporting the facts as we understand them when we recount our experiences of yesterday or ten years ago. Allowances are made – without even giving it much consideration – for differences in interpretation, for the ravages of time on the amount and accuracy of detail, particularly peripheral detail, and for other aspects of recollection that make the telling of our stories more or less exactly representative of the historical event. However, according to the norms of the discourse now being established around the issue of 'false memories,' claims of childhood sexual abuse would be viewed differently from other testimonials. Not only would they not be assumed to be generally veridical when reported by adult women, but they would be assumed to be false by reference to their context. 'She claims to have remembered being abused as a child? Was she in therapy at the time? Ah, most likely a case of false memory!'

Such a rhetorical strategy occludes the possibility that certain incest survivors can actually be incest survivors, and that women in certain cultural locations can engage in credible memory claims (Campbell, 1995). I do not think it is accidental that the women especially targeted by the FMSF are from race and class positions (white, middle and upper class) in society whose testimony regarding their life experiences would be a threat to another corresponding group of citizens (white middle- and upper-class men) who have the most to lose were their claims to be translated from personal testimony to legal testimony.

Loftus insists, in *The Myth of Repressed Memory: False Memories and Allegations of Sexual Abuse*, that 'this is not a debate about the reality or the horror of sexual abuse, incest, or violence against children. This is a debate about memory' (1994, p. xi). The location of scholars such as Loftus on the advisory board of the False Memory Syndrome Foundation belies her words. The study of memory is, indeed, an important part of developing an educated and responsible stance toward the psychotherapy client who seems to be uncovering childhood abuse experiences. However, the presentation of the issue of memory within the context of a misogynist interpretation of women (women claiming to have been sexually abused in childhood, at any rate) as 'blank canvases on which the therapist paints' (Ofshe & Watters, 1993, p. 9), victims-in-training who 'discover that playing the sexual abuse victim is both a demanding and engaging role' (p. 7), makes a joke of the claim that this is a disinterested scholarly debate. This is a battle to return women to their traditional role as false, malleable, morally irresponsible, and essentially noncredible. This is a struggle to undermine the legitimacy of our newly developed and hard-won understanding about the extent, purposes, and effects of the sexual exploitation of children in our society.

We who are engaging in the practice of psychotherapy with survivors of interpersonal abuse in childhood are in the position of attempting to help the individuals we work with build a sense of themselves as basically credible persons, deserving of the rights supposedly accorded to all people. On a personal level, individuals who were robbed of their birthright of secure self-respect find it immensely difficult to create such a radically different sense of self later in life. The social climate in which they conduct their healing process today is fraught with the same message that was continually imposed upon them in childhood – 'you do not own your body, your feelings, or your thoughts (what you think are your memories); they are mine for the taking.' This makes their task of healing from the assaults that were perpetrated upon them all the more difficult, and it makes our job as therapists harder as well.

The Canadian Broadcasting Corporation television program *the fifth estate*'s segment debunking the legitimacy of multiple personality disorder (10 November 1993) provoked powerful responses in many viewers. Some of them sent me copies of their protests to the show's producers and to the CBC. Many of these letters addressed the writer's outrage at the irresponsible way in which the program claimed that their experience of identity construction and remembering was simply an artefact of manipulative therapists.

Two weeks after the show aired, one woman spoke to me personally in a particularly poignant way about the way in which the program undermined her developing ability to come to grips with her childhood abuse. In her case, she said, there was no doubt about the events; they are documented in child welfare and court records.

But even so, I was only just beginning to believe that these horrible things happened, and that, in order not to explode completely, I divided myself up in pieces and did my best to forget much of it. Now, every time I remember something or feel something about what I am remembering, I see the condescending face of the narrator of that show, Trish Woods. I hear her say pityingly, her voice dripping with sweetness and contempt, 'You believe *that?*' And I think again what I always thought when little pieces of the abuse would come into my mind – that I have no right to think that he would do such things, and there is just something basically wrong with me.

If the goal of the false memory apologists is to undermine our society's recently developed consciousness (and conscience, perhaps) about the pervasiveness of the sexual exploitation of children and to silence the voices of adult survivors of such abuse, this woman's words show how well the strategy may be succeeding – at the private as well as the public level.

8

Ritual Abuse

Somewhere every culture has an imaginary zone for what it excludes, and it is this zone we must try to remember today.

Catherine Clément, quoted in Sandra Gilbert (1986)

Just as therapy for people with severe dissociative conditions is the same as therapy for anyone else who wants in-depth dynamic therapy – only more so – so is ritual abuse like other abuse – only more so. More so is a significant qualifier. More so means a lot. What it does not mean, however, is freakish, qualitatively different, or 'other.'

This can be a hard point to keep in mind when a therapist is working with their first client who alleges a background of ritual abuse, but it is key. The horror that the therapist has to face and feel in order to connect empathically with individuals who are recounting the annihilation of their humanity through the type of deliberate, sadistic abuse they suffered as children in cult groups can rock the therapist's existential grounding to a degree not previously experienced in encounters with more common forms of incest and battery. The temptation to escape facing one's helplessness in the face of the possibility of such evil can be great, and one of the surest ways of escape is denial. Another is through making the phenomenon of ritual abuse into something out of the human realm – framing the abuse as subhuman, perhaps, and the survivor as someone who is not like anyone else we know, whose problems demand an entirely different stance than any of the other problems we deal with as therapists.

As a defensive manoeuvre, this enables both therapist and survivor to escape the gruelling process of encountering and coping with these atrocities in much the same way, basically, that everyone struggles with coming to understand the ways in which we have all been treated badly, whether just somewhat insensitively some of the time through the ignorance and carelessness of one's caretakers, or with deliberate cruelty most of the time. Making a radical distinction between the ritual abuse survivor and everyone else may protect therapists from feeling their client's anguish personally. Unfortunately, it also stunts our capacity to help the survivor heal, for we can only reach out to someone whose experience touches ours in some way.

I have stopped teaching about ritual abuse in any context in which it is advertised as the principal topic. When representatives of the media want to interview me because they have heard that I am an expert on ritual abuse, I tell them that they have been misinformed. The reason for this is that I have found that no matter what I might say to attempt to place my thoughts about treating survivors of ritual abuse in context, agendas other than mine seem to prevail.

I remember offering a workshop on the subject at a conference that I organized myself in 1989, thinking that in those circumstances I would have some degree of control. I opened the lecture with all the caveats I could think of about the lack of data about prevalence regarding sadistic abuse perpetrated by groups, about being qualified only to talk about creating a safe and effective treatment regimen for clients who talk about these extreme kind of abuse experiences, and so on.

As soon as I stopped to take a breath, the room was flooded with questions about the FBI, law enforcement interventions, exorcism, international conspiracies, methods of intervening in kidnapping schemes, strategies for making sure people do not return to the cult, locations of cult groups in Ontario – none of which I know anything about, and none of which were the business of the members of the audience, almost all of whom were psychotherapists. I allowed the rain of questions to fall for awhile to illustrate the point I eventually made about the ubiquity and intensity of countertransference in the work with those who allege childhood experiences of ritual abuse. I expect that most of the participants at that workshop went away disappointed that I knew so little about the topics that interested them. It is very hard for many practitioners simply to do therapy with these people, rather than 'do something.' Anything.

There are a number of issues that need to be addressed in order to talk sensibly about treating ritual abuse survivors. The most obvious is the very existence of the phenomenon of ritual abuse, especially intergenerational satanic cult abuse, which is most frequently reported by individuals suffering from dissociative identity disorder. There are many legally substantiated cases of satanic activity and associated crime. Richard Ramirez, called the 'Nightstalker' and convicted of thirteen murders in California, was an avowed satanist, whose statement upon being sentenced to death row included praise for the devil. Crime with obviously satanic trappings seems to be most commonly perpetrated by adolescents, or perhaps adolescents are simply more likely to be caught. Sean Sellars, the youngest death row inmate in the United States, was convicted of three murders (including those of his mother and stepfather) committed in 1986 when he was fifteen years of age. This boy was introduced to satanic rituals when he was ten years old by a babysitter, and by the time he was a teenager – by his own report and the physical evidence used against him in court – he was deeply involved in cult activity, keeping a satanic diary, carrying out more and more elaborate rituals, and regularly and compulsively drinking his own blood (Lawson, 1990).

We have also seen numerous examples of cult groups that are dominated by a charismatic leader – Charlie Manson, Jim Jones, David Koresh – and there is a great deal of evidence that the physical and sexual abuse of both children and adults is part of the mind-control armamentarium of these groups. A group in Burnt River, Ontario, was broken up by the police in the mid-1980s, and the leader, Roch la Roch, was convicted of murder and mutilation for crimes committed against members of the cult. Twenty-three children were taken into the care of the local child welfare agency, many of them the offspring of la Roch and female cult members. The loyalty of some of these women remains with la Roch, and a group of them live not far from the maximum security penitentiary in which he is incarcerated. They are producing a new generation of children in spousal visits, and they declare that they intend to live with la Roch upon his release, despite the fact that child welfare authorities have assured them that they will once again lose their children in this event.

We live in a violent society. It is also – at least nominally – a predominantly Christian society, and Satan is the most powerful Judaeo-Christian symbol for evil. It is clear that many individuals and groups perpetrating acts of violence claim Satan as their muse and their god. This is not surprising. It does not, however, supply us with any information about a phenomenon that is more than isolated acts of social mayhem, linked by a popular religious and cultural symbol. Evidence of an international conspiracy of satanic cult groups that operate around a core of intergenerational families and practice murder, cannibalism, and ritual torture on a massive scale – or even of a plethora of individual groups that regularly rape, mutilate, and kill in the name of Satan – has not been found.

The question, 'Does satanic ritual abuse exist?' is not the same type of question as 'Does multiple personality disorder exist?' As Colin Ross (1990) points out in 'Twelve Cognitive Errors about Multiple Personality Disorder,' the second question, as phrased, is based on a cognitive error, a 'straw man error' that sets up a position no one holds and then discredits a different position by arguing against the former. According to this reasoning, because people with multiple personality do not indeed have other people living inside of them, as they believe, the condition of multiple personality does not exist.

The question 'Does ritual abuse exist?' is the equivalent of the question, 'Does child abuse exist?' Both are reasonable questions. In response to the latter, a great deal of research has been conducted, and the reality of child abuse has been convincingly documented as pervasive in our society.

We are not in the same, or even a similar but more preliminary position, regarding the documentation of ritual abuse, especially intergenerational satanic cult abuse. We are hearing survivor stories, striking in their similarity, from people who seem to have had no contact with each other. That was at one time a somewhat cogent argument in favor of the veracity of a phenomenon that had not yet been widely covered in the media. That cannot be said in the past few years. Individuals recollecting detailed experiences of satanic abuse may well have other sources besides their own life history to draw upon such that they can incorporate images and associated feelings into their consciousness and experience them as personal memories.

My opinion is that some cases of alleged ritual abuse are imagined, concocted, confabulated, or exaggerated, and that some are not. But, frankly, I am not sure my opinion about this matter is worth very much. I have not conducted any systematic research on the topic; no one has, as far as I know. It is in the nature of the problem that such research is very difficult to do. If indeed it is true that many people are being abused, tortured, and murdered each year, as part of large satanic organizations, I wish I had the information that would allow me to say so with confidence and credibility. I regret the necessity to be rigorous about what I know and what I do not know, because I am aware that my ignorance and uncertainty might well be used in the interests of those who have managed successfully to evade detection thus far. The bottom line, though – frustrating as it may be at times – is that we can only truthfully speak to what we know.

However, though I do not know much about the prevalence or even the reality of satanic cults that operate in a widespread, intergenerational way and that regularly perpetrate such atrocities as multiple human sacrifice and cannibalistic rituals, I have had experience treating some individuals who bring to the therapy context vivid images and powerful accompanying affect of being victimized within such contexts, and I can speak to that treatment. These people usually suffer from severe posttraumatic stress, and their treatment process is often even longer and more gruelling that the average therapy of a highly dissociative trauma survivor. When they have access to effective treatment and have the personal resources to complete the process, many of them get better.

I am going to employ a linguistic strategy, in discussing this topic, by using the term 'ritual abuse survivor' or 'survivor of sadistic group abuse' rather than qualifying these terms insistently and interminably. There are a number of reasons for this, but it comes down to a decision not to be more hurtful and insulting than is absolutely necessary to a group of people who have already been hurt enough. In fact, although other forms of child abuse and maltreatment of many other sorts are much more well-documented than ritual abuse, in most of the situations I deal with in treatment, I have no independent knowledge, outside of what my client reports to me about her life, that would make it proper for me to speak definitively about the veridicality of her allegations. In the therapy context, I do not make it my business to be the expert on what is historically accurate and what is not in my clients' recounting of their histories.

Just as it is crucial for therapists working with individuals suffering from multiple personality to be well grounded in general in-depth dynamic psychotherapy, so it is important for a therapist working with ritual abuse survivors to be experienced in both dynamic psychotherapy and in the treatment of severe dissociation. All ritual abuse survivors do not suffer from multiple personality, but dissociation, and often the most extreme forms of dissociation, are a major line of defence against the kind of assaults that are perpetrated on children within such milieux.

Much of the process needed to enable ritual abuse survivors to heal and lead happy, productive, responsible lives is basically the same process that all survivors of childhood trauma need to go through. Everything I talk about in terms of learning the language of the survivor, and structuring the treatment process so that grounding in everyday reality precedes, is concurrent with, and follows uncovering and processing trauma should be underscored when working with survivors of ritual abuse. There are also some issues worthy of attention because they apply specifically to the treatment of sadistic abuse perpetrated by groups. Let me frame them as some combination of commandments and caveats.

Take the same disinterested stance with memories of ritual abuse experiences as you would with any memories emerging in a psychotherapeutic process.

The word 'disinterested,' in this context, is in no way synonomous with uninterested. A disinterested stance is characterized by freedom from bias, pre-judgment. This is a difficult position to find or maintain, particularly vis-à-vis an issue as loaded as child abuse in its most extreme forms. In fact, although it is crucial to create and maintain personal and professional boundaries around our tendency to react in an emotionally-charged fashion to reports of ritual abuse from our clients, it is not possible to be utterly disinterested. We are all influenced by our personal histories and the social contexts in which we develop our perspectives and values. How we hear reports of child sexual abuse in the 1990s, for example, is an outcome of the changing social climate of the 1980s.

In the 1970s, child sexual abuse was generally understood to be a rare aberration in our society, an exception to the rule of happy, healthy families. In the 1980s, widespread child sexual abuse became an increasingly horrifying reality. Within a very short period, the general societal understanding of family life – and the experiences of children in other institutional settings such as schools – changed radically. The time when the 'click' of awareness about sexual abuse as a reality in a vast number of children's lives may have come at somewhat different times for different individuals, but between 1978 and 1988, North American societal perception changed from practically no awareness or interest in the issue to a situation in which child sexual abuse has become widely spoken of – from a variety of points of view – in almost every area of social discourse.

As a child welfare worker in the 1980s, I had to respond in practical ways to this change. Knowing that many of the children we had previously understood to be unhappy, delinquent, or exhibiting distress in any number of ways that brought them under the perview of the social systems, were being sexually assaulted by the adults who were charged with their care – parents, foster parents, teachers, clergy, coaches, babysitters, other relatives – created immediate and enormous problems for social service workers. We had rapidly to rethink our policies and interventions, and rebuild a wide array of social structures.

In Toronto, where I was practising at the time, police, social workers, judges, teachers, crown attorneys, doctors, and psychotherapists worked together to create cooperative policies and procedures that would enable us to protect these children whose needs we understood – quite correctly – to have been previously ignored and misunderstood. By necessity, changes in social policy and judicial intervention were made quickly, with little knowledge and research (Rivera, 1988b). The same efforts were made throughout North America, changing the ways in which we understood children's lives and responded to their cries for help.

At that time, I was part of a large group of therapists, representing a wide variety of agencies and private practice settings, who came together bi-monthly for a number of years in the 1980s to teach ourselves and each other about the effective and responsible treatment of children who had been sexually abused and adults who had been sexually abused as children. We were individually very different, in terms of educational backgrounds, practice disciplines, and personal and political perspectives. What we shared was a horror at the realization of how we and our professions had colluded in the social silence that had allowed children to be sexually abused for generations. A statement of implicit belief in allegations of sexual abuse that children made was the cornerstone of the philosophy of this group – and many others like it.

This made sense then. It is still applicable in a large majority of cases. But it did not reflect the complexity of the issues that were to be faced in the not too distant future when we would be listening, not only to the stories of children speaking about what happened to them when they went home from school each day, but to adults who were speaking about experiences they had had thirty years previously, the details of which were not clear even to them. Because we were appalled at the decades of incredulity that had been accorded to women who dared to speak out about their sexual exploitation as children, we declared that we would believe. We are now coming to know that it is not so simple.

The comforting simplicity of unconditional belief is not always reasonable or helpful when confronted by memories buried within layers of dissociated states of consciousness. This is especially true when the dissociation is a result of a history of deliberate torture, distortion of perception, and therefore of memory. In these cases, it is not always easy to distinguish accurate recall from dreams, fantasies, cognitive distortion, confabulation, screen memory, and sometimes deliberately induced confusion.

For example, an individual uncovers a memory of having been operated on as a child in a ceremony in the woods. The images are vivid and persuasive, and she believes she is recalling something that actually happened to her at the age of six or seven. In preparation for the operation, she is forced to witness the killing of her pet dog and to watch as the animal is eviscerated and its heart cut out. The child remembers being cut with a large knife. She remembers her heart being cut out and the dog's heart being sewn into her chest cavity. She remembers waking up with a pain in her chest, and for years she carries a scar in the area of the heart which is still faintly visible. She remembers being told that if she ever tells anyone about the cult, the dog's heart will explode inside of her, and she will die.

She remembers that, from then on, whenever she thinks about the cult experiences in a situation in which she is tempted to speak about them (at school, for example) she can feel the heart getting larger inside her chest and beating very fast, and she knows that explosion is imminent. The only way she can get the heart to shrink again is to think about something else. When she talks to her therapist about this in the state of consciousness or alter personality of the child who remembers the experience, she says, 'They cut out my heart and put my dog's heart inside me.'

How does this kind of report fit with a simple dictum to 'Believe the survivor?' We know that dog to human heart transplants are not within the realm of medical possibility. Indeed, other parts of the survivor will use the preposterousness of her claim to be living with a dog's heart inside her as proof that all of the claims of abuse and ritual torture are bogus.

From a therapist's point of view, it is easy to speculate about what might be the reality of this situation, to conjecture a maze of trickery perpetrated on a developmentally vulnerable child that effectively ensured silence and secrecy. But this is speculation; maybe it is what happened and maybe it is not. It is not something that could be taken to court.

This example illustrates the problematic nature of assessing the historical reality of many memories recovered in trance states, memories of abuse of small children by adults who had a big stake in making them confused and unbelievable – particularly in assessing some types of ritual abuse memories. It is a helpful example because it forces us to face the reality that simple rules about believing the survivor are not a useful guide to clinical practice.

Obviously, when this woman reports that she was subjected to a dog to human heart transplant at the hands of the cult, we know her recollections are contaminated. Even if we do not have such obvious impossibilities in other situations – especially when there has been no conscious recall, no corroboration, and very little ability to integrate these images with other, more mundane life experiences – there is no reason to assume that other assertions may not also represent an inaccurate picture of the historical reality. It is important to ensure that, as clinicians, we do not become wedded to a version of reality that may turn out to be significantly distorted or – with the best intentions in the world – we may reinforce the agenda of the original abusers and thus impede the healing process.

Again, many children who were abused in group settings, such as daycare centres, report that their mommies and daddies were there when they were being abused, or that they participated in the abuse in situations in which it was confirmed to be physically impossible for this to have happened as reported. Placing pieces of the puzzle together, strategies of trickery have been uncovered in which the children were convinced in a variety of ways – from animated pictures flashed on the wall of a darkened room, to conversations in which the abuser seems to be taking orders from the child's parent, to simple assertions such as, 'Your mommy told us to do this, and she said if you ever talk to anyone about it, even to her and daddy, we should kill you – that their parents' had authorized and participated in abuses that, in fact, the parents knew nothing about. These fairly simple techniques causing cognitive distortion perpetrated on young children lead them to uncover memories of their parents abusing them.

Not only is it important for therapists not to have their own agendas about the historical reality of the survivor's recollections because they may well be wrong, it is also completely unnecessary to have an accurate knowledge of a person's abuse history in detail in order to help that person. Mostly, when a client begs us to tell her whether or not she was really abused – or is she just making this all up? – the appropriate therapeutic response is an empathic reflection of her torment. 'You would like someone to settle this struggle for you once and for all.' A response that takes that struggle away from the survivor, no matter how welcomed, does not help her to claim her own life history as hers.

Even if the therapist happens to be right when she replies with an emphatic affirmative (or an attempt to persuade the client that she must face the truth about being abused if she is to heal) to the cry, 'Do you believe that these things these parts of me are talking about really happened as they say they did?' she has usurped her client's role in coming to understand and accept her own history. If the therapist happens not to be right and affirms all kinds of distortions as reliable memory, she is likely to be actively standing in the way of her client's progress in coming to grips with her life, for now the client has, not only the complexities of her own memory and meaning system to unravel, but her therapist's agendas and distortions as well.

The bottom line is that, much of the time, as therapists, we do not know exactly what happened to our clients, and we do not need to know to be helpful. Clients' transferential projections of omniscience – sometimes, unfortunately, combining with therapists' countertransferential delusions of omniscience or, more commonly, therapists' inability to confront the client's acute desire for us to be omniscient and all-powerful – make it hard for therapists to acknowledge the reality that much of the time we just do not know. This is particularly true when the memories being considered are of intergenerational satanic ritual abuse because we cannot even say – as we can about abuse experiences such as incest – that we know that they do happen to hundreds of thousands of other people.

What appears to be a deficit, however, does not need to be so. The more I, as a therapist, insist that it is only the individual who can say what happened to her and what she thinks it means, the more I reinforce the basic message of the therapy process – that her life is her own, and it does not belong to her abusers, or to me, or to anyone else.

Therapists are not parents, police officers, or priests.

Working with people who talk about being subjected to the atrocities of ritual abuse can have an extremely disorienting effect on a therapist. One of the first signs of this disorientation is often forgetting or deliberately throwing out the job description that has stood us in good stead until then. Therapists sometimes find themselves caretaking these clients in a way that, under ordinary circumstances, they would understand as disempowering rather than helpful.

Another sign of therapist role confusion can be an obsession with the details of ritual abuse, either the particular client's own history or the phenomenon in general. Further investigation of allegations of ritual abuse should undoubtedly be under-taken by law enforcement officials. But unless the therapist genuinely decides on a career change, the only effect that part-time, unofficial, untrained therapist inves-tigation will have is to derail the therapy process.

The drive to find the 'truth' often springs from two sources: protecting the survivor from ongoing abuse and supporting her as she navigates the legal system. It is common in both of these contexts for a therapist to not only forget what her job is, and therefore stop doing it, but also to start desperately trying to do things that are impossible for her.

As therapists, we know people will sometimes be hurt by others and will also engage in all kinds of behaviour that is anywhere on the self-destruction continuum from foolish to deliberately dangerous. We do not assume people in therapy will no longer be hurt in life by others or by themselves, and we do not think that we can protect them from such hurts. But when someone who reports a history of ritual abuse tells a therapist that the cult is kidnapping her every full moon and forcing her to participate in ceremonies in which she is tortured and raped, it is not uncommon for the therapist to take all kinds of extraordinary protective measures, losing sight of the fact that her job is to facilitate the client's own ability to take care of herself.

There are a number of ways in which this kind of intervention is problematic. In the first place, many survivors of ritual abuse have a great deal of difficulty distinguishing past from present, or in distinguishing personally-generated reality from consensually-validatable reality. Sometimes reports that they are being watched, abducted, or revictimized are elaborations of threats and fears from the original abuse context rather than actual dangers in the present. If the therapist not only assumes all such reports to be the literal present-day reality, but re-enforces that assumption by engaging in concrete rescuing manoeuvres, she has made it extremely difficult for the survivor to untangle past from present and to develop grounded ways of interpreting her own reality and protecting herself.

Even if the survivor is in actual danger in the present, it is the therapist's job to help her understand and learn to cope with her reality rather than to deal with it for her. There are many ways of being in danger, and therapists rarely intervene directly in their clients' lives, even when the danger is potentially life-threatening. We do not follow our sexually active clients around to make sure they engage only in safe sex practices; we help them develop their own awareness on whatever level is appropriate, whether it means offering sex education or helping them wrestle with the conflicts that cause them to behave in a way that places them in danger. If we feel like calling up the husband of a client and telling him to stop beating his wife, we would know that countertransference is at work in the situation, and we would examine our own motivations rather than act on the impulse.

This is not because active protective interventions are not entirely appropriate in certain situations, with friends or relatives, on behalf of clients who are children, or if we are police officers or child protection workers. If we assess our client as immediately likely to commit suicide or homicide, it is our professional responsibility to intervene, and if we suspect child abuse, we have a legal mandate to see that this is reported to the authorities. But as therapists, even in these situations in which we have no choice but to intervene, the more we can do to empower the client to act in a self-protective way on her own behalf, the more effectively we are doing our job. Our role as a therapist is to help an individual develop her own strengths, and we undermine those strengths when we encourage or even allow her to place the locus of control with us, no matter how much she might wish to do so in situations that confuse and terrify her.

When a therapist is working with a child, or with an adult who is reporting information that is directly relevant to the welfare of a child, the issue of the literal truth of the reports of abuse and ritualized crimes against children becomes much more urgent, but not necessarily easier to untangle. Suspected crimes of abuse against children must be reported to the child welfare authorities by all professionals, and it makes sense for the therapist to think as broadly as possible when assessing the statements and the behaviour of a disturbed child. We tend to assume that a young child's problems are a direct reflection of parent-child interaction, but children are not brought up exclusively by their parents. The majority of preschool children and virtually all older children and adolescents have a great deal of contact with adults in positions of authority outside the family.

Parents always assume that if anything as extreme as child abuse, much less severe ongoing ritualized abuse, were happening, their children would tell them. Because of the techniques of mind control that most offenders employ, and because children, in particular, are so malleable, the reality is that many children from loving, communicating families who are subjected to deliberate, sophisticated, and sadistic abuse will not – and cannot – tell. They enter into an altered state of consciousness that may preclude accurate reporting, or any reporting at all, to even the most open and sensitive adults.

However, although taking protective measures when we have professional responsibility for a minor may be entirely appropriate – if difficult to effect – our responsibilities as the therapist of an adult are significantly different. It is sometimes hard to remember that the cowering individual talking babytalk in our office about bad people coming to get her is an adult; still, we collude with her notion that she is a totally helpless child at our peril – and hers.

Trust is an ongoing issue. Try not to get impatient or take things personally.

Deliberately and purposefully perpetrated abuse is always accompanied by isolating the victim in some way and persuading her that connections with others are suspect, that no one is to be trusted. The earlier the onset of the abuse and the more sadistic its form, the more likely the conviction that trust is not only unwarranted but dangerous will be deeply embedded in the worldview of the survivor.

Children who are able to dissociate from their abuse experiences are fortunate in having the opportunity to develop states of consciousness in which they are able to reach out and make positive connections with others, and sometimes therapists will be amazed at the degree to which an individual who has experienced incredible atrocities is able to build caring relationships, including investing deeply in the therapeutic relationship. It can be all the more shocking, therefore, when a client who has seemed to be solidly connected with her therapist for a number of years, suddenly starts expressing deeply felt fears that the therapist's intentions are to suck her in by pretending to be compassionate and understanding and that exploitation of the most terrifying order is just around the corner.

Sometimes this is expressed from the point of view of a discrete personality state, and in that case it is usually easier for the therapist not to take the attack personally. 'It's only Lucifer who thinks such crazy things; I know you are trustworthy.' Often, though, in the later stages of therapy, when there is very little residual dissociation left, deep pockets of suspicion surface and take the therapist, who imagined that the basic tests had been passed long ago, by surprise. Such deep mistrust must be worked through at every level of the survivor's consciousness, and it is important that the therapist encourage its emergence in the therapeutic relationship rather than suppress it by communicating messages of impatience or injured innocence.

Spiritual issues are often very important to ritual abuse survivors.

Most therapists have been educated to see science and spirituality as two separate realms and may have a difficult time accepting their clients' need to struggle with spiritual issues as part of their healing process. Hearing a client obsess over the issue of why God allowed such terrible things happen to her and to other children, secularly trained therapists may be tempted to discount these ruminations and also to experience significant discomfort at being pushed to delve into issues outside their area of competence.

It is crucial that therapists retain their capacity for empathy, even in an area as fraught with personal prejudice as religion. In examining the lives of Holocaust survivors, Henry Krystal (1995) declares that people who are unable to complete mourning have the tendency to build monumental ecclesiastical edifices. This desperate need to construct or adapt to a simple – and often, initially, a rather inauthentic – belief system to counteract a deep and disabling distrust in the ways of humanity, nature, and God, can be exasperating to therapists who do not share in the beliefs. Their lack of empathy in this area can be extremely hurtful to the client and may eventually create a communication impasse. Therapists who share the client's religious beliefs often present their own limitations, when, deliberately or not, they influence the client in the direction of conformity and compliance rather than personal exploration and spiritual growth.

For individuals who feel the need to frame basic existential questions in religious terms, and particularly those for whom participation in organized religion is both a comfort and a necessity, it is helpful if they can be guided to a spiritual director who perceives the value of a psychotherapeutic process and is able to blend counsel about religious and spiritual matters with some knowledge of and respect for the secular aspect of the healing process. However, this referral does not absolve primary therapists from the responsibility of listening as openly, attentively, and respectfully to their clients' communications about religion and spirituality as they listen to anything else.

Many trauma survivors have been influenced by their childhood experiences to steer clear of any form of organized religion. Others are powerfully and sometimes traumatically bonded to fundamentalist religions that reinforce the dichotomous messages of the cult: God is good; you are evil. Put God first, others second, and yourself last. Your feelings are a tool of the devil that will lead you astray. Do not trust yourself and your own perceptions; trust the word of God as interpreted by His minister, and so on.

The French say that when the devil gets old, he gets pious (Krystal, 1995). For people who grow psychologically old long before they grow up – that is, weary, emotionally fragile, deeply unsure of themselves, and profoundly self-hating – simple fundamentalist religious beliefs can be compelling. The destruction of trust and helpless rage that are the consequences of merciless abuse make the evolution of a bouyant faith in a benevolent God or higher power difficult, if not impossible (Krystal, 1978). Rigid, rule-bound religion that does not challenge the survivor's self-hating mental schemata and purports to offer structure and certainty can be a very tempting prospect. Also, church members, whose religious values make them willing to take round-the-clock care of a church member in distress, but who have no training that enables them to enhance an individual's coping capacities, can provide a support system that can be very comforting while being radically disempowering.

Exorcism, a ceremony in which confusion, cognitive distortions, ego-dystonic impulses, anger – indeed, all of the feelings with which abuse survivors struggle – are framed as externally-generated evil that needs to be expelled through dramatic and intrusive means, can be an extremely seductive prospect for some abuse survivors with a religious orientation. As a therapeutic intervention, it almost always creates new problems, in addition to failing to make any positive changes that are not transient.

This is not to comment on the ontological status of spirit possession or to disallow the possibility that exorcism undertaken within the context of religious practice may sometimes have beneficial results. However, all the data currently available about the effect of exorcism on highly dissociative trauma survivors point to a mistaken identification of dissociated ego states as demons, resulting in revictimization and intense psychological and spiritual harm to the subjects of the exorcism ritual (Bowman, 1993; Fraser, 1993).

A therapist cannot offer clear answers, quick solutions, or constant care, and some therapists have found themselves in competition for the allegiance of their clients with church groups that offer rescue and actively undermine the therapy. It is important that the therapist see such groups as she would see any part of the client's life that offers a combination of benefits and problems.

It is not a therapist's business to persuade a client that she needs therapy. It is, however, the responsibility of the therapist to be aware of the ways in which aspects of the client's life are undermining, derailing, or even destroying the therapy process and to find an appropriate way to communicate this to the client. For example, in an extreme situation, a therapist may be unsuccessful in her attempts to help the client see that regularly having a therapy session in which the therapist expresses messages of acceptance to all personality states back to back with exorcism in which certain states are railed at as demonic, is not only contradictory and counterproductive but retraumatizing. In this case, the therapist may have to withdraw from a process in which she can only be part of the problem rather than part of the solution.

Ultimately, it is ideal if the survivor is able to integrate her spiritual concerns and preoccupations with those of a more obviously psychological nature and to subject both to the scrutiny of her growing sense of confidence in her own self-worth and her own evolving perceptions and values. This often leads the survivor into a place where her thinking about basic precepts and eternal verities becomes more complex and less certain. This undermining of religious beliefs that have sometimes been the only still point in a chaotic world can be frightening, and the survivor needs the support of a therapist who can respect and facilitate her quest for spiritual centredness as an important part of her healing, even when it is a stretch for the therapist to communicate in the language of a set of spiritual or religious values that may be very different from the therapist's own.

The first rule of therapy is that the therapist must survive the process.

Many of the guidelines for self-care that make it possible to work creatively with survivors of atrocities of all sorts need to be underscored when therapists work with people who have experienced sadistic and elaborate group abuse in their formative years. There is no way to build an empathic therapeutic alliance and maintain a thoroughly self-protective distance from a client. The nature of developing a therapeutic relationship with an abuse survivor is that the therapist must experience to some degree the fear, pain, rage, disillusionment, and despair that her client feels – at least enough to be able to reflect back that experience with accurate empathy. The healing power of the therapy process is the therapeutic relationship in which the client experiences her therapist responding to her from an experience-near vantage point, that is, placing herself in the inner world of the client so as to understand it from the inside out.

Heinz Kohut introduced the odd term 'self-object' (1971) to refer to the function of a relationship that enables an individual to build, maintain, or restore a vigorous sense of self.

Throughout his [sic] life a person will experience himself as a cohesive harmonious firm unit in time and space, connected with his past and pointed meaningfully into a creative-productive future, only as long as, at each stage in his life, he experiences certain representatives of his human surroundings as joyfully responding to him, as available to him as sources of idealized strength and calmness, as being silently present but in essence like him ... (Kohut, 1984, p. 52)

The heart of the therapeutic relationship is well conveyed in Kohut's words. As noted previously, the experience of therapeutic empathy is not the same as knowing what we might feel if we were in the same situation as the client, identifying with the client and becoming flooded with her feelings, magically intuiting the client's feelings, or being nice or kind to the client. The function of useful therapeutic empathy is to open up a channel for the unfolding of the client's inner world and the emergence of her developmental needs. This process allows for the evolution of a profound transference, in which the client is able to satisfy earlier unmet needs by incorporating into her sense of self her relationship with her therapist as it relates to those needs and incorporating her therapist's positive, accurate regard as reliable psychological structures that become, over time, increasingly integrated as her own.

One of the (many) problems I always had with classical psychoanalytic theory was the notion that only relatively well put-together individuals – certainly no one with a diagnosis of borderline personality disorder, that is, a great many survivors of severe and prolonged childhood trauma – have the capacity to work in the mode of an in-depth transference, and therefore, only such individuals could make the solid psychosocial change that psychoanalysis promised. It had been my experience, both professionally and in my own personal therapy, that powerful transference was indeed part of a deep psychotherapeutic process that resulted in substantial change. But I did not think it was a process only for the few and the fortunate.

I was very excited when I read Kohut's posthumously published *How Does Analysis Cure?* (1984). In his last effort to expand the envelope, Kohut speaks about the pain for the analyst in attempting to maintain an empathic connection with an individual who does not have the functional ego defenses that most of his patients have had, and he mentions particularly a borderline patient. He declares that he has come to the conclusion that it is not the patients, as the psychoanalytic literature postulates, who cannot work within the transference, but the therapists. Many cannot bear to allow the depth of chaos these patients experience on a daily basis to reverberate within them so that they are able to get and stay sufficiently close emotionally to provide the anchor that any patient needs during the course of an in-depth therapy process.

Many individuals reporting childhood histories of severe trauma illustrate his point. Working with them pushes the mental, emotional, and spiritual limits of their therapists. Many therapists find that they cannot do this work and maintain their own physical and mental health, and they give up treating survivors of severe trauma. That is certainly a better solution than continuing to treat but working ineffectively because of countertransferential, self-protective distancing from the client, or defensive boundary violations that give both therapist and client the illusion of helpfulness while simultaneously disempowering the client and rendering the therapy useless or, indeed, harmful. In order to avoid either giving up the work or working badly, therapists who wish to create a healthy, professionally viable empathic bond with survivors of severe trauma must be able to care, first and foremost, for themselves.

As I see it, there must be two aspects to this self-care regimen. Therapists talk a great deal about issues such as proper diet and exercise, a calm personal life, consistent collegial support, rituals to clear out toxic energy between sessions, and so on, and all of these are important. But the bottom line aspect of self-care in this business is the ability to process the material that a therapist is taking in from a client, so that it is not hitting up against areas of the therapist's psyche that are as yet unexplored and therefore defensively closed off.

We are not different from our clients. When we sense danger we avoid, and we put a lot of energy into the effort to avoid knowing that we avoid. There are therapists who have never had much personal therapy. Sometimes, if they are fairly stable individuals, they can get away with this – up to a point. There are very few individuals hearing terrible stories of the systematic torture and terrorization of young children, however, who are not shaken to their depths and who do not have to acknowledge that the precepts and values that are the underpinnings of their existence are called into question by what they are experiencing in their work (Steele, 1989).

Defenses that have never been tampered with in the therapist who has not experienced in-depth therapy often crumble in such situations, and the personal and philosophical issues that lie beneath them must either be processed rigorously, or the therapist must leave the field in order to rebuild her defence system. Even therapists who have completed a regimen of therapy that both they and their own therapists considered pretty thorough often find untouched areas and need to return periodically to treatment to ensure that they remain a relatively clear and clean vessel for the use of their trauma survivor clients.

This commitment to scrupulous personal honesty is the least glamorous but most basic of the self-care strategies. It provides the best insurance (there are no perfect insurance policies in this area) that therapists will neither burn out nor act out by unconsciously trying to resolve personal conflicts or satisfy unmet needs of their own under the guise of treating trauma survivors, whose needs and conflicts are so obvious.

Supportive contact with other clinicians working in the same field and wrestling with the same kind of issues is the next way in which therapists can create a healthy self-care context. Facing trauma alone is too stressful – not only for the client, but for the therapist as well. If the client is the only person who is aware of her therapist's engagement in the arena of the terror and anguish that is her client's daily life, it is only her client to whom the therapist will be able to look for support, to the obvious detriment of the therapeutic relationship.

Especially in professional contexts in which the therapist is working alone or in which the therapist's work with trauma survivors is unsupported or undermined by colleagues, the likelihood of the therapist/client dyad becoming isolated and turned in on itself is high. This isolation creates a climate in which excesses and exploitation of the client are more likely to occur than a treatment context that is open to at least partial scrutiny by a professional community. In such situations, the therapist must be particularly rigorous about finding both consultation from a professional with more experience in the field and a peer support group.

Different levels of support are needed at different stages of the therapist's experience. When working with one's first cases of severe abuse/fragmentation/multiple personality/ritual abuse, it is ideal if the therapist has the opportunity for case consultation and also for peer support after almost every session until the therapist develops her own sea legs. A supportive peer or a few colleagues who offer the therapist the opportunity to talk in detail about what she is hearing, seeing, and experiencing in the sessions (with suitable care taken to maintain confidentiality) can make it possible for the therapist to use consultation efficiently.

I have had experienced therapists, in consultation sessions, telling me all the details of the abuse their clients endured as children. When, after a few minutes of this flow, I would interrupt and suggest that we move on to discuss the therapy process, they would agree and then continue talking compulsively about the details of the terrible things their clients were telling them. I understand and point out that what is transpiring in the process is countertransferential flooding, overidentification, secondary posttraumatic stress reactions, and so on, and it is my job as consultant to help the therapist see this and deal with it appropriately. In some, perhaps many cases, it may be a matter for personal therapy.

In almost all cases, though, it is also a completely human need to process with others the shock, horror, fear, anger, and despair that is our inescapable response to hearing in detail and experiencing the attendant affect that accompanies the narratives of atrocity that are the life stories of this group of suffering people. It is crucial that, as their therapists, we do whatever it is we need to do to take care of ourselves so that we do not become one more person who must distance or must reject them because we cannot tolerate the affect they stir up in us.

Even more importantly, we must create a personal and professional life for ourselves that enables us to attend to our own needs, so that we do not ask our clients to care for us. When this happens, it is generally in a way that is subtle, or at least out of the conscious awareness of both therapist and client, although some therapists do engage in dual roles with clients that serve this purpose in an obvious way. Sexual exploitation is one of the most damaging ways in which therapists manipulate clients to meet their needs, but there are also many other, often less obvious ways of placing the burden of our care upon our client because we are not tending conscientiously to our own needs. If the client is caring for the therapist, this experience significantly weakens the therapeutic context and makes it impossible to construct a strong enough container for the client's projections – not only her desperation, needs, and longings, but also her rage, her mistrust, and her deep and abiding fear.

Working within the context of a long-term therapy process with an individual who talks a great deal about abuse and torture of the most extreme sort provides special challenges to the therapist. But they are not challenges to learn the dates of satanic holidays or fancy new techniques like deprogramming, special accessing codes, or the use of four-point leather restraints to deal with problems that are qualitatively different from the problems all abuse survivors and, to some degree, most human beings experience. There is an obvious secondary gain potential in re-enforcing the notion that some clients have the most heavy-duty, most extreme, and most implacable psychopathology. For people whose sense of themselves as special and unique in the basic and positive way every child is special and unique has been systematically destroyed, it is therapeutically counterproductive to offer them the seductive option of being considered special and unique by an important person in their lives, their therapist, because they exhibit such high-level programming, have so many personalities, or have been subjected to atrocities that the therapist has never heard of before.

Therapists of ritual abuse survivors do indeed have a particular needs. For one, we need to develop our comfort level with all that we do not know. We also need to enhance the personal qualities and the skills that make us helpful to all of our clients – empathy, compassion, and disinterest.

9

Treating the Lesbian and Gay Survivor of Abuse

No one had turned to us and held out a handful of questions: How many ways are there to have the *sex* of a girl, boy, man woman? How many ways are there to have *gender* – from masculine to androgynous to feminine? Is there a connection between the *sexualities* of lesbian, bisexual, heterosexual, between desire and liberation? No one told us: The path divides, and divides again, in many directions. No one asked: How many ways can the *body's sex* vary by chromosomes, hormones, genitals? How many ways can *gender expression* multiply – between home and work, at the computer and when you kiss someone, in your dreams and when you walk down the street? No one asked us: What is your dream of who you want to be?

Minnie Bruce Pratt (1995)

It ain't ignorance that causes all the trouble. It's knowing things that ain't so.

J. Zubin (1987)

Sexuality is often a key area of conflict for abuse survivors. People who were sexually abused and exploited from early in childhood often find sex an area of confusion and pain. They are the same in this regard as everyone else who is socialized in a society in which sex is simultaneously privileged and denigrated beyond reason. The difficulties experienced by anyone raised in an anti-sex and sex-preoccupied society in attempting to create a healthy, integrated sexuality are also experienced by survivors of sexual abuse, often only more so.

Similarly, people – with sexual abuse histories or not – who are moved to explore sexual practices that are not widely accepted in all areas of this society, such as gay, lesbian, bisexual, or transgendered individuals (men who experience themselves as women or women who experience themselves as men), usually find themselves struggling with both external and internal prejudice as part of their journey to construct their sexuality. Conflicts that are difficult enough to manage for someone who has not been sexually abused in childhood become even more fraught with anguish when an individual is the heir to the deep shame imposed on the sexually abused child.

Few individuals grow to maturity without having incorporated some degree of the homophobia that is endemic in our culture. Homophobia – although usually understood as a fear, from its Latin root – is more often about hostility than blatant fear. The clinical-sounding term, as Claudia Card (1995) points out, is generous to anti-gay individuals and institutions, who may or may not be deeply afraid but often choose to express themselves in self-righteous hatred and open efforts to oppress those they hate by depriving them of their basic civil rights, and, in all too many cases, physically violating them.

'Gay bashing' is common on the streets of large urban centres and in any small town in which lesbians and gay men dare to be open about their love for each other. Transgendered men and women are also frequent targets of violence, no matter what their sexual orientation. The righteous hatred and contempt that fuels the energy of packs of predators beating up a gay man walking down a street alone or two women holding hands as they enter their home all too often leads to murder.

I picked up the *San Francisco Examiner* during a California stopover on a recent trip to Southeast Asia. The front-page headline read: 'Oregon Killing Suspect: "It's the American Way." ' The article recounted an interview with Robert James Acremont, who admitted to kidnapping, confining, and killing two lesbians, Roxanne Ellis and Michelle Abdell. These women lived together with their family, including a young grandchild, in Medford, Oregon. They were open about their twelve-year relationship and were accepted in the business and social life of the town. Acremont was quoted as declaring:

I don't care for lesbians ... I couldn't help but think that she was fifty-four years old and had been dating that woman for twelve years; isn't that sick? That's someone's grandma, for God sake ... I couldn't believe that. It crossed my mind a couple of times – lesbo grandma, what a thing, huh? (p. A-18)

A defence strategy commonly used to prevent the conviction of those accused of assaulting or murdering lesbians or gay men is the 'homosexual panic' defence. By the same logic, if every woman who had unwanted sexual advances made to her by a male had the right to murder the man, the streets would be littered with the bodies of heterosexual men (Freiburg, 1988).

Internalized homophobia is a fear and hatred of oneself as a sexual being with same-sex sexual desires and affectional preferences that is an understandable response to prejudice, hatred, and violence. Sometimes this emotional response is reactive to very obvious and immediate dangers in the environment. For example, Laura Brown (1994) describes how many lesbians rushed to therapists' offices during the 1992 campaigns in Oregon and Colorado to repeal the civil rights of lesbians and gay men. Fears, self-doubts, eroded self-esteem, shame, mistrust of people in whom one previously felt some confidence – all regarding sexual orientation – resurfaced, or even emerged for the first time, under these threatening circumstances, in which employment, housing, and child custody were all named as areas where it would be legal to discriminate against lesbians and gay men. Issues many individuals had considered resolved to their satisfaction were resuscitated as polititions, employers, religious leaders, and others harboring an anti-gay bias worked fiercely and publicly to destroy the lives of lesbians and gay men.

The virulent rhetoric about the homosexual agenda to seduce schoolchildren and spread AIDS to God-fearing heterosexuals was aired daily during these campaigns, in the media, from church pulpits, at county fairs, charity bazaars, and PTA meetings. This kind of exposure is bound to incite not only the hateful response that is its overt goal (the repealing of the basic civil rights of lesbians and gays), but also righteous, muderous rage in those individuals looking for a target for their free-flowing violence. Widely publicized examples of genocidal malice were Pat Robertson's 'AIDS is God's way of weeding his garden' and Pat Buchanan's 'The homosexuals have declared war on nature and nature is exacting an awful retribution' ('An Assault,' 1988).

Internalized homophobia is usually the long-term outcome of coming up against such frightening situations repeatedly, with few weapons with which to retaliate. Just as a child who is maltreated by the adults in her life must internalize the shame and the blame for what she cannot control and cannot escape, so lesbians, gays, and transgendered individuals often incorporate into their self-definition and sense of self-esteem the shame and hatred that is spewed in their direction. They are then further silenced, disabled in terms of being able to struggle for the preservation of their own basic freedoms, and sometimes in their capacity to lead fulfilling, joyful personal lives as well.

In many communities in North America, the state of seige felt in Colorado and Oregon is business as usual. Many lesbians would lose their children if their sexuality became public; many more would lose their jobs. Many do lose children, jobs, social standing, and the support of those they love. Relationships with families are often shattered or changed forever when individuals decide they cannot keep such an important secret from people whose acceptance and love has always been central to their lives. Some lesbians and gay men are fortunate enough to be able to structure our lives so that we are relatively protected from continuous anti-gay sentiment and activity. We can therefore be open about our lives with some degree of impunity much of the time. For most, however, this is not possible. The emotional consequences of this suppression and oppression are often intense. Therapists must be aware of this context, or they will be inclined to slip easily into disease terminology, discounting the reality of the threat and pathologizing anxious or angry responses.

People with a history of abuse in childhood are even more vulnerable to the psychological effects of coping with pervasive homophobia. Some of the Vietnam veterans who suffered the most severe posttraumatic stress reactions were individuals who brought with them to the battlefield a history of childhood trauma. This does not mean their responses to the horrors of combat could be dismissed as some kind of flashback. Their war was as real as any other soldier's war. However, they incorporated their adult experiences into a cognitive, emotional, and somatic framework that was already fragile and fraught. They brought a battlefield with them into the war, and the effects of adult terrors often overloaded a system that was already barely holding together.

Lesbian and gay adults who were exploited, assaulted, and oppressed as children bring the experience of being a child who is singled out, made to feel different, and hated and hurt by people in authority to the adult experience of being singled out as different and hated and hurt by many people, including people in authority. It is no wonder that some of their coping strategies for dealing with anti-gay prejudice are childlike and not particularly adaptive. Only a therapist who can recognize the reality of both oppressions – the childhood abuse and the homophobia faced by the adult (or adolescent) – can help such an individual face and deal with each as it is reinforced by the other.

All too often survivors of childhood abuse who are lesbian, gay, bisexual, and/or transgendered encounter no such understanding when they reach out to mental health professionals for help. Not only are they compelled to cope with the ignorance and hatred of society in general and their own internalized homophobia. Very often they must also face some degree of prejudice from those to whom they look for healing. Therapists working with survivors of abuse in childhood are socialized in their formative years to stereotypic beliefs about sexuality, and particularly lesbian and gay sexuality, in the same way everyone else growing up in our society is. Even if we are not obviously homophobic, mental health professionals are no more likely than anyone else to be free from heterosexism, the worldview that assumes heterosexuality to be the norm (indeed, the ideal) against which everything else is measured. This worldview necessarily obscures and distorts different experiences of sexuality.

Selective blindness to homophobia and heterosexism is not only suffered by professionals leading heterosexual lives, but also by most gay, lesbian, and bisexual professionals as well. We may know more about the reality of life as a lesbian or gay man – or a bisexual or transgendered woman or man – but we learned about the world in a culture that frames heterosexuality as the only choice in almost all home, school, church, and community contexts. The vast majority of us were children who saw nothing but heterosexual images of couples and families in the media, and who only came to hear of lesbian and gay sexuality through dirty jokes and rude name-calling by our peers. Even now, we and our children must watch – and even enjoy watching – children's entertainment like Raffi, Sesame Street, and Barney, which conscientiously incorporates images of different races, cultures, customs, and family constellations into their educational format, but never includes two mommies or two daddies and their children as one of the many types of families they celebrate. We cannot help being influenced by all the insults of commission and omission that are an integral part of our life in this culture. Our choice is to live in a constant state of heightened awareness, or to indulge in a more comfortable state of denial.

Unfortunately, there is very little education in professional programs about sexuality, including and particularly lesbian, gay, and bi sexuality, that would be likely to challenge, enrich, or offer some balance to the narrow and distorted values we incorporate as children and which are reinforced every day in our lives as adults. Therapists' prejudices are, therefore, rarely challenged in their training. They can easily go unnoticed and then be enacted in ways that are profoundly harmful to psychotherapy clients. Lesbian, gay, and bisexual abuse survivors are particularly vulnerable to being damaged by the limitations of their therapists' thinking about issues related to sexuality.

It is important to touch on the issue of our cultural responses to lesbian and gay sexuality before looking at the subject in relation to the treatment of individuals with dissociative conditions, because the cultural context within which lesbian and gay sexuality is situated is particularly evocative of the taboos, mixed messages, double-binding constraints, and gross and pervasive oppression that are familiar to the survivor of childhood sexual abuse. If we replicate, in our treatment milieux, the homophobic and heterosexist environments of our clients' childhoods, the harm we do may well outweigh the good.

In our cultural labeling process, both personal and so-called scientific, we are rarely focused on understanding what males and females actually do, but rather on what males and females should do, and why they don't. As John Money (1988) states, 'We are heirs to a long history of cultural fixation on sex divergency rather than sex sharing.' Kinsey's data (1948, 1953) make it clear that large numbers of individuals experience same-sex sexual attraction and engage in same-sex sexual activities. Some of these people have only, or more commonly, predominantly sexual relations with members of the same sex. Many of them have sexual experiences with members of both sexes. Individuals' labelling of themselves at a given time in their life history of sexual expression does not appear to have all that much to do with the kind of sexual activities they engage in and their object choices throughout their lives.

In fact, in all of us, monosexuality is secondary and a derivative of primary bisexual or ambisexual plasticity that varies greatly from one person to another – and can vary for each individual at different stages of the lifespan. The widespread practice and ideology of heterosexual monosexuality are created and maintained by the socialization of children from the earliest ages. Theorists and researchers from Freud

(1905/1949) onward have demonstrated that the boundaries between sexualities are fluid and that many people (Kinsey, 1948, 1953; Bell & Weinberg, 1978) manage to follow fluid patterns of sexual behaviour despite our cultural dictates and institutional arrangements.

However, the statistical norm yields to the ideological norm, and ideologically, there is little place for the ambisexual within our culture (Money, 1988). In practice, the twentieth century has been a time of multiplication of forms of sexuality, but the prevailing discourse of 'compulsory heterosexuality' (Rich, 1980) enjoins male-female sexual coupling as the only natural, healthy, and socially sanctioned expression of sexuality. This is a sexuality understood as having no historical or social constituents, an obvious and simple manifestation of the laws of nature.

In the past twenty years, popular and earlier medical attributions of gay and lesbian sexuality as deviant or wicked have been thoroughly refuted, and there is now a body of social science literature that makes it clear that individuals who are lesbian, gay, or bisexual are no more likely to have psychological problems or to create difficulties for their children than the average person (Lewis, 1980; Gottman, 1989; Green & Bozett, 1991). In 1973, the disorder of 'homosexuality' was deleted by the American Psychiatric Association from its *Diagnostic and Statistical Manual*, and over the next twenty years, the first clinical books were published that presented a positive view of gays and lesbians as well as direction for counselling them in evolving a healthy sexuality and a happy, productive life (for example, Gonsiorek, 1982; Hetrick & Stein, 1984; Stein & Cohen, 1986; Boston Lesbian Psychologies Collective, 1987; Coleman, 1987; Silverstein, 1991; Dynes & Donaldson, 1992; Garnets & Kimmel, 1993; Augelli & Patterson, 1995). A more rational and humane perspective has evolved in some sectors of the culture, and there have been many remarkable successes won by ordinary people that have affected the lives of millions of other ordinary people in the contemporary movement for lesbian and gay rights, which is usually dated as beginning with the Stonewall riots in New York City in June 1969.

However, despite important changes in knowledge and in tolerance, we do not live in a society in which the basic rights of a worker or a family member to have access to the benefits accorded to everyone else in a similar social category are automatically accorded to lesbian and gay adults and their children. There have been many court cases in the past decade about family status, spousal benefits, and same-sex relationship recognition. Karen Andrews (1995) litigated for same-sex health benefits for her partner from 1985 to 1991 and saw the Ontario health insurance plan redesign its entire structure in such a way that every Ontario citizen received an individual health number and card, and the category of 'family member' was obliterated. Although the argument that the organization of the health plan according to family status was necessary to support the institution of the family in Ontario was advanced in defense of its structure when its exclusion of lesbian and gay families was challenged in court, politicians and government bureaucrats were swift to reorganize when they were ordered to right this obvious inequity, rather than offend their constituents by officially recognizing gay and lesbian partnerships as families.

Many of the challenges to oppressive practices against lesbians and gays have been made and won on the terrain of the workplace. Since the initiation of Andrews' action, there have been many others, and increasing numbers of large insurance companies in North America now offer same-sex benefit packages to employers who request them and the federal government has been ordered by the Canadian Human Rights Tribunal to extend benefits to all same-sex partners of its employees. Most people in a capitalist society can understand the analogy between same-sex and opposite-sex partners regarding benefits that are contracted for and are part of the compensation package of all employees (Ursel, 1995). Even some of the most conservative can understand the unfairness of a particular class of employees paying for benefits not received.

Despite progress in extending some of the rights that our society guarantees to most of its citizens to lesbians and gays in the workplace, and some change in the pervasiveness of the most virulently homophobic assumptions about lesbian and gay lifestyles and mental health, the area of 'family' – particularly as it relates to the care of minor children – is still bound by deep-seated fear and prejudice. There is no evidence that lesbian and gay parents harm their children to any greater degree than heterosexual parents (and much evidence that they do not), and it is obvious that hundreds of thousands of lesbian and gay families would be strengthened and supported as they raise millions of children by being accorded the respect and rights of their heterosexual counterparts, but any extension of a conversation about lesbian and gay rights into the area of adoption, for example, often rips the veneer off the civilized discussion. 'Why can't you people realize that you are just asking for too much? We do not intend to hand over our children to you.'

The assumption that lesbians and gay men do not have children is pervasive, and legal case after case singles out the fact that gay sex is not procreative sex as the factor that distinguishes gay couples from everyone else – including, somehow, infertile heterosexual couples, old couples, and couples who choose childlessness – and thus justifies denying them social benefits (Andrews, 1995). In fact, many lesbians and gay men are raising children from previous heterosexual relationships. Lesbians, in particular, are choosing to conceive, bear, and raise their own children in the context of committed relationships. In all of these situations, the biological parent of the child is in some danger of losing custody in many jurisdictions, simply because of her sexual orientation. Prior to 1970, few lesbian mothers contested custody in court. Most relinquished custody if challenged, sometimes in exchange for liberal access – or any access at all. Most lied about or hid their sexuality. The outcome of a contested custody case is no longer guaranteed if the mother is a lesbian, but there are still many cases throughout North American in which women lose their children because a 'lesbian lifestyle' is deemed to be, by definition, not in the best interests of a child.

The plight of the non-biological parent of a child is even more difficult. She or he almost never has any legally sanctioned rights to or responsibilities for the children that may have been parented from birth. Heterosexual men and women can adopt the children of a new partner, after relatively little contact with them, gaining all the rights of a biological parent. Non-biological parents who are lesbian or gay usually have no official standing in the lives of their children, in terms of medical care, even in emergencies, travel, and, most crucially, custody. Upon the death of one parent, the children in these families can face losing both parents.

Bill 167 was introduced in 1994 by the provincial government of Ontario to eliminate discrimination against lesbian and gay individuals and families, following the September, 1992, decision of the Ontario human rights board that the provincial government could not withhold benefits from the spouses of its lesbian and gay employees. Although the bill was eventually defeated, the conversation about what 'family' actually means was opened up throughout Ontario in a way that has changed the way we live. Families came out in newspapers in small towns throughout the province, and members of the provincial legislature – and all the other neighbors who read the letters sent to the local MPP (member of Provincial Parliament) and copied to the local newspaper – learned that 'those people' lived next door to them, and that their children played hockey on the teams they coached.

The struggle for basic recognition and human rights for lesbians and gays has not been won, and that creates much suffering every day, but it is an issue that is much less likely to be silenced in the 1990s than it was previously, and changes in policy and practise are taking place frequently. It is, therefore an issue that is likely to come up in therapy in a variety of ways, directly and indirectly, and it is encumbent on therapists to develop an educated perspective if they intend to take on the treatment of lesbians, gay men, bisexuals, or transgendered individuals.

A therapist will need to be aware of the ways in which lesbians and gay men are, to some degree, outsiders, and how that is demonstrated every day of their lives through systemic discrimination in all cases, and physical assault, emotional battery, and social ostracization in all too many cases. Whatever level of denial about this reality clients bring to the psychotherapy context (and denial of the extent of the problem is a *sine qua non* of adaptation when escape or immediate transformation of the threatening situation are not options), it is helpful if they are not faced with a therapist who has an even greater need than they do to deny. Lesbian and gay practitioners should explore their own denial level, and heterosexual therapists should find a path of education for themselves that will enable them to be an informed and empathic container for the full range of their lesbian and gay clients' experiences – their rage and anguish, the joy in their own sexuality that they may not allow themselves to feel, and ways in which living in a homophobic culture can effect every aspect of their lives.

Another issue that is quite likely to arise in the therapy of lesbian and gay abuse survivors is the origins of their sexual orientation. Some individuals who have been sexually abused in childhood and find themselves attracted to members of the same sex frame their sexuality – in a reductionist and self-degrading way – in terms of their abuse experiences, at least some of the time, and, unfortunately they are likely to be encouraged in this way of thinking by relatives, friends, clergy, and, all too often, mental health professionals.

The following scenario is not uncommon. A woman reports to her therapist that she has been having strong sexual feelings towards another woman, and she is sure that this is only because she was abused by her father and therefore is afraid of men (or was abused by her mother and therefore turned on to women, or abused by everyone and therefore just plain perverted). The therapist listens and nods and eventually helps her client develop strategies to extinguish her feelings toward women and direct them more appropriately. Although the therapist never says to the client that her feelings are the outcome of her abuse, her actions indicate that she agrees with the client's interpretation. This is a mild version of the scenario that is repeated with damaging effects in countless treatment rooms.

I once gave a presentation at an international conference, with much the same point that I am making here. At the end of the short talk, a woman approached me, as people do, and told me she came to my talk because she was counselling a lesbian who had been sexually abused by her father in childhood, and that she had found my session very useful. She had only one question, she said, she wanted to ask me. 'How can I make my client understand that her sexual feelings for other women are an unhealthy result of her abuse?' She went on to explain that she had tried every way she could think of to convince her client to try to change, without success. This anecdote is neither an invention nor an exaggeration. The two other people waiting to speak to me were open-mouthed witnesses.

Therapists of lesbians and gay men have the responsibility to have an educated and independent perspective, in the same way that a therapist who works with sexual abuse survivors needs to understand all the levels of meaning that might be encompassed by a sexual abuse survivor's interpretation of her own experiences. A client might declare with utter conviction and sincerity, 'My father was not an abusive man. The only reason he started having sex with me when I was five was that I was so needy and seductive, and he was too soft-hearted and couldn't say no.'

Can you imagine a therapist responding to such a statement with the offer to help her write a letter of apology to her father for putting him in such an awkward position and then create strategies to help her change from being so needy and seductive? I guess it is not entirely unimaginable, but very few professionals would see it as helpful or responsible to reinforce the client's initially necessary but eventually self-defeating cognitive distortions in this way. I have heard many professionals, however, justify their ignorant and homophobic therapeutic strategies by declaring that they were simply responding to their client's request for a particular direction in treatment.

Therapists who are working with lesbian and gay abuse survivors who are tormented to some degree by their sexual desires and wish they were different, or who find it difficult or do not wish to develop stable, long-term relationships, can, in their own ignorance of any sexual lifestyles but the most socially sanctioned, easily interpret this pattern as a sign that their clients' attraction to people of the same sex is abuse-related and pathological. These therapists therefore assume, imply, or even clearly counsel that to find happiness, individuals must cure their deviant patterns of arousal. This can only reinforce the internalized homophobia that is a common problem for lesbians and gays with damaged self-esteem. It is not only incompetent treatment, but re-traumatizing as well.

Even if therapists do not go so far as to openly advocate a change in sexual desire and object choice, they may see any fantasies, desires, and practices of the client that are different from those with which they are familiar as deviant, thus colluding in the disciplining of the client to conform to certain narrow social standards. A wide array of sexual activities, most notably sado-masochism, but also many other variations on the norm of securely coupled monogamous relationships, even when they are intentionally and caringly practised by consenting adults, are often discounted as de facto pathological. Again and again, sexual desire is naturalized and simplified, its overdetermined quality hidden, as well as the political and prescriptive purposes of the way its stories are told and its meanings constructed.

I would like to think that the experienced therapist working with a gay abuse survivor is likely to notice the self-hatred and internalized homophobia in the cry, 'I know my compulsive sexual feelings for other men only exist because of the sexual abuse by my uncle. I really need your help in getting rid of those feelings he put in me, so that I can enjoy normal sex with my wife.' I am afraid that in many cases, however, the liberal, humanistic framework of supporting clients' own framing of their experience rationalizes a profound heterosexism on the part of the therapist, who then can easily collude with the client in denigrating his own sexuality. The man who is pained about his relationship with his wife and shamed about his sexual desires has a complicated set of life problems with which to wrestle. He needs a therapist who can hear his torment – and his longings – at many levels, rather than accepting his simplistic, and probably largely inaccurate, interpretation of his situation and his prescription for health.

Many people – gays and lesbians included – have a high level of certainty about the origin of sexual orientation, both their own and that of others. So far, however, research does not support sweeping statements about any one source for variations in the ways in which sexual desire and the longing for affiliation manifest themselves in different people. There is some data about neuroanatomical differences between heterosexual and gay men in the brain region involved in the regulation of sexual behaviour, the anterior hypothalamus (Le Vay, 1991; Swaab, Gooran & Hofman, 1992). The results do not allow one to decide, however, if the differences in brain morphology are the cause or the consequence of an individual's sexual orientation, or if both the brain and sexual orientation co-vary under the influence of another, unidentified variable (Le Vay, 1991). Research on the role of genetics in the evolution of sexual orientation found one sub-type of male homosexuality to be genetically influenced (Hamer, Hu et al., 1995), but the same linkage was not discovered in lesbians (Hu, Pattatucci et al., 1995). When familial clustering (often considered a measure of the genetic loading of a trait) is studied regarding lesbians and their families, there is elevation in rates of non-heterosexuality among female relatives (Pattatucci & Hamer, 1995), but the study states clearly that the current data are not sufficient to distinguish between inherited and cultural sources of influence.

There is definitely some interesting research in three biological disciplines – neuroanatomy, endocrinology, and genetics – that is exploring the ways in which biology plays a part in the development of an individual's sexual orientation. The responses to the research, however, exaggerate both the scope and the certainty of the results. Every new finding is greeted as if it offers the answer to a simple question, rather than a piece of a large and complicated puzzle. 'In Search of the Gay Gene' was the title of the cover story in the December 26, 1995, issue of *The Advocate*, a U.S. gay and lesbian publication. The table of contents described the article as follows: 'A new study fuels a growing consensus that when it comes to sexual orientation, biology is destiny' (p. 3). Not only is this a wild exaggeration from a scientific point of view, this kind of simplification is probably as helpful to the cause of gay rights as its original formulation has been to the liberation of women.

Some researchers make honest attempts to protect their work from being misused against gays and lesbians: 'We believe that it would be fundamentally unethical to use such information to try to assess or alter a person's current or future sexual orientation, either heterosexual or homosexual, or other normal attributes of human behavior' (Hamer, Hu et al., 1995, p. 326). Others have no such scruples:

The discovery that a nucleus differs in size between heterosexual and homosexual men illustrates that sexual orientation in humans is amenable to study at the biological level, and this discovery opens the door to studies of neurotransmitters or receptors that might be involved in regulating this aspect of personality. (Le Vay, 1991, p. 1036)

In any case, researchers do not retain control over the knowledge they contribute to the body of science. Philip Reilly, a clinical geneticist, declares that once a gene that influences sexual orientation in some people is found and further work accomplished, there is no doubt that the information will be used to alter the development of same-sex sexual orientation. 'To think about a biological intervention (in essence a drug) ... to return the person to the quote-unquote standard orientation ... biomedically, this is the logical outcome of the research' (Burr, 1995, pp. 37–8). His view reinforces the legitimacy of Eve Sedgwick's fear that 'there currently exists no framework in which to ask about the origins or development of individual gay identity that is not already structured by an implicit, transindividual Western project or fantasy of eradicating that identity' (1990, p. 41).

Lesbian and gay sexuality – as with every other aspect of life – is not an abstract and universal category of the erotic or the sexual, a simple, fixed, inherited nature. There may be aspects of a particular individual's sexual desire that are influenced by genetics. One person may, indeed, from early in childhood, find only members of the same sex sexually attractive, and such experiences may in some cases be reflected in brain morphology. How this plays itself out in terms of the sexual life this person creates will be very different from another person who also finds people of the same sex attractive. These differences are at least as important as some possible similarities that are suggested by research that is at an early stage. Also, the similarities – whether genetic or neuroanatomical – likely only apply to a subgroup of individuals who call themselves lesbian, gay, bisexual, or transgendered. There is no indication – as yet – that most lesbians or many gay men are like each other and different, genetically or neuroanatomically, from their heterosexual peers, except insofar as we are all different from one another.

Therapists of clients who present themselves as lesbian, gay, bisexual, or transgendered (or who are struggling with questions in this area) would be more helpful if their minds were open, not closed, to the complexities of the phenomenon of human sexuality. Our discourse is simplistic, on the whole, and we would be wise not to inflate our feelings of self-importance or to take ourselves too literally when we use the only language we have to help our clients explore their hopes, their desires, their secret shames – all of the ways in which their lives show them that to be human is to be sexual.

The construct of multiple personalities challenges the simplicities of categories of sexuality the same way it does the many other categories that uphold the status quo in a patriarchal society. Dualisms such as body-mind and victim-oppressor have a hard time maintaining their credibility when viewed through the kaleidoscope of a highly dissociative configuration of consciousness. The binary thinking central to most of our understandings about gender and sex (these two so consistently conflated in most conceptualizations about sexuality), woman-man and gay-straight, and even woman-man-transexual-transgendered, and gay-straight-bi, meet the same fate. Simplistic taxonomies such as these can rarely withstand the onslaught of multiply constructed consciousness. The language of multiple personality often shows us the irony of taking an experience as complicated as an individual's expression of sexuality and treating it as an 'it,' rather than an outpouring of the person's energy from birth to death.

Women, for example, who develop highly dissociative states of consciousness as a way of coping with experiences of child abuse usually evolve personality states they perceive as male and personality states they perceive as female. These personality states often endorse different culturally stereotypic and polarized values about many things. Their perceptions about gender identity and sexual orientation open up and destabilize the more reductionistic reference points against which the issues of gender and sex are usually considered and studied (Rivera, 1988a). Some of this is simple – or not so simple – posttraumatic confusion that may be set straight, so to speak, through proper therapeutic intervention. Much less of it, however, is disposable in this way than is comfortable, if therapy is to be something other than one more oppressive regulatory mechanism in a life more than normally full of them.

Here again multiple personality illustrates that the ways in which we are constrained to think about ourselves are narrower (and different from) the reality of what we are really like. In the life experience and self-expression of an individual who sees the world through the eyes of a plethora of dissociated ego states, the person's ongoing presentation in the world may simultaneously (or almost simultaneously) be that of macho heterosexual man, vulnerable child, nurturing woman, sensitive gay man, domineering woman, playful, carefree child, child bowed with grief, woman desperate to conform who cannot figure out how to do so, executive female who is antagonistic to men and contemptuous of women, lesbian with butch presentation, lesbian with femme presentation, and many other effects of a complexly constructed subjectivity.

Some of the responses that I received from a questionnaire I distributed in 1989 to a small number (n=100 questionnaires passed out) of individuals self-identifying as suffering from multiple personality disorder, about issues related to gender identity and sexual orientation, illustrate the richness and diversity of the pathways that these people travelled in developing their understanding of themselves as sexual beings.

Respondents were asked to explore in some detail their views, attitudes and actions regarding sexuality as expressed in altered states of consciousness. Only individuals who experienced this as a significant issue for them would have been likely to have filled in the questionnaire. Given that I did not select by sexual orientation, it is interesting that all of questionnaires that were returned were from individuals who either identified as lesbian (n=10) or gay male (n=2), or who identified as bisexual and reported a predominance of same-sex sexual partners in consensual sexual activity (n=8, all female).

I did not conclude that more severely dissociative abuse survivors were gay than straight from this small and not particularly randomly selected group of individuals seen in my practice, the practices of a few colleagues, or who attended a local multiple personality self-help group or attended a forum 'For Multiples Only' at a dissociation conference held in Toronto. In fact, research indicates that the same percentage of women who self-identify as lesbians have a history of childhood sexual abuse – 38 per cent – (Loulan, 1987) as women in studies in which sexual orientation was not noted (Russell, 1986). I hypothesized that, for individuals struggling to understand their sexual desires, same-sex sexuality needed more explaining – and from severely dissociative people, more dividing up – to make it manageable than heterosexual sexuality.

The rich and detailed life stories that were written in response to the questionnaire illustrated the complexity of the construction of sexuality as it plays itself out in the lives of lesbian, gay, and bisexual abuse survivors. Common configurations were child personality states who wanted affection and were horrified when the affection turned sexual; anhedonic states in which individuals experienced themselves as asexual and sometimes non-gendered as well; hypersexual teenagers, sometimes promiscuous; stereotypically heterosexual female personalities who voiced conventional desires for security, safety, and a vine-covered cottage and saw sex as a means to those ends; male-identified personalities in women's bodies who were actively sexual with other women but framed the behaviour as heterosexual; female personalities in men's bodies who were passively sexual with other men but framed the behaviour as heterosexual; sexually aggressive personalities in both lesbians and gay men, usually experienced as male by both women and men; personalities who knew they were lesbian or gay and were comfortable with that awareness; and personalities who thought it was silly to choose the people to whom you wanted to relate intimately by whether they were men or women, rather than by what they were like in so many other ways.

There were scores of permutations and combinations of personality states with different self-understandings about their gender and sexual identity in the twenty questionnaires that were fully filled out. The respondents (n=5) who had had a lot of therapy and appeared to have resolved a great deal of the most dysfunctional aspects of their dissociative coping mechanisms described the evolution of their understandings about their sexuality. Some personalities who had endorsed stereotypical (and often viciously intolerant) perspectives about same-sex sexual expression as an unnatural (and usually ungodly) abomination became more accepting of the desires and the practices of the others. Eventually, in the less rigidly divided person, earlier self-loathing about same-sex relationships was replaced with general accep-tance and only the occasional deprectory self-judgment. Child personalities were gradually subsumed into the general category of childlikeness or vulnerability, and those aspects of the individual, as described by some individuals, disappeared during sexual activity or, as described by others, became a playful aspect of sexual expression.

Gender, interestingly, seemed less of an issue than sexuality to the group of people who responded to this particular questionnaire. There were no resounding cries of joyous acceptance of gender identity in the way that there were sometimes about sexuality. The issue of 'Am I a boy or a girl?' – a thorny one in the experience of many individuals who are severely dissociated and often expressed in ongoing conflict among personality states about issues such as what clothes to put on each day – either is not mentioned by the individuals who had resolved many of these issues, or is given only passing mention, as in 'I am still not comfortable in dresses and other obviously feminine clothing, but that doesn't mean I am a man. To be honest, I don't feel particularly like a man or a woman, but it is not a problem for me anymore. I'm just me, and that seems to be good enough.' One woman wrote tersely about the conflicts about gender at her workplace; she is a police officer. 'It pays not to be particularly feminine where I work. The other woman officer I work with closely gets a lot more hassle than I do.'

What do these individuals' personal struggles demonstrate about gender identity and sexual orientation? First of all, that it is individual and complicated – no one person's process is exactly like another's. It is also a process that takes place within a field of multileveled social and historical influences, which are both personal and idiosyncratic to individual life circumstances and much wider than that. Above all, it illustrates that the development of gendered sexuality is not a simple, so-called natural process and shows us that most of our questions, our studies, and certainly the simplistic conclusions we often come to, are driven by ideology rather than a desire to know, understand, or explore.

Reductionism of any sort in the area of human sexuality – whether to biology, psychodynamics, sociology, religion, or politics – may be expedient for any number of reasons – to gain funding, to teach Bible study classes, to fight bigots, to make hypotheses for research projects, to create catchy slogans to carry in gay pride day marches, and so on. A relatively simple stance may also be the deeply felt reality for many people trying to place their life experience in a manageable cognitive frame. It is more common for gay men than lesbians to make declarations like, 'I knew from the time I was four years old that I was attracted to little boys rather than little girls and that never changed.' Explanatory models of sexual identity that privilege the notion of a fixed, unchanging sexual self that is primarily biologically determined are therefore particularly compelling for many gay men. Many lesbians, though, also frame their sexual desire for women as a clear and non-changing element in their life experience, unmediated by other influences.

Other lesbians, many of whom came to an acceptance of lesbian sexuality through involvement with the women's movement, claim that their sexual practice is a matter of political choice. In her autobiography, *From Housewife to Heretic* (1989), Sonia Johnson talks about her determination to give up heterosexual sex because of her conviction that it was inevitably a site of oppression for women. She describes her gradual transformation from a woman whose sexual desires were strongly and viscerally heterosexual to a woman who became open to the pleasures of sex with women.

Rather than understand their sexuality as lesbian initially, a great many women experienced their affectionate bonds with other women evolving into a more consciously sexual passion. Such women tend to insist on a broad definition of their lesbian identity, as relating to the primary status of their social and affiliative connections with other women, rather than focusing narrowly on sexual arousal or acts.

Although I have been listing 'lesbian, gay, bisexual, and transgendered' as though there were a significant degree of similarity among individuals who identify with these labels, there are many differences. Lesbian sexuality, for example, cannot be understood apart from an understanding of women's development in a particular cultural context. Lesbians and gay men have sexual minority status in common, but other aspects of the development of their experience of themselves as sexual beings may be sufficiently different to render suspect any model that purports to describe both lesbians and gay men (Brown, 1995). Individuals who experience themselves as bisexual challenge the adequacy of dichotomous frameworks for describing the diversity of human sexual experience.

Transgendered women and men present even greater challenges to the way we invent categories, pigeonhole people, and try to force reality to conform to our simplistic theories. The question of sex and the question of gender, although inextricably bound to each other, are not the same question (Sedgewick, 1990). We need a multidimensional view of sexual orientation that takes into consideration the many factors that are part of living life as a sexual person, including emotional and sexual preferences, the complexities of gender identity, lifestyle, self-identification, changes in identity over the lifespan, as well as sexual attraction, fantasy, and behaviour (Fox, 1995).

The hegemony of the field of medicine in the study of sexuality influences us to see sexuality as an individual thing, as something inside us, rather than as a construct that emerges in interaction as a result of expectations and negotiation. The development of our sexuality, including our object choice and the ways in which we fantasize and enact our desires, is an overdetermined process. People become sexual the way they become anything else, as Foucault says, 'gradually, progressively, really and materially constituted through a multiplicity of organisms, forces, energies, desires and thoughts' (1980, p. 97).

There is significant opposition to the notion of nuancing the prevailing dogma that sexual orientation is inate and fixed. The vocabulary of sexual preference or choice is considered dangerous by some crusaders for equal civil rights for lesbians and gays. If one can choose to be gay, the same person can choose to be straight. It implies that it is possible – and from there it is not too big a leap to desirable or imperative – to enforce heterosexuality through either legal statute or moral force. It is becoming increasingly obvious, however, that the research supporting a biological base to sexual orientation can be used the same way the Bible is used by some Christian fundamentalists – as both tool and justification for wiping out the scourge of lesbian and gay sexuality. Simplifying sexuality will not serve as effective protection.

It is not our responsibility to educate our clients so that they embrace a complex and multilevelled understanding of their sexuality. It is our responsibility to educate ourselves so that we do not promote or reinforce simplifications, and so that we are able to be a helpful and challenging travelling companion if our clients choose to explore the territory beyond simple answers and soothing rationalizations.

Opening up the issue of the construction of sexual orientation has important clinical implications. We are offering treatment within the context of a patriarchal, heterosexist, homophobic society. The less aware we as practitioners are of that reality, the more likely it is that our practices will be profoundly influenced by the very reality that is so easily obscured. Foucault (1981) has thoroughly explored and convincingly documented the role of science, and particularly psychiatric medicine, in supporting the hidden social and moral agenda of the status quo in a culture. Psychiatry and psychology's use of disease terminology to characterize socially and politically deviant behaviour functions as a powerful tool of social control (Kitzinger, 1987). With the best intentions in the world, it is relatively easy for therapists to be one more oppressive force in our clients' lives, especially those of our lesbian, gay, bisexual and transgendered clients, through the unconscious or rationalized incorporation of heterosexist and homophobic attitudes.

Another way we can discount the complexity of our clients' lives is through the emphasis we place on the categories of their experience that interest us and the way in which we notice not at all what lies beyond or beneath or intertwined with them. Audre Lorde's ironic cry could be that of anyone on a healing journey who has to choose – or, more likely, does not even get to choose – which of her identifications and which of her oppressions will be dignified with informed and respectful focus.

But I who am bound by my mirror
as well as my bed
see cause in color
as well as sex.

and sit here wondering
which me will survive
all these liberations   Audre Lorde
                                                  'Who Said It Was Simple'

The separation of the site of sexuality from all of the other places in which an individual learns to be the person she bring into the therapist's office is common in therapy as well as many other locations. The rich and complicated life of any individual is too often simplified in the articulation of the life story of the client, both as she herself tells it and as the therapist hears and rearticulates it. Sexuality, and all the other categories through which we name and dismiss ourselves and others, need to be 'excavated from the inside' (Allison, 1994). Our sexual desire is created in the crucible of our experience of class, our experience of race, of gender, of religion, of physical strengths and limitations, our experience of family, traumatic and otherwise – our experience of our life with its many blessings and many burdens (Rule, 1994).

Understanding ourselves and others is not a matter of adding together race, sexuality, gender, and class, as if they are separable axes of power, in an ever-expanding enumeration that effectively separates what it purports to connect. Neither is it a question of appropriating all differences – between individuals or groups or within one individual – into an illusory embrace of unity 'by way of a romantic, insidious, all-consuming humanism' (Butler, 1993). It is a matter of honouring the person in her many identifications and coming to understand, slowly and with respect, how these identifications are all vehicles for each other, each influencing the others in a spiraling momentum.

If we wish to offer our clients as wide a range of options as possible so that they are able to express themselves fully and freely, personally and socially, particularly in the arena of sexuality, which is so often a core area of struggle for them, we would do well to be open to acknowledging and challenging our culturally limited and limiting preconceptions. The rich, complicated, and contradictory multiplicity that is so often vividly expressed in the multiple personality construct can open up new ways of looking at the complex and ongoing process that is the creation of sexual desire for everyone.

This openness can help us encourage our clients to celebrate their same-sex sexual desire as a victory over the constraints of a heteronormative (and often viciously homophobic) culture, and at the same time, if they wish, to disorganize – at least a little bit – tidy categories like 'straight' and 'gay,' thus avoiding the necessity for the fictive certainty that is too often demanded by the notion of a coherent and stable 'sexual identity.' Such an openness can broaden our understanding of how our identifications, including our race, class, ethnic, religious, and sexual identifications, are invariably imbricated in one another in the ongoing creation of an ever-evolving, unique, and radically constructed subjectivity.

10

The Politics of Child Abuse and Dissociation

Le Sage ne rit qu'en tremblant. (The Sage does not laugh without trembling.)

Charles Baudelaire

There is a lot of talk in the clinical community about the secondary PTSD (post-traumatic stress disorder) symptoms that often affect therapists treating individuals suffering from severe dissociation. This is generally attributed to the empathic connection with trauma survivors as they reveal and sometimes relive terrible experiences beyond the usual life experience of the therapist. Intrusive thoughts, sleep disturbance, numbing of emotions, hypervigilance, pervasive lack of trust, lability – all can be signs that the therapeutic work is taking a toll on the therapist as well as the client.

In the first years of my work with severely dissociative individuals, I sometimes had bouts of what, in retrospect, would be called secondary PTSD. I did what was called for in the circumstances – mostly dealt with my own countertransference issues in a variety of ways and contexts and created more of a balance in my practice so that I was doing some assessment, some teaching, some consulting, some administration, and some research, along with direct service to clients in long-term therapy. On the whole now, I rarely feel burned out vis-à-vis my work. The only exception to my being able to keep my work in perspective is my limited ability to approach the politics of dissociation (which overlap with the politics of child abuse and the politics of contemporary feminism) with the detachment and disinterest that I consider appropriate.

I appear to have a great capacity for being objective about my clients' rage and destructive feelings towards themselves, towards other people, and towards me. Yet I become incredibly angry and hurt, and am somehow always naively surprised, when other professionals take virulent stands against the work of enabling vulnerable people to get back the lives that were taken away from them at such an early age.

This is a complex and difficult time to be working in the field of dissociation. In its first ten years the field encompassed many people who would not ordinarily have collaborated professionally. We developed an *esprit de corps* based on our commitment to finding effective ways to reach out to a group of people who had been previously ignored by the rest of psychiatry and psychology. Although we recognized our differences, they seemed less important than this commonality.

This was especially true because, no matter how mainstream and respectable any of us had been in our professional lives, there was almost always resistence, and more often than not a great deal of resistence, in our professional contexts to this new work in which we were so engrossed. So the camaraderie of those under seige was often part of the professional networking of the first decade of widespread clinical work with individuals suffering from dissociative conditions. The same can be said for both of the other areas I noted in which internecine struggles between partisans have since become fierce and constant – child abuse and feminism.

The most recent upsurge of the feminist struggle for liberation emerged in North America in the early 1960s and, out of women's grassroots effort to speak honestly and analytically with each other about their life experiences in a patriarchal society came the realization that, not only were women, by the millions, being raped on the streets and beaten and raped in our homes by our male partners as adults, but vast numbers of us had been sexually assaulted as girls and as teenagers in our childhood homes. The feminist analysis of child sexual abuse as a solution to training young girls for their subservient role in a misogynist culture was less likely to be taken up by the child abuse specialists than the awareness that the sexual abuse of children is a serious and widespread problem, but the attention to the issue of child sexual abuse in both the mental health profession and in the awareness of the general public evolved directly from the consciousness-raising efforts of the women's movement.

The field of dissociation evolved directly from the sexual abuse field. There are some obvious links among these struggles to liberate oppressed people, and there are obvious and important differences and discontinuities. One thing they have in common at this point in history is a fierce resistance to their positions from outside their movements and powerful efforts to destroy gains made over the past decade(s) by retrogressive social forces concerned with maintaining the status quo of power inequality between men and women, and adults and children.

The 1970s and 1980s, particularly in North America, saw the awareness of the widespread abuse of children rise in a way unparalleled in history. Sexual abuse was the type of maltreatment most likely to be highlighted in school prevention programs, in media accounts, and in first-person survivor stories. For the first time in recorded history, academic research documented the reality that child sexual abuse was the oppressive childhood experience of millions of children each year (Badgely, 1984; Russell, 1986; Finkelhor et al., 1990).

With the advent of the 1990s, our social tolerance for facing this cultural corruption seems to have peaked, and a reaction of pervasive denial of this reality is often the prime-time news topic. There are very few people who read the daily newspaper or watch any documentary television who could not venture a good guess at what the catchphrase 'false memory' refers to – allegations of childhood sexual abuse brought against loving parents by misguided and vindictive adult children, usually influenced by a therapist. Over the course of two or three years, it has become common knowledge that we are engaged in a 'witch-hunt,' and thousands of innocent adults are being victimized by what is sometimes termed in the media 'the sexual abuse industry.'

It is also common for stories, programs, and even some scholarly articles (Loftus, 1993) that characterize child sexual abuse investigations as witch-hunts to pay lip service to the reality of some few cases of *real* child abuse. The tone of much media coverage of the issue of false allegations of child sexual abuse creates the impression that, as a society, we have recognized a serious problem, we have responsibly dealt with it by way of child protection efforts, and now some zealots are taking advantage of our social responsibility.

What is the reality in terms of our efforts to protect children in the 1990s from adult sexual exploitation? A thorough documentation of reported and investigated incidents of sexual abuse, conducted by Ontario children's aid societies and police in 1993 in the province of Ontario, found that 5 cases of sexual abuse were reported and investigated per thousand children, and 1.57, 29 per cent of them, were substantiated (Trocme, 1994). These statistics are not significantly different from U.S. figures in which 1.65 cases of sexual abuse are substantiated per thousand children in the general population. If, based on incidence studies that have been replicated repeatedly, a minimum of 25 out of 100 children, male and female, are sexually abused before they are 18 years of age, our child protection efforts appear to be picking up fewer than 0.2 per cent of the actual incidence of child sexual abuse activity for intervention of any kind.

This is not to say that some investigations are not undertaken with more enthusiasm than skill or that there are no examples of mistaken allegations or even malicious accusations. But contrary to the now current belief that we are caught up in a conspiracy to label every man a sex offender, or that we are engaged in mass hysteria in the witch-hunt of child sexual abuse investigations, as a society we are barely scratching the surface of the problem of protecting our children from sexual exploitation.

However, despite the reality that the vast majority of children who are currently being sexually abused are afforded no protection at all, the child welfare movement, the women's rights movement, and the professionals who tend to the healing of adults sexually abused as children are all being assailed as biased zealots in arenas from the tabloid press to the academy. However, although it is upsetting to see massive retrenchment in a society that seemed to be beginning to accept, at least in principle, the notion of equal rights for children and women, the reality of slow and dialectical social change allows us to make sense of what has come to be called the 'backlash.'

Historical perspective is of little comfort when one's work is interfered with, one's clients are emotionally damaged, and one is personally subjected to irresponsible attack. Still, it is important to keep some form of perspective and to recognize that it is naive to imagine that work in support of the liberation of women and children would result in universal acceptance in a society in which the self-interest of the powerful may well be threatened by such work. The backlash against the work of healing the wounds of abuse survivors and struggling to make a society that is radically different from the one that inflicted those wounds is likely to get worse before it gets better.

As well as beseiged from without, individuals and groups working against the oppression of children and women are also divided from within. The horizontal dissention, the in-fighting within groups and among individuals who espouse many of the same basic values, is even harder to bear than opposition from those with whom one was never aligned and from whom one never received or expected to receive support.

'If you think you were abused you probably were' or 'We always see women going from suspicion to confirmation of abuse; it never goes the other way' (Bass & Davis, 1988) were always simplistic statements that did not take the vagaries of memory and the phenomenon of influence into consideration, but they were much more likely to represent the reality in many cases at the date of the publishing of the first edition of *The Courage to Heal* than they are now. At this point in time, it is probably truer to say that if an individual, especially a woman, has life problems like sexual difficulties, an eating disorder, problems developing or maintaining intimate relationships, low self-esteem in general, mood swings, addictions, suicidal thoughts, self-mutilation, pervasive dissatisfaction with her life, and so on, and she has never wondered whether childhood sexual abuse might have been a factor in the evolution of these problems, then either she has been exposed to exceptionally little popular culture or she is suspiciously defended against even considering such a possibility. The psychological effects of child sexual abuse have been widely promulgated, not only in specialist books and scholarly journals, but in made-for-tv movies, widely available survivor stories, news programs, and magazine and newspaper reports, and very few people who are struggling with these kind of problems are not asking themselves a desperate 'why?'

I am not suggesting that it is a bad thing that the possibility of a history of sexual abuse be widely considered by people suffering from life problems or by the professionals that help them. In a society where so many children are abused and where the psychological sequelae are so serious, closing our eyes to such a possibility would be similar to not taking an HIV test because you might get a negative result and therefore have wasted the energy being worried, or, more frighteningly, a false positive. It is important to explore all the possibilities one can think of when dealing with physical and emotional problems, even when the exploration itself may be fraught with some degree of fear and distress.

In the 1980s, when little was widely known about the HIV virus, people were much more relaxed. We were also not actively protecting ourselves and those we loved from a deadly disease. The knowledge that we have now is painful and frightening, and it does not ensure protection or effective treatment. It does, however, offer a chance to protect ourselves and others that we did not have before we were burdened with this awareness. In the case of AIDS, this awareness also offers society the opportunity to invest its energies in the scientific search for effective treatment and inoculation.

The analogy is certainly imperfect. Prevention in the area of the sexual abuse of children is a matter of restructuring a social system that promotes their exploitation (not that AIDS prevention is a simple and concrete matter either). But the key point of the analogy is that knowledge is a blessing, but not an unmixed blessing. An awareness of the prevalence and the psychological effects of child sexual abuse can open the door to taking practical steps for prevention and engaging in effective treatment, but public awareness has brought with it some devastating consequences.

I have seen the harm done by individuals, professional and otherwise, who replace common sense or sound clinical judgment with ideology and impose their agendas upon others. I have seen cases taken to court long before the complainant was in a position to swear with any degree of certainty as to the identity of her abuser. I have seen clinical judgment – and common sense – abandoned in favour of adhering to outmoded principles like 'Always believe the child' and 'The woman's perception of her own experience should be believed at all times,' no matter what the harm might be to other people.

The False Memory Syndrome Foundation – as is no doubt clear from my previous disquisition on the topic – is not my favourite group. I do not respect their tactics, and I suspect their motives. I do think, however, that they have made a contribution by forcing the therapeutic community to face the degree to which some helping professionals in all disciplines have not been paying enough attention to the complexities of memory and have been underestimating the power of suggestion and influence of many sorts on the narratives that our clients either bring to therapy with them or develop in the course of their treatment.

One of the reasons for the adversarial and essentially anti-scientific atmosphere surrounding most professional discussions about memories of childhood abuse recovered in psychotherapy is the shift of the arena of investigation from the laboratory, the library, or the treatment room into the courtroom. The rules of evidence and the conventions of communication are quite different in the legal context, and the need to prove one's point often outweighs one's inclination to consider all sides of an issue in a curious and open-minded fashion.

An increase in successful criminal and civil cases against perpetrators of child sexual abuse is one of the most obvious causes of the upsurge in resistance against the veridicality of childhood memories uncovered or reconstructed in therapy. Many a frightened perpetrator is looking for an effective defence against accusations that would never have seen the inside of a courtroom even ten years ago, when crimes against children were committed in privacy with no witnesses, or at least no witnesses brave enough to talk or credible enough to be taken seriously by the authorities.

This criminalization of offences that were once considered a private matter has been a goal and a gain of the women's movement's insistence on taking violence against women and children out of the home and into the public and political arenas. Again, as with our awareness of the prevalence of child sexual abuse, the removal of issues of sexual violence perpetrated against children from the realm of personal suffering, therapeutic exploration, and healing (at best) – or, more commonly, personal silent suffering – into that of legal accountability is not an unmixed blessing. It is a blessing with a cost.

Perhaps there has always been a tendency toward counterproductive polarization in this area. In the 1980s, I certainly heard many therapists of sexual abuse survivors say that they would never treat a perpetrator and that they viewed with suspicion those who did. And there were enough professionals who discounted the reality, the prevalence, or the powerful psychological effects of child sexual abuse to keep the gulf between professionals working for what should have been one goal, child abuse prevention, deep and wide. An assessor in a prestigious mental health centre in a university-affiliated hospital in Toronto sent an admitted sex offender – who was not interested in treatment and not particularly remorseful – home to live with his terrified nine year-old victim, my client, because, as he wrote in his assessment report, 'I see no evidence that sexual abuse is necessarily harmful to children, and I see plenty of evidence that family breakdown is.'

Now that the courts are more open, however, to hearing allegations of child sexual abuse, the stakes are much higher, and everyone – victims, survivors, and professionals alike – are forced into playing by the rules of the judicial system. These are rarely the structures most conducive to revealing the multilevelled reality of human life experiences, much less facilitative of the deep healing desired by survivors of childhood trauma.

There are wonderful exceptions, and it is too bad that they cannot be the rule. I have seen adults, and particularly teenagers and children, whose rights to protection were confirmed in a judicial context, have their faith in caring individuals and a basically just society reaffirmed. The legal process in these cases reinforced their therapy process. They returned to their social milieux as confident fighters for justice, for themselves and others. When the public and the private aspects of an individual's struggle can integrate in this way, the empowerment of the individual is great.

Sometimes a word spoken by a person with obvious authority – wearing judicial robes or a police uniform – can be more powerful than many well-meaning reassurances from helping professionals. I will never forget the look on the face of a teenager who was being interviewed by two burly police officers about the sexual abuses perpetrated on her and a number of her classmates by her school principal. When asked why she had not told anyone about what was happening, she replied that the man had said that she would get in a lot of trouble if she told anyone, because, although there was nothing wrong with what they were doing, it was technically illegal.

One of the police officers looked the young woman straight in the eyes for a moment, and then he said, slowly and deliberately, 'He is the one who was commiting the crimes, and we intend to arrest him for those crimes. You did absolutely nothing illegal.' From that moment, a burden seemed to be lifted from her spirit. She and the only one of her classmates willing to testify against their assailant were further empowered by the outcome of a long and gruelling trial, in which the principal's lawyer did everything possible to undermine the adolescents' straightforward testimony, to no avail.

This offender spent some time in a federal penitentiary. The young women had to struggle for a much longer time to recover the sense of self-worth and emotional bouyancy he had stolen from them. This is not fair and will never be fair. It was, however, a much more positive outcome than that which the majority of abuse survivors experience when they interact with the judicial system, and I always thought that the clear and unequivocal statement by the policeman – who pointed out the difference between a criminal and a victim of crime – was an important milestone in the struggle of those young women.

Unfortunately, the more common scenario, especially when adults are engaged in the accusation of a childhood perpetrator, is one in which survivors must choose between a process of deeply personal exploration and healing in which they can acknowledge the complexities and, in some cases, the uncertainties of their search for truth and meaning, or involvement in a court process that may take years out of their lives. In court, premature conviction and defensive certainty are positive attributes, and the vagaries of memory are the enemy of legal victory rather than the rich and fruitful vein to mine for personal growth and the making of meaning. This makes the choice of legal validation one that is all too often revictimizing for adults who were sexually abused as children.

Even in those cases in which there is no uncertainty about the historical facts of the abuse, the adverserial nature of the court process is such that the goal of telling one's story in public, as fully and honestly as possible, becomes secondary to goals and means generated by the rules of what still remains – efforts and exceptions nonwithstanding – a bastion of the patriarchal protection of the powerful. Too many survivors come out of an engagement in the judicial process feeling reabused and more cynical than when they began.

In the past ten years or so I have noticed something that has saddened me. People whom I would have been aligned with years ago in the struggle against a wide variety of social injustices have become my adversary in the area on which I am most often focused, the sexual abuse of children. One of the most gruelling trials I have ever been a part of was one in which my connection with the complainants was not professional but personal, and because of that personal relationship, in combination with my professional experience, I was closely involved in the development of the case from the legal perspective.

The defense lawyer pontificated to the judge and the jury throughout the trial in such a way that it appeared she believed her client to be an innocent man, maliciously accused, and in this case I knew with certainty that this was not true. It was my impression, however, that she may well have believed it; at least, she put on a performance that had me convinced that she did. In any case, she went well beyond what would have been required to mount a fair defence for her client in terms of attempting to undermine the credibility and the emotional stability of the young victim witnesses, and she came close to slander in her representations of their families. I experienced a strong bond with the crown prosecutor over the course of this case, and I came to experience the defence lawyer, not just as someone who was doing her job, but as a person who was joined with her client in his project of the destruction of children.

I later learned that these two lawyers had, in 1982, conducted a prolonged and bitter court battle over the case of the notorious bathhouse raids in Toronto, during which more than 200 citizens were arrested in a police raid on the venues in which gay men met for sexual encounters. The zeal with which the crown attorney (whose conviction I shared that the sexual abuse perpetrator in the case we worked on together had harmed the innocent and would continue to do so unless he was punished to the full extent of the law) prosecuted these men is one of the blots on the page of the history of civil rights in Canada. I found myself disoriented as I realized how differently I would have seen both lawyers had I observed them in the bathhouse trial. I tried to understand what has happened to the clarity with which the sides once seemed to be drawn – those who champion the rights of the marginalized and those who support systemic oppression.

The answer is far from simple, and I sometimes harken nostalgically for the times – even just ten years ago – when I could believe that the radical feminist project of eradicating the sexual oppression of women and children was a clear and clean vehicle for justice, and any person or force that opposed or even attempted to nuance the principles it stood for and the practice of those principles, was, by definition, part of the problem rather than part of the solution.

Some feminists would argue that postmodernism is another masculine invention to exclude women (Modelski, 1986), but I think the core of the feminist project is a quintessentially postmodern challenge to the dualisms central to patriarchial culture – body-mind, sexuality-spirituality, inside-outside, victim-aggressor, public-private, and even woman-man. We need rough-hewn separatist strategies and fairly crude ideological positions to tackle oppression in some contexts. Holding on to their appealing simplicities, however, can land us in the very position we have struggled to escape. A mature feminism struggles to evolve a more subtle elucidation of the differences among women – and among men – and in the experience of being a woman or man in culture.

Much of the early (and in some contexts, ongoing) radical feminist position, in pointing to sexuality of a particular kind as the heart of women's experience of oppression, was unintentionally and maybe even necessarily anti-sex. It is not in the nature of revolutionary rhetoric to be overly concerned with the finer points of analysis, and wide brush strokes were needed – still are needed, in fact – to paint slogans on placards. However, when our slogans take the place of rigorous analysis of the complexities and the differences that inhere in both individual situations and cultural phenomena, we become the problem we are trying to solve. We have simply moved from the position of being decided over to the position of deciding over others, with little change in the methodology or the goals.

Because of its grounding in the personal, feminism has the potential to challenge the anti-sex bias that is fundamental to Western culture. The intensely individual and utterly constructed nature of sexuality as the site of fantasy, conflict, power, and desire places it at the centre of the conversation about who we are and who we might be. The complexities that emerge when we allow ourselves to engage deeply in the exploration of ourselves as sexual beings challenge the dualisms upon which traditional politics – including much feminist politics – depend.

At this time in history, conflicts over sexual values have taken on the fervor of religious disputes and are often embedded in fundamentalist rhetoric. This can be seen in the passionate conviction of the religious right as they attempt to repeal the civil rights of lesbians and gays and to return the United States to the culture of Joe McCarthy's 1950s, in which the merest suspicion of any unorthodox political or sexual belief (much less practice) was ground for enthusiastic investigation, and any hint of confirmation resulted in the most severe discrimination sanctioned by the highest authorities in the country.

Unfortunately, the spirit of fascism as it has re-surfaced in today's political climate is not confined to the reactionary right. Social and political movements like the women's movement and the children's rights movement often seem to forget that we developed our strength and our moral force from refusing to accept the authority of those in power to define our reality. When, having made some gains into the centres of power ourselves, we begin to use the same tactics we deplored when we were marginalized, we contaminate any cause we espouse.

The atmosphere of the Inquisition often pervades the courtroom when there is an accusation of the sexual abuse of a child, even when there is very little evidence that the allegations are veridical. I have been railed at righteously on the witness stand, 'Don't you always believe the child?' in a context in which the child herself, who refused to testify, was highly conflicted, extremely unsure, and profoundly influenced by her environment. We do not do any cause – including the most worthy, such as the protection of children from adult sexual exploitation – any service when we construct ideological simplicities to tame the disturbing complexities of reality.

As I pointed out in the discussion about boundaries in the therapy relationship, the feminist and humanist therapy movements seem to be participating in this left-wing form of conservative politics, designed to protect the incursions that outlaws have made into the corridors of power by denying our heritage of challenge to the status quo. The rush of professional regulating bodies, for example, to make sweeping proscriptions about post-therapy relationships between therapist and client, outlawing sexual and sometimes social and business relationships with ex-clients for the duration of the therapist's lifetime, is an example of crude legislative posturing replacing difficult analysis and dialogue. The result is the construction of the image of an 'ethical professional' and the imposition of it over the reality a group of professions that have barely begun to wrestle in any deep and genuine way with ethical issues. This exercise serves only to protect the power of the profession rather than genuinely respecting and protecting the consumer from exploitation.

Each of these areas represents examples of a pendulum swing in which one reactive simplicity is replaced with another. This is historically understandable but nonetheless a betrayal of the struggle for social change that, in part at least, drove the process. There is no doubt that many adults sexually abuse children, far more than are ever caught or accused. There is no doubt that there are many predatory professionals, including therapists, who exploit their clients and ex-clients. However, pretending we can wipe out problem of the strong abusing the weak by imposing moral martial law ignores the depth and the complexity of the problem. It also paints an us and them scenario that does not accurately reflect the reality of 'patriarchy in the blood and bones of each of us,' as Juliet Mitchell (1974) eloquently puts it. In the guise of protecting the defenseless, we protect ourselves from what we do not wish to see about ourselves. In doing so, we undermine the civil rights of those we claim to champion and eventually our own civil rights as well.

I am reminded Robert Bolt's play, *A Man for All Seasons*. Thomas More responds passionately to his son-in law's declaration that he would tear down all the laws in England in order to serve his God.

Roper: So now you'd give the Devil the benefit of law!

More: Yes. What would you do? Cut a great road through the law to go after the Devil?

Roper: I'd cut down every law in England to do that!

More: (Roused and excited) Oh? (Advances on Roper) And when the last law was down and the Devil turned on you – where would you hide, Roper, the laws all being flat? This country's planted thick with laws from coast to coast – man's laws, not God's – and if you cut them down – and you're just the man to do it – do you really think you could stand upright in the winds that would blow then? (Quietly) Yes, I'd give the Devil the benefit of law, for my own safety's sake. (1962, p. 147)

Partisan politics, the most obvious and crude aspect of what I understand as political, also effects the lives of severely dissociative survivors of childhood trauma and the ways in which they continue, as adults, to be denied the resources routinely provided for other citizens. I have seen this play out in the attempts in the past few years to create and implement a system of mental health services for individuals suffering from dissociative conditions in the province of Ontario.

A needs assessment was funded by the Ontario Ministry of Health, which clearly documented the need for such services and the financial and social costs of not providing them (Rivera, 1992a). Approval in principle was given for a government-funded program to fill the current gap. A proposal was developed, with the assistance of Ministry of Health personnel, for a continuum of community-based resources, including self-help initiatives, assessment/treatment resource centres in five geographical ares of the province, and a provincial day hospital and inpatient program for the most severe cases. A vigorous evaluation component was incorporated into the model, to ensure both treatment and cost effectiveness (Rivera & Leichner, 1994). Significantly, in these fiscally challenging times, the program was almost guaranteed to save money, not only in the long run but immediately, by cutting off the flow of Ontario dollars from the provincial health insurance fund to profit-making U.S. inpatient programs. In fact, almost the exact sum of money that would have financed this comprehensive program at home, was being spent each year to send a few Ontario residents to the U.S. treatment centres because of the lack of appropriate resources in Ontario.

Just weeks before a decision about the funding of this program was to be announced, an episode of *the fifth estate* was aired characterizing the treatment of dissociative conditions as a money-making scheme of fringy mental health professionals taking advantage of gullible consumers. The decision about funding was postponed, and eventually the Ministry of Health announced that massive cutbacks made it impossible to fund any services at all for this group of people.

Canadians are justly proud of our commitment to seeing that all citizens can be assured of the highest standard of health care and that economic and social status does not influence access to medical services. An Ontario physicians' strike in the mid-1980s on the issue of the right to extra-bill above provincial insurance rates was one of the actions least publicly-supported in recent labor history, and it took the medical profession a while to recover its image as caring and compassionate. Canadians are even perhaps a little smug, as we observe our neighbours in the United States having a difficult time implementing even very narrow measures to extend the right to health care to its citizens. Unfortunately, the principle of universally accessible health care that most citizens take for granted does not apply to some of the most needy of Canadian citizens – individuals suffering from dissociative conditions.

The Ontario Health Insurance Plan did not want to continue to send Ontario consumers to the United States; they backed the proposal to create Ontario services strongly. The public service unions who see Canadian jobs lost also supported the proposal vehemently. Above all, Ontario consumer/survivors do not wish to have to leave the country to get a few weeks of inpatient treatment with no follow-up. They want appropriate services in their own communities, and their families and friends want to be able to be close to them and provide them with support as they engage in the arduous treatment they need to recover. For all that, millions of dollars were spent to send people to the out of the country when there are trained professionals who are eager to treat them for a fraction of the cost in Canada. This is the politics of dissociation at its most irrational.

These are not easy times. They are adversarial and litigious times. A sense of history – oppression is not a recent phenomenon and has not been transitory – can offer some perspective when we, survivors and mental health and social service professionals alike, are in danger of becoming mired in our own intense and absorbing difficulties, which make it obvious how hard it is, in a society entrenched in patriarchal power, to create grounded and lasting change. We live in a social order that is structured for the benefit of affluent white males and those who are able and willing to fit ourselves into that pattern, and most of us are implicated in the forces of oppression as well as struggling in our personal and professional lives to transform the structures that entrap some people more than others and that diminish us all.

Children who are abused are violated and discounted during childhood, and as adults they continue to be excluded from participating in the richness that our society has to offer. Individually, many professionals reach out to these suffering people – sometimes at considerable personal cost. Individually, many survivors find a way to access the resources they need to heal from the damage inflicted upon them – always at great personal cost. But neither our individual efforts nor our good intentions make a dent in the reality and the pervasiveness of the systemic violence that destroys those who are less influential in our society – children, women, people of colour, lesbians and gays, poor people – in the interests of those who seek to establish and secure their bases of power, whether that power is financial, political, or psychological. It is only in struggling together on all fronts – the personal, the professional, and the political – for the transformation of institutional power and the wider extension of the principles of social justice, each of us using, with honour, compassion, and humour, our own particular gifts, that we can hope to build a movement that will generate creative and liberating change.

Conclusion: Who Are You?

'Who are you?' said the Caterpillar.

This was not an encouraging opening for a conversation.

Alice replied, rather shyly, 'I – I hardly know, Sir, just at present – at least I know who I was when I got up this morning but I think I must have been changed several times since then.'

'What do you mean by that?' said the Caterpillar, sternly. 'Explain yourself!'

'I can't explain myself, I'm afraid, Sir,' said Alice, 'because I'm not myself, you see.'

'I don't see,' said the Caterpillar.

'I'm afraid I can't put it more clearly,' Alice replied very politely, 'for I can't understand it myself, to begin with; and being so many different sizes in a day is very confusing.'

'It isn't, said the Caterpillar.

'Well, perhaps you haven't found it so yet,' said Alice; "but when you have to turn into a chrysalis – you will someday, you know – and then after that into a butterfly, I should think you'll feel it a little queer, won't you?'

'Not a bit,' said the Caterpillar.

'Well, perhaps *your* feelings may be different,' said Alice: 'all I know is, it would feel very queer to *me*.'

'You!' said the Caterpillar contemptuously, 'Who are you?'

Lewis Carroll, *Alice's Adventures Through the Looking Glass* (1922)

The dialogue between Alice and the caterpillar is evocative of the encounters many women suffering from severe posttraumatic dissociative symptomatology experience with mental health professionals. In *Madness and Civilization* (1972), Michel Foucault traces the changes in conceptualizations of illness – both physical and mental – throughout history. During the Middle Ages, lepers were scattered in colonies on the edges of European cities. They were considered dangerous and wicked, punished through their sickness by God. During the Renaissance, those who were considered mad were loaded onto ships and sent off to sail down Europe's rivers in search of their sanity. The seventeenth century marked the first wide-scale internment of the mad, the poor, and the wayward. Until this time, the theme of disorder was cast in terms of excess and irregularity, not in terms of medical dysfunction (Dreyfus & Rabinow, 1982). With the rise of industrial capitalism, the population began to be conceptualized as a component of the nation's wealth and by the nineteenth century, widespread confinement of large classes of people was considered to be a gross economic mistake (Foucault, 1972). The mad must be returned to health and economic productivity as quickly as possible.

Changing conceptualizations of mental illness have more to do with the shifting relationships of power and discourse than they do with any objective scientific advance. Foucault documents that what we call psychiatric practice is a moral attitude and tactic of disciplinary technology that emerged to support capitalism at the end of the eighteenth century. Once women who displayed multiple personalities would have been considered under the power of the devil, and they would have been punished – usually burned – for their sinfulness. Twentieth century ideology frames that as ignorant and barbaric. We call 'dissociative identity disorder' a 'mental health problem.' Mental health problems are the gap through which reason – our god and the basis on which our culture rests – threatens to topple into irrationality. Madness has now become something to be tamed and silenced through medical intervention rather than on the stake (Foucault, 1972). Social definitions and strategies around any deviation from the norm in the behaviour of the population have increasingly been toward the goal of amplifying and disciplining the capacities of individuals so that they can function as efficient workers within the capitalist mode of production (Foucault, 1981).

'Who are you?' – that impatient, demanding, unbearable question for women with multiple personalities – has all too often come to mean, 'Where do you fit?' in relation to the model which fixes the norms – that is, the white male rational individual who behaves in a fashion beneficial to the state. Psychology and psychiatry, with their focus on psychopathology, have been among the most powerful instruments the State has developed for normalizing and disciplining its population.

Cross-cultural mental-health theorists and practitioners are the exception. Like social constructionists and many feminists, they insist that psychological generalizations cannot be uniformly applied across different cultural contexts. Dissociation, for example, including the most extreme forms of trance experience, is not seen as pathological in many cultures. Even sudden and dramatic shifts in consciousness, behaviour, and identity, with little ability to remember them afterwards, are interpreted in a pro-social and extremely positive light in a variety of social contexts in all parts of the world (Krippner, 1994).

In Bali, for example, the experience of being taken over, psychologically and behaviourally, by a force experienced as a god or spirit, is common and seen as desirable and socially valued. It is positively reinforced by society, and the individuals so transported are pleased with themselves afterwards (Suryani & Jensen, 1993).

When I visited Bali in 1995, I saw adults and children slip into trance states during processions, religious ceremonies, and ritual performances that are a part of everyday life. One man danced repeatedly through a roaring fire kicking burning sticks into the audience until there were only embers where the fire once burned. As his frenzy peaked, a couple of other men held him gently, and he gradually shifted into a more tranquil trance state and slipped to the ground. After a few minutes, he began to emerge from the trance, and sat, smiling peacefully next to the remains of the fire. When most people had left, he showed some of us his feet, which were covered with ashes, but not burned.

There are some North American religious sects in which trance phenomena, such as speaking in tongues, are valued, but, on the whole, we see the more extreme forms of dissociation as de facto pathological, a sign of mental illness.

Giving serious consideration to the cultural, social, and political framework within which psychiatry and psychology operate is rarely a part of their functioning. Medicine and the social sciences have cut themselves off from metaphysics and politics in order to vest their explorations with the authority of science. They function, by and large, as if it were both possible and desirable to operate separately and autonomously from cultural complexity, philosophical speculation, and a political perspective.

Both the positivists, who imagine their task to be the scientific and neutral examination of the psychic machinery of the human being, and the humanists, who revolt against the positivist principles dominant in most of medicine and psychology, partake in a fundamental premise that the ideal human being is a unitary, rational subject. Almost all types of psychiatry and psychology and most brands of psychotherapy tend to operate from this position of centring the individual subject as if she were the agent of all social phenomena and productions (Henriques et al., 1984). Although much of our mental health theory throughout the nineteenth and twentieth centuries has been built on this philosophy of individualism, we rarely acknowledge this or recognize its powerful implications for our practice.

Psychiatry and psychology generally concern themselves, not so much with universal processes as with the systematic study of variations, with an emphasis on those that are dysfunctional to the social order. Practitioners and researchers in the area of mental health are mainly concerned with the calibration of error – with what we frame as pathology. We rarely analyse or challenge the norms we prescribe. The norms thus reproduced are those consistent with the dominant sociality, the relations of power as they are played out in society as a whole (Henriques et al., 1984).

Psychoanalysis, that rebel child of psychology and medicine, can be – although it often is not – a challenge to medicine's common-sense acceptance of these understandings about human beings. The most revolutionary aspect of Freud's work was that it de-centred the rational cogito (Mitchell, 1974). Psychoanalysis supports the view of subjectivity as produced through contradiction and conflict, uneasily inserted into the social structures of civilization. It contradicts psychiatry and psychology's assumptions about the accessibility of the machinery of the individual through its emphasis on the subterfuges of the unconscious.

The phenomenon of multiple personality – that plethora of self-states, tenuously united in the trauma survivor – also consistently and pressingly challenges these hegemonic assumptions about the individual's behavior and make-up. A severely dissociative individual – the unitary subject that medicine and psychology usually construct as a pre-given object – presents herself, often chaotically and intrusively, as deconstructed. The process of psychotherapy proceeds through her further deconstruction.

The therapeutic journey is through an exploration of the various discourses that have produced this individual who does not appear to be an individual in the unified and basically non-contradictory sense in which we are used to conceptualizing ourselves and others. The individual is encouraged to experience and exhibit the idiosyncratic feelings and behaviour she has compartmentalized within more or less dissociated states of consciousness. In considering their intense and antipodal claims, she traces the development of her history, both internal and external, the evolution of the person she has come to be through innumerable complex interactions between herself and her social surroundings.

Individuals are most securely and consensually regulated through their identifications with particular subject positions within particular discourses, and this is both a conscious and a subconscious process. This process works most efficiently for the status quo in society when the individual identifies her own interests fully with her position(s) within a dominant discourse. When there is a space between the subject position offered by a discourse and the individual's self-perceived interest, a resistance to that position is produced. This is part of the wider social play of power (Weedon, 1987). Power needs resistance as a fundamental condition of its operation. It is through the articulation of points of resistance that power spreads through the social field, so that resistance is both an element of the functioning of power and a source of its perpetual disorder (Dreyfus & Rabinow, 1982).

The personalities within the severely dissociative trauma survivor are a living theatre of these plays of desire, knowledge, and power. For every state in which she identifies with one subject position in one particular discourse (the compliant girl, for example), there is another state in which she ferociously resists that subject position (the anti-social boy). Both social control and resistance to that control can be clearly seen in the ongoing drama of her life. The dynamic of power and powerlessness inheres in their differences and in the shifts from one state to another, from one subject position to another, depending on the circumstances and her responses to those circumstances at any given moment. Each self-state, each subject position, also demonstrates aspects of social regulation and resistance to that regulation, and they all influence each other. Thus, subjectivity continues to be constructed and reconstructed within the social context of the individual and within the larger social order.

The goal of treatment informed by a feminist perspective is not to change this continuous process of the construction of subjectivity, but to open it up to examination, so that, in eroding the dissociative barriers between the states with their often contradictory subject positions, the woman who had relatively little control over her life can reflect upon the discursive relations that constitute her and the society in which she must live and work. The opening up of previously hidden, disguised, or inaccessible discourses offers her – not unlimited freedom – but an opportunity to choose from a wider range of options and to produce new meanings for herself that are less rigidly constrained by the power relations of her past.

In witnessing and participating in the therapeutic journey of a severely dissociative woman, the notion of identity undergoes a shift. The search for identity does not appear to be a digging for an essential self, the 'true self' of the object relations psychoanalysts that is hidden beneath protective layers of socialization. What emerges is a multiple, shifting, and often self-contradictory identity made up of heterogeneous and heteronomous representations of gender, race, class, and culture (deLauretis, 1986). This is not a denial of personal identity for a woman, but the affirmation of an agential subjectivity that can confront the hierarchical relations of power in an oppressive society and, at the same time, remain aware that she is being constituted within the contexts that she is challenging.

It is this central insight about the multiplicity of our subjectivity (and our sexuality as an inextricable part of our constructed subjectivity) and its conflicted and contradictory insertion into culture, that makes postmodernism useful for feminism. However, feminism differs from philosophical anti-humanism in that its desire to understand how individuals and their social situations are constructed is rooted in the drive to change these conditions in concrete and practical ways.

Feminism is a political movement as well as a conceptual framework in which some women share assumptions – such as the centrality of gender to an account of social processes. The understanding of women's individual experience as a political reality is the most basic principle of the feminist movement in its many diverse manifestations. Feminism may sometimes use the tools of psychoanalysis and postmodernism to analyze how women have become subjected and oppressed – and the ways in which we have both reproduced and resisted that oppression. But the stated goal of feminism is always to facilitate not only individual, but also social change.

It is very common to encounter in feminist politics an active hostility to theory, which is accused of being the refuge of the elite who can afford to take time out from the trenches to speculate and to write, and who then take all the credit that rightfully belongs to those who are transforming the material conditions of women's lives. Postmodernism, with its often inaccessible and self-referential discourse, understandably comes in for more than its share of this sort of attack. However, despite the serious problems in the production and dissemination of theory as we know it, it is crucial that, in attempting to transform social structures, including the ways we engage in the project of psychotherapy with abuse survivors, we simultaneously tackle the basic questions of how these structures have been produced, or we shall be certain of reproducing them in our own work.

The tension between theory and practice – between the experiential that is completely embedded in its own position and the theoretical perspective that overlooks personal history, between an analysis that destabilizes the notion of identity and our lived and felt experience of our own identities – is enacted and re-enacted throughout feminist theory, including theorizing feminist therapy, and in feminist political practice, including the practice of psychotherapy by feminist practitioners. It is a tension with which we must learn to live, for it does not lend itself to any easy resolution.

It is crucial that we continue to develop an analysis that is large enough to encompass the contradictions of our experiences as gendered subjects in our society. We need to develop theoretical frameworks that transcend the victim/heroine, domination/resistance dualisms that are often part of our myths (Gordon, 1986; Hooks, 1984). New vocabularies are needed to explore the complexities of our situations and the many levels on which power operates in our lives, so that our engagement with the material and spiritual conditions of oppression will be as effective as possible.

We also need our myths. We need places from within which to speak and to act. Feminism has always been a politics of everyday life, and it is important not to lose this grounding in the personal, the material, even as we come to recognize the complexities that are involved in the construction of this amazing creature, the individual woman, and the exclusions and denials upon which our myths are predicated.

The story of the dissociative woman as she works and re-works her identity demonstrates the importance of narrative and historical specificity in our attempts to develop new ways of understanding our experiences. The shifts and changes in her sense of identity and her interpretation of reality point to the interminable boundary confusions we all face. Her struggles against the oppressive forces that threaten her integrity and her survival embody the struggles of all women.

There are many more women with multiple personalities than we would ever have suspected only a decade ago, but they do not make up a large percentage of the population. We cannot say – as we can about survivors of incest and child sexual abuse – that every woman either is one or knows one well. But, although we may not be acquainted with a woman who has multiple personalities, we can all identify with many aspects of her way of life. We are all well acquainted with the scrambling to find the appropriate face in an oppressive or abusive situation – to protect us from harm, or to hide our fear, our anger, or our shame when we have been harmed. All women have had the experience of hardening ourselves so that we can lash out in self-protection or to protect those who are dependent on us.

We have all submitted – and pretended it was fine to submit – to things that would have made us shrink with shame if we had allowed ourselves to feel them. The child clamours within all of us, and we suppress, mock, and torment her almost every day of our lives. Most of the time, we succeed in being entirely unaware of these struggles that rage inside of us. We work hard at keeping these mutually contradictory voices silent, or at least out of touch with each other. And we do this for the same reasons severely dissociative women do. We want to survive. We don't want to be hurt.

The same process of suppression, denial, and extrusion that we exercise over the differences within us we extend to the world around us – and everything in it that is not us. We create our identity through the exclusion of those who are not like us; whose race makes them see the world from a different angle; whose class location inspires them to want something different; whose sexuality allows them to feel what we do not feel. We have a terribly hard time appreciating differences and negotiating and re-negotiating connectedness. We find it easier to draw clear – if often unacknowledged – boundaries and to build our identities within the enclosure. This fear and exclusion among women is probably the single most powerful weapon our patriarchal culture has developed for undercutting a revolutionary women's movement.

Minnie Bruce Pratt's autobiographical essay, "Identity: Skin Blood Heart" (1984), is the testimony of a woman who struggled with this notion of an identity bought at the price of others' oppression. It is the narrative of a woman who identifies herself as white, middle-class, southern, Christian-raised, and lesbian. Pratt explores the exclusions and repressions that support the apparent homogeneity and stability of her identity, which is derived from and dependent on the marginalization of differences from both without and within. The form of the personal narration forces her to anchor herself repeatedly in positions at the same time as she is working to expose the illusory coherence of those positions.

She problematizes her own sense of identity by juxtaposing the assumed histories of her family, which are predicated on the invisibility of the histories of people unlike her in one way or another, black people, for example, or poor people, and to the exploitation and struggles of those people who lived in the same place she called home. The price of the illusion of a stable identity for her is also based on the exclusion, secured by terror, of her own personal experience of her sexuality (Martin & Mohanty, 1986). In embracing her sexuality, she lost the home she thought was hers and safe, and the two little boys she gave birth to and loved.

Minnie Bruce Pratt was not a victim of obvious, sadistic child abuse. She was a woman who could declare that she was 'raised to believe that I could be where I wanted and have what I wanted' (p. 25). But, although the concrete manifestations of her oppression – and her particular adaptation to and protest against that oppression – are different from those of survivors of sadistic child abuse, there are similarities that we are able to see because Minnie Bruce Pratt had the courage to deconstruct her safe, privileged, relatively comfortable life to illustrate 'how much of my memory and my experience of a safe space to be was based on places secured by omission, exclusions or violence, and on my submitting to the limits of that place' (p. 26).

The question that is so urgent for women with multiple personalities – who am I?' – becomes a critical question for all women in a patriarchal culture. We all have – someplace within us – a deep desire for home, for acceptance and self-acceptance, for a sense of mastery over this uncertain and dangerous world. We long to capture our identity, join with others with the same identity, and call the enclosure we have created a community. Because we do not call this home the Ku Klux Klan or REAL Women does not insulate us from the likelihood that all too often we are defining our space by what we are excluding.

There is no easy answer, no simple way to break out. Our lives are socially and historically constructed so that we build with the set of materials we have at any given moment. Scrambling to pretend that this is not so is just using the energy needed to transform the situation to deny that it exists. Becoming mired in a highly personalized guilt is another self-indulgent dynamic that drains individuals and groups so that they cannot exercise what Martin and Mohanty, in their powerful essay about Pratt's narrative, call 'the responsibilities of working through the complex historical relations between and among structures of domination and oppression' (1986, p. 199).

. For the trauma survivor who comes eventually to a place where she can claim all of her voices as her own and allow them to speak in unison, or sometimes separately when need be, there is no final escape from the struggle to build and re-build continuously a self she can live with honestly and joyfully. There is no final escape from the struggle, no new identity that she can comfortably assume to replace the chaotic self that was created during childhood. This is no less true for the rest of us who find it easier to escape from that insistent question, 'Who are you?' The past is always part of our present, and we must continually challenge the lessons we learned as infants, as children, as adolescents, and as adults – unlearn them, reframe them, and relearn how to be ourselves again and again.

   We do not like this one bit. Much of the time we do not accept it and cry out that it is not fair – there must be a new, safe, unchanging home someplace where we can rest and not have to keep struggling. Our protests echo those of women throughout history. We build homes for ourselves – and often for each other, for children, and for men – hoping we will be protected from the differences that are built into us and into the enclosures we create. There is no such safe place, and we pretend there is at our peril. Only through our courage in continually facing our differences and our contradictory positions – both from others and within ourselves – only by challenging the barriers we construct between these differences and by rebuilding connections anew all the time – within ourselves, in intimate relationships, and in larger and larger groups of people – will we be able to work together to change the structures of our society that allow children – and all the rest of us – to be hurt and diminished the way we are.

References

Abel, G., Becker, J.V., Cunningham-Rathner, J., Kaplan, M., & Reid, J. (1984). *The treatment of child molesters.* New York: SBC-TM.

Allison, D. (1994). *Skin: Talking about sex, class and literature.* Ithaca, New York: Firebrand Books.

Andrews, K. (1995). Ancient affections: Gays, lesbians and family status. In Arnup, K. (Ed.). *Lesbian parenting: Living with pride and prejudice.* Charlottetown, PEI: Gynergy Press, 358–77.

Armstrong, L. (1978). *Kiss Daddy Goodnight.* New York: Hawthorn Press.

Armstrong, L. (1983). *The home front: Notes from the family war zone.* New York: McGraw-Hill.

An assault on the nature of the individual. (1988, November 28). *Los Angeles Times.*

Badgley, R. (1984). *Sexual offences against children.* Ottawa: Canadian Government Publishing Centre.

Badgley, C., & King, K. (1990). *Child sexual abuse.* New York: Tavistock/Routledge.

Baker-Miller, J. (1976). *Towards a new psychology of women.* Boston: Beacon Press.

Bass, E., & Davis L. (1988). *The courage to heal.* New York: Harper and Row.

Ballou, M., & Gabalac, N. (1985). *A feminist position on mental health.* Springfield, IL: Charles C. Thomas.

Barach, P. (1991). Multiple personality disorder as an attachment disorder. *Dissociation, 4 (3),* 117–23.

Barach, P. (1994). *ISSD guidelines for treating dissociative identity disorder (multiple personality disorder) in adults (1994).* Skokie, IL: The International Society for the Study of Dissociation.

Barthes, R. (1977). *Image-music-text.* (S. Heath, Trans.). London: Fontana/Collins.

Baudelaire, C. (1976). Essay on laughter. *Oeuvres completes.* (Vol. 2). Paris: Gallimard, Bibliotèque de la Pleiade.

Baudrillard, J. (1988). *Selected writings.* (M. Poster, Ed.). Stanford, CA: Stanford University Press.

Beebe, B., & Lachmann, F. (1988). Mother-infant mutual influence and precursors of psychic structure. In Goldberg, A. (Ed.). *Frontiers in self psychology: Progress in self psychology.* (Vol. 4). Hillsdale, NJ: Analytic Press, 5–25.

Bell, A., & Weinberg, M. (1978). *Homosexualities: A study of diversity in women and men.* New York: Simon and Schuster.

Bernstein, E., & Putnam, F. (1986). Development, reliability and validity of a dissociation scale. *Journal of Nervous and Mental Disorders, 174,* 727–735.

Beskind, H., Bartels, S., & Brooks, M. (1993). Practical and theoretical dilemmas of dynamic psychotherapy in a small community. In Gold, J., & Nemiah, J. (Eds.). *Beyond transference: When the therapist's real life intrudes.* Washington, DC: American Psychiatric Press, 1–20.

Bettleheim, B. (1962). *Dialogues with mothers.* New York: Hoon Books.

Bliss, E. (1986). *Multiple personality, allied disorders and hypnosis.* New York: Oxford University Press.

Bolt, R. (1960). *A man for all seasons.* In *Three plays.* (1963). London: Mercury Books, 87–208.

Boon, S. (1995, September). Unpublished data quoted in Ross, C. Imitation and simulation of dissociative identity disorder: A diagnostic challenge. Paper presented at the Twelfth International Conference on the Study of Dissociation, Orlando, FL.

Boon, S., & Draijer, N. (1991). Diagnosing dissociative disorders in the Netherlands. *American Journal of Psychiatry, 148,* 458–462.

Boon, S., & Draijer, N. (1993). Multiple personality disorder in the Netherlands: A clinical investigation of 71 patients. *American Journal of Psychiatry, 150 (3),* 489–94.

Bornstein, R., & Pittman, T., (Eds.). (1992). *Perception without awareness.* New York: Guilford.

Boston Lesbian Psychologies Collective (Ed.). (1987). *Lesbian psychologies: Explorations and challenges.* Chicago: University of Chicago Press.

Boswell, J. (1990). Categories, experience and sexuality. In Stein, E. (Ed.). *Forms of desire.* New York: Routledge, 133–74.

Bouhoutsos, J., Holroyd, J., Lerman, H., Forer, B., & Greenberg, M. (1983). Sexual intimacy between psychotherapists and patients. *Professional Psychology: Research and Practice, 14.* 185–196.

Bowman, E. (1993). Clinical and spiritual effects of exorcism in fifteen patients with multiple personality disorder. *Dissociation. 4 (4),* 222–238.

Bowman, E. (1995, May). The reality of repressed memories: A review of the research. Paper presented at the Fifth International Spring Conference of the International Society for the Study of Dissociation, Amsterdam.

Braude, S. (1995). *First person plural: Multiple personality and the philosophy of the mind.* Lanham, MD: Rowman & Littlefield.

Braun, B. (1983). Psychophysiologic phenomenon in multiple personality and hypnosis. *American Journal of Clinical Hypnosis, 26*, 124–137.

Braun, B. (1986). *Treatment of multiple personality disorder*. Washington DC: American Psychiatric Press.

Bremner, J., Scott, T., Delaney, R., Southwick, S., Mason, J., Johnson, D., Innis, R., McCarthy, G., & Charney, D. (1993). Deficits in short-term memory in posttraumatic stress disorder. *American Journal of Psychiatry, 150 (7)*, 1015–1019.

Bremner, J., Steinberg, M., Southwick, S., Johnson, D., & Charney D. (1993). Use of the structured clinical interview for DSM-IV dissociative disorders for systematic assessment of dissociative symptoms in posttraumatic stress disorder. *American Journal of Psychiatry, 150 (7)*, 1011–1014.

Briere, J., & Conte, J. (1993). Self-reported amnesia for abuse in adults molested as children. *Journal of Traumatic Stress, 6 (1)*, 21–31.

Brodkey, L. (1987). Writing ethnographic narratives. *Written Communication, 4*, 25–50.

Brown, L. (1994). *Subversive dialogues: Theory in feminist therapy*. New York: Basic Books.

Brown, L. (1995). Lesbian identities: Concepts and issues. In D'Augelli, A. & Patterson, C. (Eds.). *Lesbian, gay and bisexual identities over the lifespan: Psychological perspectives*. New York: Oxford University Press, 3–23.

Brown, L., & Ballou, M. (Eds.). (1992). *Personality and psychopathology: Feminist reappraisals*. New York: Guilford Press.

Brownmiller, S. (1975). *Against our will: Men, women and rape*. New York: Simon and Schuster.

Burr, C. (1995). The destiny of you: Once a gay gene is found, can gene 'therapy' be far behind? *The Advocate*. December 26, 1995, 36–42.

Butler, J. (1993). *Bodies that matter: On the discursive limits of 'sex'*. New York: Routledge, Chapman, and Hall.

Butler, S. (1978). *Conspiracy of silence: The trauma of incest*. San Francisco: New Glide Publications.

Campbell, S. (1995). Women/memory/persons. Paper presented at the Philosophy Colloquium: Queen's University, Kingston, ON.

Card, C. (1995). *Lesbian choices*. New York: Columbia University Press.

Carlson, E., & Armstrong, J. (1994). The diagnosis and assessment of dissociative disorders. In Jay, S., & Rhue, J. (Eds.). *Dissociation: Clinical and theoretical perspectives*. New York: Guilford Press, 159–174.

Carlson, E., Putnam, F., Ross, C., Torem, M., Coons, P., Dill, D., Loewenstein, R., & Braun, B. (1993). Validity of the dissociative experiences scale in screening for multiple personality disorder: A multicenter study. *American Journal of Psychiatry, 150 (7)*, 1030–1036.

Carroll, L. (1922). *Alice's adventures in Wonderland*. London: Bracken Books.

Carter, D., & Rawlings, E. (Eds.). (1977). *Psychotherapy for women*. Springfield, IL: Charles C. Thomas.

Caruth, C. (1995). (Ed.). *Trauma: Explorations in memory*. Baltimore: Johns Hopkins University Press.

Chodorow, N. (1978). *The reproduction of mothering: Psychoanalysis and the sociology of gender*. Berkeley, CA: University of California Press.

Cixous, H. (1976). The laugh of Medusa. *Signs: Journal of Women in Culture and Society, 1 (4)*, 875–893.

Cixous, H. (1986). Exchange. In Cixous, H., & Clément, C. *The newly born woman*. Minneapolis: University of Minnesota Press, 135–160.

Clément, C. (1986). The guilty one. In Cixous, H., & Clément, C. *The newly born woman*. Minneapolis: University of Minnesota Press, 1–62.

Comstock, C., & Vickery, D. (1992). The therapist as victim: A preliminary discussion. *Dissociation, 5 (3)*, 155–158.

Coons, P. (1986). Treatment progress in 20 patients with multiple personality disorder. *Journal of Nervous and Mental Disease, 174*, 715–721.

Coons, P., & Milstein, V. (1994). Factitious or malingered multiple personality disorder: Eleven cases. *Dissociation, 7 (2)*, 81–85.

Crabtree, A. (1992). Dissociation and memory: A 200-year perspective. *Dissociation, 5 (3)*, 150–154.

Crabtree, A. (1993). *From Mesmer to Freud: Magnetic sleep and the roots of psychological healing*. New Haven, CT: Yale University Press.

Creet, J. (1991). Daughter of the movement: The psychodynamics of lesbian s/m fantasy. *Differences: A Journal of feminist cultural studies, 3 (2)*, 135–159.

Danieli, Y. (1989). Mourning in survivors and children of survivors of the Nazi holocaust: The role of group and community modalities. In Deitrich, D., & Shabad, R. (Eds.). *The problem of loss and mourning: Psychoanalytic perspectives*. New York: International Universities Press, 436–437.

D'Augelli, A., & Patterson, C. (Eds.). (1995). *Lesbian, gay, and bisexual identities over the lifespan: Psychological perspectives*. New York: Oxford University Press.

Dawson, D., & MacMillian, H. (1993). *Relationship management of the borderline patient: From understanding to treatment*. New York: Brunnel Mazel.

De Bellis, M., Chrousos, G., Dorn, L., Burke, L., Helmers, K., Kling, M., Trickett, P., & Putnam, F. (1994). Hypothalamic-pituitary-adrenal axis dysregulation in sexually abused girls. *Journal of Clinical Endocrinology and Metabolism, 78 (2)*.

De Bellis, M., Lefter, L., Trickett, P., & Putnam, F. (1994). Urinary catecholamine excretion in sexually abused girls. *Journal of the American Academy of Child and Adolescent Psychiatry, 33 (3)*, 320–327.

deLauretis, T. (1986). Feminist studies/critical studies: Issues, terms and contexts. In deLauretis, T. (Ed.). *Feminist Studies/Critical Studies*. Bloomington, IN: University of Indiana Press.

deLauretis, T. (1994). *Practice of love: Lesbian sexuality and perverse desire*. Bloomington, IN: University of Indiana Press.

Deleuze, G., & Guattari, F. (1977). *Anti-Oedipus: Capitalism and schizophrenia*. New York: Viking.

Dent-Brown, K. (1993). Child sexual abuse: Problems for adult survivors. *Journal of Mental Health, 2*, 329–338.

Dominelli, L. (1986). Father-daughter incest: Patriarchy's shameful secret. *Critical Social Policy, 16*, 8–22.

Dreyfus, H., & Rabinow, P. (1982). *Michel Foucault: Beyond structuralism and hermeneutics*. Chicago: University of Chicago Press.

Dunn, G., Paolo, A., Ryan,J., & Van Fleet, J. (1993). Dissociative symptoms in a substance abuse population. *American Journal of Psychiatry, 150 (7)*, 1043–1047.

Dynes, W., & Donaldson, S. (Eds.). (1992). *Lesbianism*. New York: Garland Publishing.

Eichenbaum, L., & Orbach, S. (1982). *Understanding women: A feminist psychoanalytic approach*. New York: Basic Books.

Ellenberger, H. (1970). *The discovery of the unconscious*. New York: Basic Books.

Erdelyi, M. (1994). Dissociation, defense, and the unconscious. In Spiegel, D. (Ed.). *Dissociation: Culture, mind, and body*. Washington, DC: American Psychiatric Press, 3–20.

Erdelyi, M. (1993). Repression: The mechanism and the defense. In Wagner, D., & Pennebaker, J. (Eds.). *The handbook of mental control*. Engelwood Cliffs, NJ: Simon and Schuster, 126–148.

Felman, S. (1995). Education and crisis, or the vicissitudes of teaching. In Caruth, C. (Ed.). *Trauma: Explorations in memory*. Baltimore: Johns Hopkins University Press, 13–60.

Finkelhor, D., Hoting, G., Lewis, I., & Smith, C. (1990). Sexual abuse in a national study of adult men and women: Prevalence, characteristics and risk factors. *Child Abuse and Neglect, 14*, 19–28.

Fisher, S. (1995, February). De-rigidifying the biological approach. Paper presented at Trauma, Loss and Dissociation: Foundations of 21st Century Traumatology, Alexandria, VA.

Fitzgerald, F. (1945). *The crack-up*. (E. Wilson, Ed.). New York: New Directions Books.

Fortune, M. (1994a). Therapy and intimacy: Confused about boundaries. *The Christian Century, May 18–25*. 254–526.

Fortune, M. (1994b). Boundaries or barriers. *The Christian Century, June 1–8*, 579–82.

Foucault, M. (1972). *Madness and civilization: A history of insanity in the age of reason*. New York: Vintage Books.

Foucault, M. (1981). *The history of sexuality: Vol. 1. An introduction*. Harmondsworth: Pelican Books.

Foucault, M. (1982). The subject and power. *Critical Inquiry, 8 (4)*, 777–789.

Fox, R. (1995). Bisexual identities. In D'Augelli, A., & Patterson, C. (Eds.). *Lesbian, gay and bisexual identities over the lifespan: Psychological perspectives*. New York: Oxford University Press, 48–86.

Fraser, G. (1993). Exorcism rituals: Effects on multiple personality disorder patients. *Dissociation, 4 (4)*, 239–244.

Freedman, A., Kaplan, H., & Saddock, B. (Eds.). (1975). *Comprehensive Textbook of Psychiatry*. (2nd ed.). Baltimore: Williams and Williams.

Freedman, A., Kaplan, H., & Saddock, B. (Eds.). (1975). *Comprehensive Textbook of Psychiatry*. (2nd ed.). Baltimore: Williams and Williams.

Freiberg, P. (1988). Blaming the victim: New life for the 'gay panic' defense. *The Advocate*, May 24, 1988.

Freud, S. (1949) *Three essays on the theory of sexuality*. (J. Strachey, Trans.). London: Imago. (Original work published 1905)

Freud, S. (1958). The dynamics of transference. In J. Strachey (Ed. and Trans.), *The standard edition of the complete psychological works of Sigmund Freud* (Vol. 12). London: Hogarth Press (Original work published 1912)

Freud, S. (1962). Charcot. In J. Strachey (Ed. and Trans.), *The standard edition of the complete psychological works of Sigmund Freud* (Vol. 3). London: Hogarth Press. (Original work published 1893)

Freud, S. (1974). Female sexuality. In J. Strachey (Ed. and Trans.), *The standard edition of the complete psychological works of Sigmund Freud* (Vol. 21). London: Hogarth Press. (Original work published 1931)

Freud, S., & Breuer, J. (1974). *Studies on hysteria*. Harmondsworth: Penguin Books. (Original work published 1896)

Fyer, M., Frances, A., Sullivan, T., Hurt, S., & Clarkin, J. (1988). Suicide attempts in patients with borderline personality disorder. *American Journal of Psychiatry, 145 (6)*, 358–1352.

Gallop, J. (1982). *The Daughter's seduction: Feminism and psychoanalysis*. Ithaca, NY: Cornell University Press.

Garnets, L., & Kimmel, D. (Eds.). (1993). *Psychological perspective on lesbian and gay male experiences*. New York: Columbia University Press.

Gartrell, N., Herman, J., Olarte, S., Feldstein, M., & Localio, R. (1986). Psychiatrist-patient sexual contact: Results of a national survey, I: Prevalence. *American Journal of Psychiatry, 143 (9)*, 1126–1131.

Gazzaniga, M. (1985). *The social brain*. New York: Basic Books.

Gergen, K. (1985). The social constructionist movement in modern psychology. *American Psychologist, 40 (3)*, 266–275.

Gergen, K. (1987, August). Self-disclosure and the emergence of pan-cultural identity. Paper presented at the American Psychological Association, New York, NY.

Gilbert, S. (1986). Introduction: A tarantella of theory. In Cixous, H., & Clément, C. *The newly born woman*. Minneapolis: University of Minnesota Press.

Gilligan, C. (1982). *In a different voice*. Cambridge, MA: Harvard University Press.

Gill, D. (1975). Unravelling child abuse. *American Journal of Orthopsychiatry. 45 (3)*, 346–356.

Glass, J. (1993). *Shattered selves: Multiple personality in a postmodern world.* Ithaca, NY: Cornell University Press.

Goodwin, J. (1985). Credibility problems in multiple personality disorder patients and abused children. In Kluft, R. (Ed.). *Childhood antecedents of multiple personality.* Washington, DC: American Psychiatric Press, 1–20.

Gonsiorek, J. (1991). The empirical basis for the demise of the illness model of homosexuality. In Gonsiorek J., & Weinrich, J. (Eds.). *Homosexuality: Research implications for public policy.* Newbury Park, CA: Sage Publications, 115–136.

Gonsiorek, J., & Rudolph, J. (1991). Homosexual identity: Coming out and other developmental events. In Gonsiorek J., & Weinrich, J. (Eds.). *Homosexuality: Research implications for public policy.* Newbury Park, CA: Sage Publications, 161–176.

Gordon, L. (1986). What's new in women's history? In deLauretis, T. (Ed.). *Feminist Studies/Critical Studies.* Bloomington, IN: Indiana University Press, 20–30.

Gottman, J. (1989). Children of gay and lesbian parents. *Marriage and Family Review, 14,* 177–196.

Greaves, G. (1980). Multiple personality: 165 Years after Mary Reynolds. *Journal of Nervous and Mental Disorders, 168,* 577–596.

Green, D., & Bozett, F. (1991). Lesbian mothers and gay fathers. In Gonsiorek, J. & Weinrich, J. (Eds.). *Homosexuality: Research implications for public policy.* Newbury Park, CA: Sage Publications.

Greenspan, M. (1983). *A new approach to women and therapy.* New York: McGraw-Hill.

Grosz, E. (1994). Refiguring lesbian desire. In Doan, L. (Ed.). *The lesbian postmodern.* New York: Columbia University Press, 67–84.

Grumet, M. (1987). The politics of personal knowledge. *Curriculum Inquiry, 17 (3),* 319–329.

Gunderson, J., & Sabo, A. (1993). The phenomenological and conceptual interface between borderline personality disorder and PTSD. *American Journal of Psychiatry, 150 (1),* 19–27.

Gunderson, J., & Zanarini, M. (1987). Current overview of the borderline diagnosis. *Journal of Clinical Psychiatry, 48* (Supplementary), 5–11.

Hacking, I. (1995). *Rewriting the soul: Multiple personality and the sciences of memory.* Princeton, NJ: Princeton University Press.

Hamer, D., Hu, S., Magneson, V., Hu, V., & Pattatucci, A. (1995). A linkage between DNA markers on the X chromosome and male sexual orientation. *Science, 261,* 321–327.

Henriques, J., Hollway, W., Urwin, C., Couze, V., & Walkerdine, V. (1984). *Changing the subject: Psychology, social regulation and subjectivity.* London: Methuen.

Herman, J. (1992) *Trauma and recovery: The aftermath of violence from domestic abuse to political terror*. New York: Basic Books.

Herman, J., Gartrell, N., Olarte, S., Feldstein, M., Localio, R. (1987). Psychiatrist-patient sexual contact: Results of a national survey, II: Psychiatrists' attitudes. *American Journal of Psychiatry, 144 (2)*, 164–169.

Herman, J., & Schatzow, E. (1987). Recovery and verification of memories of sexual trauma. *Psychoanalytic Psychotherapy, 4*, 1–14.

Heyward, C. (1993). *When boundaries betray us: Beyond illusions of what is ethical in therapy and life*. San Francisco: Harper.

Hilgard, E. (1977). *Divided consciousness: Multiple controls in human thought and action.* New York: John Wiley and Sons.

hooks, b. (1994). *Feminist theory: From margin to center*. Boston: South End Press.

Hu, S., Pattatucci, A., Patterson, C., Li, L., Fulkes, D., Cherny, S., Kruglyak, L., & Hamer, D. (1995). Linkage between sexual orientation and chromosome Xq28 in males but not in females. *Nature Genetics, 11(3)*, 248–256.

Hunt, M. (1994). Degrees of separation: Good boundaries support good relationships. *On The Issues*, Summer, 18–21.

Institute for Family Research. (1982). Cited in Dunwoody, E. Sexual abuse of children: A serious widespread problem. *Response, 5*.

Irigaray, L. (1985a). *Speculum of the other woman*. Ithaca, NY: Cornell University Press.

Irigaray, L. (1985b). *This sex which is not one*. Ithaca, NY: Cornell University Press.

James, W. (1902). Varieties of religious experience. In 1987. *Writings: 1902–1910*. New York: Library of America, 20.

Janet, P. (1889). *Psychologique l'automatisme*. Paris: Felix Alcan.

Jardine, A. (1986). Opaque tests and transparent contexts. In Miller, N. (Ed.). *The poetics of gender*. New York: Columbia University Press, 96–116.

Jefferies, S. (1985). *The spinster and her enemies: Feminism and sexuality, 1880–1930*. London: Pandora Press.

Johnson, S. (1989). *From housewife to heretic: One woman's spiritual awakening and her excommunication from the Mormon church*. (rev. ed. Barrett, L. (Ed.). Albuquerque, NM: Wildfire Books.

Kempe, C., Silverman, F., Steele, B., Droegemuller, W., & Silver, H. (1962). The battered child syndrome. *Journal of the American Medical Association, 18 (1)*, 105–112.

Kendall-Tackett, K., Williams, L., & Finkelhor, D. (1993). Impact of sexual abuse on children: A review and synthesis. *Psychological Bulletin, 113(1)*, 164–180.

Kinsey, A., Pomeroy, W. & Martin, C. (1948). *Sexual behavior in the human male*. Philadelphia, PA: W.B. Saunders.

Kirmayer, L. (1992). Social constructions of hypnosis. *International Journal of Clinical and Experimental Hypnosis, 40*, 276–300.

Kirmayer, L. (1994). Pacing the void: Social and cultural dimensions of dissociation. In

Spiegel, D. (Ed.). *Dissociation: Culture, mind, and body.* Washington, DC: American Psychiatric Press, 91–122.

Kitzinger, C. (1987). *The social construction of lesbianism.* London: Sage Publications.

Kitzinger, C., & Perkins, R. (1993). *Changing our minds.* New York: New York University Press.

Kluft, R. (Ed.). (1985). *Childhood antecedants of multiple personality.* Washington, DC: American Psychiatric Press.

Kluft, R. (1988). Postunification treatment of multiple personality disorder: First findings. *American Journal of Psychotherapy, 42 (2),* 212–28.

Kluft, R. (1990a). Educational domains and andragogical approaches in teaching psychotherapists about MPD. *Dissociation, 3(4),* 188–194.

Kluft, R. (Ed.). (1990b). *Incest-related syndromes of adult psychopathology.* Washington, DC: American Psychiatric Press.

Kluft, R. (1995a, September). True lies and false truths: Meditations on elective misperceptions. Paper presented at Twelfth Annual Conference on the Study of Dissociation, Orlando, FL.

Kluft, R. (1995b, May). Hospital-based treatment of DID patients. Paper presented at the Fifth Annual Spring Conference of the International Society for the Study of Dissociation, Amsterdam.

Kohut, H. (1971). *The analysis of the self.* Madison, CT: International Universities Press.

Kohut, H. (1977). *The restoration of the self.* Madison, CT: International Universities Press.

Kohut, H. (1984). *How does analysis cure?* Goldberg, H., & Stepansky, P. (Eds.). Chicago: University of Chicago Press.

Kopp, S. (1972). *If you meet the buddha on the road, kill him! The pilgrimage of psychotherapy patients.* Ben Lomond, CA: Science and Behavior Books.

Krippner, S. (1994). Cross-cultural treatment perspectives on dissociative disorders. In Lynn, S., & Rhue, J. (Eds.). *Dissociation: Clinical and theoretical perspectives.* New York: Guildford Press, 338–361.

Kristiansen, C., Allard, C., Felton, K., & Hoodestad, W. (1996). *The Ottawa survivors study of recovered memories of child abuse.* Ottawa, ON: Department of Psychology, Carleton University.

Krystal, H. (1978). Self-representation and the capacity for self-care. *Annual of Psychoanalysis, 6,* 209–46.

Krystal, H. (1995). Trauma and aging: A thirty-year follow-up. In Caruth, C. (Ed.). *Trauma: Explorations in memory.* Baltimore: John Hopkins University Press, 76–99.

Kullgren, G. (1988). Factors associated with completed suicide in borderline personality disorder. *Journal of Nervous and Mental Disease, 176,* 40–44.

Lacan, J. (1975). *Le seminaire livre xx: Encore.* Paris: Editions du Seuil.

Lanzmann, C. (1990). Hier ist kein Warum. In *Au Sujet de Shoah: Le film de Claude Lanzmann.* Cuar, B., et al. (Ed.). Quoted in English in Shoshana Felman's Introduction to Claude Lanzmann's address to the Western New England Institute of Psychoanalysis, Yale, April, 1990. Reproduced in Caruth, C. (Ed.). (1990). *Trauma: Explorations in memory*. Baltimore: Johns Hopkins University Press, 204.

Laub, D. (1990). Truth and testimony: The process and the struggle. In Caruth, C. (Ed.). *Trauma: Explorations in memory*. Baltimore: Johns Hopkins University Press, 61–75.

Lawson, B. (1990). *In the name of Satan*. Denver: Compassion Connection.

Lerman, H. (1986). *A mote in Freud's eye: From psychoanalysis to a psychology of women*. New York: Springer.

Le Vay, S. (1991). A difference in hypothalamic structure between heterosexual and homosexual men. *Science, 253*, 1034–1037.

Levi-Strauss, C. (1956). Sorciers et psychoanalyse. *Courrier de l'Unesco, IX*, 8–10.

Levi-Strauss, C. (1963). *Structural Anthropology*. (C. Jackson & B. Grundfest, Trans.). New York: Basic Books.

Lewandowsky, S., Dunn, J., & Krisner, K., (Eds.). (1989). *Implicit memory: Theoretical issues*. Hillside, NJ: Erlbaum.

Lewinberg, E. (1994). Personal communication.

Lewis, K. (1980). Children of lesbians: Their point of view. *Social Work, May*, 198–203.

Lindsay, D., & Read, J. (1994). Psychotherapy and memories of childhood sexual abuse: A cognitive perspective. *Applied Cognitive Psychology, 8*, 281–338.

Linehan, M. (1993). *Cognitive behavioral treatment of borderline personality disorder*. New York: Guilford Press.

Loftus, E. (1979). *Eyewitness testimony*. Cambridge, MA: Harvard University Press.

Loftus, E. (1993). The reality of repressed memories. *American Psychologist, 48*, 518–537.

Loftus, E. (1994). The repressed memory controversy. *American Psychologist, 49*, 443–445.

Loftus, E., Garry, M., & Feldman, J. (1994). Forgetting sexual trauma: What does it mean when 38% forget? *Journal of Consulting and Clinical Psychology, 62(6)*, 1177–1181.

Loftus, E., & Ketchum, K. (1994). *The myth of repressed memory: False memories and allegations of sexual abuse*. New York: St Martin's Press.

Loftus, E., Polonsky, S., & Fullilove, M. (1994). Memories of childhood sexual abuse: Remembering and repressing. *Psychology of Women Quarterly, 18*, 67–84.

Lorde, A. (1992). *Undersong: Chosen poems old and new*. New York: Norton.

Loulan, J. (1987). *Lesbian passion: Loving ourselves and each other*. Duluth, MN: Spinsters Ink.

Martin, B., & Mohanty, C. (1986). Feminist politics: What's home got to do with it? In deLaurentis, T. (Ed.). *Feminist Studies/Critical Studies*. Bloomington, IN: Indiana University Press, 191–212.

McGlashan, T. (1986). The Chestnut Lodge follow-up study: III. Long term outcome of borderline personalities. *Archives of General Psychiatry, 40*, 1319–1323.

McHugh, P. (1993). Do patients recovered memories of sexual abuse constitute a 'false memory syndrome'? *Psychiatric News, 28 (23)*, 8.

Mitchell, J. (1974). *Psychoanalysis and feminism: Freud, Reich, Laing and women.* New York: Random House.

Mitchell, S. (1993). *Hope and dread in psychoanalysis.* NY: Basic Books.

Modell, A. (1990). *Other times, other realities: Toward a theory of psychoanalytic treatment.* Cambridge, MA: Harvard University Press.

Modleski, T. (1986). Feminism and the power of interpretation: Some critical readings. In deLaurentis, T. (Ed.). *Feminist Studies/Critical Studies.* Bloomington, IN: Indiana University Press, 121–138.

Money, J. (1988). *Gay, straight and in between.* New York: Oxford University Press.

Money, J. (1989). Personal communication.

Morgan, R. (1974). Theory and practice: Pornography and rape. In (1994). *The word of a woman: Feminist dispatches.* (2nd ed.). New York: W.W. Norton.

Nicholson, L. (1990). Introduction. In Nicholson, L. (Ed.). *Feminism/Postmodernism.* New York: Routledge.

Neill, A. (1960). *Summerhill: A radical approach to childrearing.* New York: Hart Publishing.

Ofsche, R., & Watters, E. (1993). Making monsters. *Society, 30 (3),* 4–16.

Ofsche, R., & Watters, E. (1994). *Making monsters: False memories, psychotherapy and sexual hysteria.* New York: Scribner's.

Oregon killing suspect: 'It's the American way'. *San Francisco Examiner.* Sunday, December 17, 1995, pp. A-1 & A-18.

Paris, J., Brown, R., & Nowlis, D. (1987). Long-term follow-up of borderline patients in a general hospital. *Comprehensive Psychiatry, 28,* 530–535.

Paris, J., Nowlis, D., & Brown, R. (1989). Predictions of suicide in borderline personality disorder. *Canadian Journal of Psychiatry, 34,* 8–9.

Parker, I. (1992). *Discourse dynamics: Critical analysis for social and individual psychology.* London: Routledge.

Parsons, T. (1951). *The social system.* Glencoe, IL: Free Press of Glencoe.

Pattatucci, A., & Hamer, D. (1995). Development and familiarity of sexual orientation in females. *Behavioral Genetics, 25(5),* 407–420.

Pope, K., & Bouhoutsos, J. (1986). *Sexual intimacy between therapists and patients.* New York: Praeger Press.

Poulantzas, N. (1980). *State power socialism.* Trowbridge and Esher, UK: Redwood, Burn Ltd.

Pratt, M. (1984). Identity: Skin blood heart. In Bulken, M., Pratt, M., & Smith, B. (Eds.). *Yours in struggle: Three feminist perspectives on anti-Semitism and racism.* Ithaca, NY: Firebrand Books, 9–64.

Pratt, M. (1995). *S/he.* Ithaca, NY: Firebrand Books.

Putnam, F. (1985). Dissociation as a response to extreme trauma. In Kluft, R. (Ed.).

Childhood antecedents of multiple personality. Washington, DC: American Psychiatric Press, 65–98.

Putnam, F. (1989). *Diagnosis and treatment of multiple personality disorder.* New York: Guilford Press.

Putnam, F., Buchsbaum, M., Howland, F., Braun, B., & Post, R. (1982). Evoked potentials in multiple personality disorder. Paper presented at the Annual Meeting of the American Psychiatric Association. New Research Abstract #137.

Putnam, F., Curoff, J., Silberman, E., Barban, L., & Post, R. (1986). The clinical phenomenology of multiple personality disorder: Review of 100 recent cases. *Journal of Clinical Psychiatry, 47,* 285–293.

Putnam, F., Loewenstein, R., & Silberman, E. (1984). Multiple personality disorder in a hospital setting. *Journal of Clinical Psychiatry, 45,* 172–75.

Rich, A. (1980). Compulsory heterosexuality and lesbian existence. *Signs: Journal of Women in Culture and Society, 5 (4),* 631–660.

Ritter, P., & Ritter, J. (1959). *The Free Family.* London: Victor Gallancy.

Rivera, M. (1988a). Am I a boy or a girl? Multiple personality as a window on gender differences. *Resources for Feminist Research/Documentation Recherche Feministe, 17 (2),* 41–46.

Rivera, M. (1988b). Social systems' intervention in families of victims of child sexual abuse. *Canadian Journal of Community Mental Health, 7 (1),* 35–51.

Rivera, M. (1989). Linking the psychological and the social: Feminism, poststructuralism and multiple personality. *Dissociation. 2 (1),* 24–31.

Rivera, M. (1991). Multiple personality and the social systems: 185 cases. *Dissociation. 4 (2),* 79–82.

Rivera, M. (1992a). *Multiple personality: A needs assessment.* Ontario Ministry of Health.

Rivera, M. (1992b). *Multiple personality: A training model.* Toronto: Education/ Dissociation.

Rivera, M., & Leichner, P. (1994). The dissociation network: A proposal for assessment, treatment and research re dissociative disorders in Ontario. Submitted to the Ontario Ministry of Health.

Rose, J. (1983). Femininity and its discontents. *Feminist Review, 14,* 5–21.

Rosewater, L., & Walker, L. (Eds.). (1985). *Handbook of feminist therapy: Women's issues in psychotherapy.* New York: Springer.

Ross, C. (1989). *Multiple personality disorder: Diagnosis, clinical features and treatment.* New York: John Wiley and Sons.

Ross, C. (1990). Twelve cognitive errors about multiple personality disorder. *American Journal of Psychotherapy, 44 (3),* 348–56.

Ross, C. (1991). The epidemiology of multiple personality disorder and dissociation. *Psychiatric Clinics of North America, 14 (3),* 503–517.

Ross, C. (1995a). *Satanic ritual abuse.* Toronto: University of Toronto Press.

Ross, C. (1995b, September). Imitation and simulation of dissociative identity disorder: A diagnostic challenge. Paper presented at the Twelfth International Conference for the Study of Dissociation, Orlando, FL.

Ross, C., Fraser, G. (1987). Recognizing multiple personality disorder. *Annals of the Royal College of Physicians and Surgeons of Canada, 20 (5)*, 357–360.

Ross, C., Norton, C., & Wozney, K., (1989). Multiple personality disorder: An analysis of 236 cases. *Canadian Journal of Psychiatry, 34 (5)*, 413–418.

Ross, C., & Pam, A. (1995). *Pseudo-science in biological psychiatry: Blaming the body.* New York: John Wiley.

Rubin, G. (1993). Thinking sex: Notes for a radical theory of the politics of sexuality. In Abelove, H., Ainabarale, M., & Halperin, D. (Eds.). *Lesbian and gay studies reader.* London: Routledge, 3–44.

Rule, J. (1994). Acceptance speech on receipt of Doctor of Letters Honoris Causa, University of British Columbia. In *Fiction and other truths: A film about Jane Rule.* Fernie, L., & Weissman, A. (Directors). TV Ontario.

Ruse, M. (1988). *Homosexuality.* Oxford: Basil Blackwell.

Rush, F. (1974). The sexual abuse of children: A feminist point of view. In Connell, N., & Wilson, C. (Eds.). *Rape: The first sourcebook for women.* New York: New American Library.

Rush, F. (1977). The Freudian cover-up. *Chrysalis, 1*, 31–45.

Rush, F. (1980). *The best kept secret: Sexual abuse of children.* New York: McGraw-Hill.

Saussure, F. (1974). *A course in general linguistics.* London: Fontana.

Saxe, G., van der Kolk, B., Berkowitz, R., Chinman, G., Hall K., Lieberg, G. & Schwartz, J. (1993). Dissociative disorders in psychiatric inpatients. *American Journal of Psychiatry, 150 (7)*, 1037–1042.

Sedgwick, E. (1985). *Between men: English literature and male homosocial desire.* New York: Columbia University Press.

Sedgwick, E. (1990). *Epistemology of the closet.* Berkeley, CA: University of California Press.

Snowdon, R. (1982). Working with incest offenders: Excuses, excuses, excuses. *Aegis, 35*.

Southwick, S., Yehuda, R., & Giller, E. (1993). Personality disorders in treatment-seeking combat veterans with posttraumatic stress disorder. *American Journal of Psychiatry, 150 (7)*, 1020–1023.

Spiegel, D. (Ed.). (1994). *Dissociation: Culture, mind, and body.* Washington, DC: American Psychiatric Press.

Steele, K. (1989). Sitting with the shattered soul. *Pilgrimage: Journal of Personal Exploration and Psychotherapy, 15 (6)*, 19–25.

Steinberg, M. (1993). *The structured clinical interview for DSM-IV dissociative disorders (SCID-D).* Washington, DC: American Psychiatric Press.

Stolorow, R., & Atwood, G. (1995). *Contexts of being: The intersubjective foundations of psychological life.* Hillside, NJ: Analytic Press.

Stolorow, R., Brandchaft, B., & Atwood, G. (1987). *Psychoanalytic treatment: An intersubjective approach*. Hillsdale, NJ: Analytic Press.

Stone, M. (1989). Long-term follow-up of narcissistic/borderline patients. *Psychiatric Clinics of North America, 12*, 621-641.

Stone, M. (1990). *The fate of borderline patients: Successful outcome and psychiatric practice*. New York: Guilford Press.

Stone, M. (1992). Suicide in borderline and other adolescents. *Adolescent Psychiatry, 18*, 289-305.

Stone, M., Hurt, S., & Stone, D. (1987a). The P.I.-500: Long-term follow-up of borderline inpatients meeting DSM-III criteria. 1. Global Outcome. *Journal of Personality Disorders, 1*, 291-298.

Stone, M., Stone, D., & Hurt, S. (1987b). Natural history of borderline patients treated by intensive hospitalization. *Psychiatric Clinics of North America, 10*, 185-206.

Sturdivant, S. (1980). *Therapy with women: A feminist philosophy of treatment*. New York: Springer.

Suryani, L., & Jensen, G. (1993). *Trance and possession in Bali: A window on western multiple personality, possession disorder and suicide*. Kuala Lumpur: Oxford University Press.

Svrakic, D. (1985). Emotional features of narcissistic personality disorder. *American Journal of Psychiatry, 142*, 720-724.

Swaab, D., Gooran, L., U Hofman, M. (1992). Gender and sexual orientation in relation to hypothalmic structures. *Hormone Research, 38*, 51-61.

Taylor, W., & Martin, M. (1944). Multiple personality. *Journal of Abnormal and Social Psychology, 39*, 281-300.

Trickett, P., McBride-Chang, C., & Putnam, F. (1994). The classroom performance and behavior of sexually abused females. *Development and Psychopathology, 6*, 183-194.

Trocme, N. (1994). *Ontario incidence study of reported child abuse and neglect*. Toronto: Ontario Institute for the Prevention of Child Abuse.

Ulman, R., & Brothers, D. (1988). *The shattered self: A psychoanalytic study of trauma*. Hillsdale, NJ: Analytic Press.

Ursel, S. (1995). Bill 167 and full human rights. In Arnup, K. (Ed.). *Lesbian parenting: Living with pride and prejudice*. Charlottetown, PEI: Gynergy Press, 341-351.

van der Kolk, B. (1995, February). When experiential interventionism is not enough: Psychopharmacology and the psychobiology of complex PTSD. Paper presented at Trauma, Loss and Dissociation: Foundations of 21st Century Traumatology, Alexandria, VA.

van der Kolk, B., & van der Hart, O. (1995). The intrusive past: The flexibility of memory and the engraving of trauma. In Caruth, C. (Ed.). *Trauma: Explorations in memory*. Baltimore: Johns Hopkins University Press, 158-182.

Vermeule, B. (1991). Is there a Sedgwick school for girls? *Qui Parle?, 5 (1)*.

Wakefield, H., & Underwager, R. (1992). Recovered memories of alleged sexual abuse: Lawsuits against parents. *Behavioral Sciences and the Law, 10*, 483–507.

Walkerdine, V. (1984). Someday my prince will come: Young girls and the preparation for adolescent sexuality. In McRobbie, A., & Mica, N. (Eds.). *Gender and generation.* London: MacMillan.

Weedon, C. (1987). *Feminist practice and poststructuralist theory.* Oxford: Basil Blackwell.

Williams, L. (1994a). Recall of childhood trauma: A prospective study of women's memories of child sexual abuse. *Journal of Consulting and Clinical Psychology, 62 (6),* 1167–1176.

Williams, L. (1994b). What does it mean to forget child sexual abuse? A reply to Loftus, Garry, & Feldman (1994). *Journal of Consulting and Clinical Psychology, 62 (6),* 1182–1186.

Williams, L., Siegal, J., & Jackson-Graves, J. (1993). Women's reports of documented child sexual abuse: Implications for retrospective research. In Williams, L. Siegal, J., Hyman, B., & Jackson-Graves, J. (Eds.). *Recovery from sexual abuse.* Durham, NH: Family Research Laboratory, 8.1–8.22.

Wolf, E. (1988). *Treating the self: Elements of clinical self psychology.* New York: Guilford Press.

Wolff, P. (1987). *The development of behavioral states and expression of emotion in early infancy: New proposals for investigation.* Chicago: University of Chicago Press.

Wyatt, G. (1985). The sexual abuse of Afro-American and white women in childhood. *The International Journal of Child Abuse and Neglect, 9*, 231–240.

Wyckoff, H. (1977). Radical psychiatry techniques for solving women's problems in groups. In Rawlings, E., & Carter, D. (Eds.). *Psychotherapy for women.* Springfield, IL: Charles C. Thomas.

Wyckoff, H. (1980). *Solving problems together.* New York: Grove Press.

Zubin, J. (1987). Closing comments. In Hafner, H., Gattaz, W., & Janzarik, W. (Eds.). *Search for the causes of schizophrenia.* Berlin: Springer-Verlag, 359–365.

Index